BONE AND JOINT
DISEASES

BONE AND JOINT DISEASES

*Pathology Correlated
With Roentgenological and Clinical
Features*

J. VERNON LUCK
M.S. (Ortho.), M.D., F.A.C.S., F.I.C.S.

*Assistant Clinical Professor of Orthopedic Surgery, University
of Southern California. Senior Attending Physician, Department of Orthopedic Surgery, and Consultant in Orthopedic
Pathology, Los Angeles County Hospital. Member, Subcom-
mittee in Orthopedic Surgery, National Research Council.
Member, Board of Associate Editors, Journal of Bone and
Joint Surgery.*

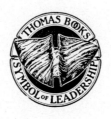

CHARLES C THOMAS · PUBLISHER
Springfield · Illinois · U.S.A.

CHARLES C THOMAS • PUBLISHER

BANNERSTONE HOUSE

301-327 East Lawrence Avenue, Springfield, Illinois, U.S.A.

Published simultaneously in The British Commonwealth of Nations by
Blackwell Scientific Publications, Ltd., Oxford, England

Published simultaneously in Canada by
The Ryerson Press, Toronto

Printed in the United States of America

To

ARTHUR STEINDLER

WITH GRATITUDE, AFFECTION, AND
RESPECT

Preface

This book has been ten years in preparation. It began as a set of mimeographed lectures prepared at the requests of graduate students, interns, and resident physicians in Doctor Arthur Steindler's Department of Orthopedic Surgery at the State University of Iowa. Seminars, given throughout the year, emphasized the correlation of pathologic anatomy with the associated roentgenologic and clinical findings. Since no textbook of the pathology of bones and joints was in existence, it occurred to Doctor Steindler and Mr. Charles C Thomas that I should prepare such a book. Impressed by the great need for a book on this subject and having a large store of the needed materials from which to draw, I agreed to undertake this arduous task. The preparation of the manuscript took ten years in place of two as planned; and while it was laborious and protracted it was never monotonous or uninteresting. Four years in military service delayed completion of the manuscript but at the same time led me to the Army Institute of Pathology and an opportunity to study its magnificent collection of bone and joint specimens and histologic sections.

In the study of bone and joint diseases there is an urgent need for further correlation of the reflections of these diseases in pathologic anatomy, roentgenograms, and clinical symptoms. This book has been written with this need ever in mind. A constant effort has been made to help bridge the chasm that has existed between the laboratory and the clinical practice of medicine. Emphasis has been placed upon the "dynamic quality of pathologic events" and upon the fact that "disease is not a *thing* but a *process.*"

The study of surgical pathology is not limited to the examination of dead tissues. It is, of course, essential to study the characteristics of the various entities as portrayed by surgical and autopsy specimens, but our goal is to visualize and understand the abnormal physiological functions that terminated in the changes observed in the specimen. No one claims that this is an easy task. The explanation of so many living processes ever eludes us, but this does not excuse us when we lose sight of the fact that the structural organization of the body is a living process.

Many physicians have excused themselves from learning more about bone and joint pathology by the erroneous belief that our knowledge of this subject is hopelessly cloaked in uncertainty and controversy. This view, and the complacency it breeds, needs to be uprooted. Even in the most controversial of subjects there is much that is understood. For example, the subject of bone tumors is little understood in the realm of the etiology. Yet the pathologic anatomy and much of the pathogenesis are well defined and a clear knowledge of them is of real practical value to the clinician.

An orthopedic surgeon lifts himself above the technician class by his knowledge of physiology and pathology. As Joseph Nash stated so well; "Operative technique is only the apex of the great pyramid of surgical knowledge; it is the broad and heavy base that is most needed and most difficult to construct." The roentgenologist rises above seeing mere shadows on his roentgenograms when his knowledge of physiology and pathology enable him to visualize the shadows unfolding before him as living tissue undergoing their kaleidoscope of changes.

It was formerly considered ideal for clinicians to acquire a knowledge of pathology but was not looked upon as either essential or entirely practicable. A knowledge of pathology is now deemed a practical necessity, and in becoming so, the practice of medicine has stepped upward on its ladder of achievement. Even in the field of fracture therapy, so often viewed as being entirely mechanical, Sir Reginald Watson-Jones stated: "The surgeon who attempts to treat fractures without a full knowledge of the pathology of bones and joints is faced with insuperable difficulties."

One cannot engage in a long and detailed study of the pathology of bones and joints without acquiring a profound admiration for the magnificent manner in which the skeleton frequently carries on its functions in the face of seemingly insurmountable obstacles. For example, to watch an entire diaphysis of a long bone succumb to the ravages of a pyogenic osteomyelitis and then be rebuilt without ever an interruption in continuity of the bone is so impressive. We do well, in our study of living pathology, when we attempt to determine what nature is seeking to achieve in her defensive responses to the onslaughts of disease processes. Arthrodecing operations for tuberculous arthritis were founded upon the observation that nature was striving to fuse the involved joint and was in need of help. Nature was attempting to fuse the joint for the good reason that bony fusion would bring the complete immobilization necessary for an arrest of the infection.

Obviously it is impossible to present a comprehensive dissertation on so vast a subject in so few pages. It is not often that the earnest student will find all that he seeks within these covers. A textbook style of presentation has been necessary, and, although didactic, it is not intended to be dogmatic and certainly not judicial. I have felt no obligation to supply a theory to explain each of numerous unanswered questions in the field of bone and joint pathology. The old chinese proverb comes to mind: "To be uncertain is to be uncomfortable, but to be certain is to be ridiculous."

Acknowledgments

I hold a keen appreciation of the fact that it is the contributions of my contemporaries and the works of countless investigators who, through the centuries, have contributed to our knowledge of bone and joint diseases that gives this volume whatever value it possesses. The greater portion of the illustrative material herein presented is from the departments of orthopedic surgery, pathology, roentgenology, general surgery, and pediatrics of the State University of Iowa. When illustrations were used from sources other than the State University of Iowa and my private practice, the source is mentioned beneath the illustration. I shall feel apologetic if there is an instance in which proper credit has not been given.

This book is dedicated to Doctor Arthur Steindler as a token of my gratitude to him for the great privilege of having been his student and for the pleasure and inspiration that comes from having him for a friend.

I also owe a debt of gratitude to the late Ernst Freund. His knowledge and enthusiasm for the study of bone and joint pathology were great indeed. I am indebted to him for several of the gross specimens portrayed in the chapters on the malacic diseases. These valuable specimens, collected by him while he was associated with Erdheim, were bequeathed to the State University of Iowa when his untimely passing robbed the world of an outstanding physician and teacher.

In the actual preparation of the manuscript for a book such as this, an author needs a host of generous friends, a patient and enthusiastic publisher, well trained medical librarians, professional photographers, and, I might add, a tolerant family. I have had the advantages of all these.

I must, and do with pleasure acknowledge my indebtedness to the following contributors to this volume:

Physicians—V. L. Andrews, Colonel J. E. Ash, Ray A. Carter, Edward L. Compere, William Cooper, Colonel R. O. Dart, Hugh A. Edmondson, Jerome G. Finder, Carl L. Gillies, Earnest M. Hall, C. Howard Hatcher, Phillip C. Jeans, H. Dabney Kerr, Ralph E. Knutti, M. Pinson Neal, Dallas B. Phemister, Ignacio Ponseti, Alfred R. Shands, Jr., Albert R. Smith, Harry P. Smith, Sophie Spitz, A. Purdy Stout, Robert T. Tidrick, Emory D. Warner, John C. Wilson, and Angus Wright.

Librarians—Miss N. A. Frohwein, Mrs. B. P. Wallace (who also read the manuscript), Miss Frances Glaeser, Mrs. Mary Irish, and the late Hazel Granger.

Photographers—Messers Fred and Gordon Kent (photographers for the State University of Iowa), Daryl Davis, Julius Weber, Edward Hamilton, Lloyd Matlovsky, and Roy M. Reeves.

Histologic Technician—Mrs. Geraldine Sheridan.

Publisher—And last but by no means the least, I owe a debt of gratitude to Mr. Charles C Thomas and his son Mr. Payne Thomas for their continuous interest and help in the years of preparation of the manuscript, and for their expert handling of the physical qualities of the book.

Contents

BONE AND JOINT
DISEASES

CHAPTER I

The Normal Skeletal System

Contents

INTRODUCTION

The skeleton is far more than the articulated framework for the body. It is the "great storehouse" of calcium, the center for the production of red blood cells and granulocytes, and an armor for the brain and thoracic viscera. Bone and cartilage, the principal tissues through which these purposes are so well achieved, are low in metabolism but very much alive, and remarkably sensitive to internal and external influences.

Bone is a connective tissue modified for the special function of forming a rigid framework; hyaline articular cartilage is a connective tissue modified to form articular surfaces. The rigidity of bone is attained through the deposition of calcium salts in a dense network of collagenous fibrils; the lime salts serving the dual purpose of conferring rigidity and offering a readily available store of calcium and phosphorus for bodily needs.

Its inert appearance and its hardness long led investigators into the error of believing bone to be a nonviable, inorganic structure. Even Virchow is said by McCrudden to have looked upon bone as "a finished product." Cohnheim, in his classical report in 1889, refuted the previous teachings and demonstrated anabolism and catabolism in bone. This pioneer work touched off innumerable investigations into the character of bone in health and disease, but it is only in recent years that the subject has received the widespread interest and attention it justly deserves.

EMBRYOLOGY OF THE SKELETON

At the fifth week of embryonic development, the first evidence of what is destined to become a skeletal system appears in the form of axis condensation of the mesenchyme in the extremity anlagen. The mesenchyme forming the anlagen is a part of the mesoderm growing between the ectoderm and endoderm. Mesenchymal cells, creating the skeleton, differentiate first into precartilage and then into hyaline cartilage. At the periphery of the cartilaginous core a connective tissue sheath forms and serves as a perichondrium. There are mother cells in the deep layers of the perichondrium, and through these more cartilage is deposited, layer upon layer, increasing the dimensions of the cartilaginous core by appositional growth. In the beginning the cartilaginous cells have an angular shape and large nuclei, and are closely packed; with increasing maturity the cells lose their angular shape, become rounded and develop capsules. During the sixth week of embryonic life, transverse segmentation appears in the cartilaginous cores, these zones of segmentation representing sites of future joints (Fig. 1).

Differentiation of the upper extremities proceeds ahead of the lower extremities, and the proximal aspect of the extremities precedes the differentiation in the distal aspect. This embryonic process, in which proximal aspects of the skeleton and of other parts of the body differentiate prior to the distal aspects, is known as the law of proximo-distal differentiation.

By the ninth week of embryonic life, the perichondrium in the middle one-third of the future diaphyses transforms to periosteum and forms

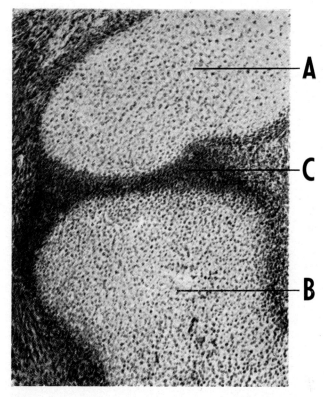

FIGURE 1. The knee of a human foetus at the sixth week. Section includes the lower femur A, upper tibia B, and the transverse zone of demarcation C, that marks the site of the knee joint. Skeleton is entirely cartilaginous.

a thin sleeve of bone. This sleeve of periosteal bone advances proximally and distally toward the transverse zones of demarcation which are being transformed into joints. At this same time a nucleus of calcification appears in the center of the cartilaginous core. Blood vessels are attracted to the nucleus and erode their way to it from the periphery passing through the periosteum and the sleeve of periosteal bone. Having reached the nucleus, a process of enchondral ossification is established in which the calcified cartilage is absorbed and a primitive, spongy type of bone is laid down. A nucleus of ossification thus forms, gradually enlarges in all directions, fuses with the sleeve of periosteal bone at the periphery, and extends proximally and distally to ossify the diaphysis.

During the third and fourth months, joint cavities appear in the transverse zones of demarcation. Periosteum and perichondrium, crossing the joint sites, differentiate into joint capsules and peripheral ligaments. Such ligaments as the anterior and posterior cruciates of the knee move into the joint from the periphery after the joint has formed, explaining the presence of their synovial covering. While the major portion of the skeleton ossifies by enchondral ossification in the manner described, the bones of the cranial vault, the face, and the major portion of the clavicles ossify by intramembranous ossification. By this method the preosseous membrane structure, which forms the original skeleton, becomes ossified by direct ossification of the primitive fibrous tissues forming the membrane. Ossification of the membrane bones appears between the sixth and eighth weeks of embryonic life. The processes of enchondral and intramembranous ossification will be described in detail later in this chapter under *Histogenesis*.

Many congenital abnormalities develop during the first month of embryonic life. Such conditions as polydactylism, lobster-claw hand and complete loss of parts or entire extremities develop during this time. Such deformities as club feet usually appear considerably later, occurring in most instances during the second trimester of pregnancy.

HISTOLOGY OF BONES AND JOINTS

BONE

Bone, a dense calcified tissue, contains cells termed osteocytes which lie in microscopic cavities called lacunae. Fine processes project in all directions from the cells through minute canals, termed canaliculae. There is a free branching and anastomosis of the canaliculae as well as the processes that pass through them. Bone differs from other types of connective tissue in that it contains a large inorganic component. The phosphates and carbonates of calcium in bone give it hardness and rigidity. When this element of bone is removed by an acid, the organic element may be studied. The organic collagenous bundles are similar to those in other forms of connective tissue and form a dense network which serves as a receptacle for the inorganic element.

Bone is divided on a microscopic basis into two types, depending on the pattern and arrangement of the collagenous fibers: (1) fibrous bone, (2) lamellar bone. Fibrous bone (Fig. 3). is more primitive phylogenetically, and is characterized by the collagenous fibers forming an irregular network, visible on histologic sections, ramifying through the homogeneous interstitial substance. This type of bone, always spongy in structure, is usually replaced by mature lamellar bone. Lamellar bone, in striking contrast to fibrous bone, has a regular lamellar arrangement of the collagenous fibers. The lamellations are made visible by the alternating direction of collagenous fibers in adjacent lamellae. A lamellar structure is found in both compact and spongy types of mature bone; however, the lamellations are more clear cut in compact bone where they form haversian systems. Haversian system lamellae (Fig. 4) encircle the haversian vascular canals in a manner that gives the bone maximum resistance to mechanical stresses; the systems tend to run in a longitudinal direction. Another system of canals, Volkmann's canals, may be identified in long bones on the internal and external surfaces, forming communicating canals between the bone surfaces and the haversian canals. Volkmann's canals carry blood vessels, nerves, and lymphatics from the periosteum peripherally and from the marrow spaces centrally into the network of haversian systems. Lamellar plates do not encircle Volkman's canals.

Three types of lamellae may be seen in compact bone: (1) haversian, (2) interstitial, (3) general or circumferential. Haversian lamellae have been described. Interstitial lamellae may be seen connecting adjacent haversian systems. General or circumferential lamellae run longitudinally in the long bones and form a confining bony plate on both the internal and external cortical surfaces of the bone.

Collagenous fiber bundles form perforating fibers known as Sharpey's fibers. It is through the mechanism of these fibers that periosteum, tendons, and ligaments receive their anchorage into bone. The collagenous bundles that form Sharpey's fibers run perpendicular to the surface but do not penetrate the haversian systems or the lacunae. In tendon anchorage into bone, there is a narrow, transverse zone of calcified cartilage which is perforated by Sharpey's fibers before

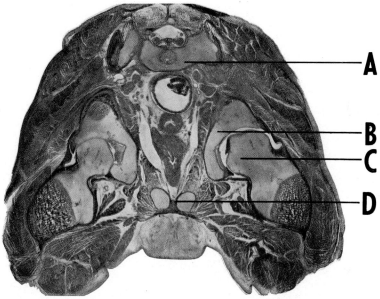

FIGURE 2. A section from a human foetus at the 20th week. A. Sacrum. B. Acetabulum.
C. Head of femur. D. Symphysis pubis.

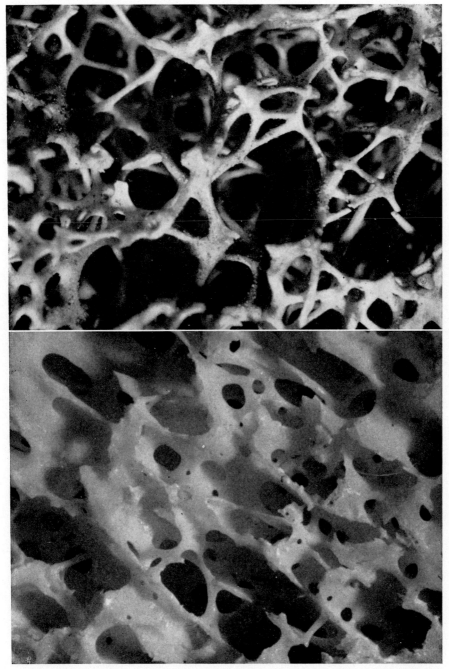

FIGURE 5. Normal cancellous bone. A. (*Above*) Porotic. B. (*Below*) Dense.

layer remains with the bony cortex. The part played by the periosteum in osteogenesis will be taken up later.

Endosteum

The endosteum appears as a thin layer of connective tissue lining the larger but not the smaller marrow cavities bordering the cortex. It is not often a well-defined layer as compared with the periosteum. However, it can be stirred into considerable proliferation with injury or disease, and thereby play an important part in the stage of repair.

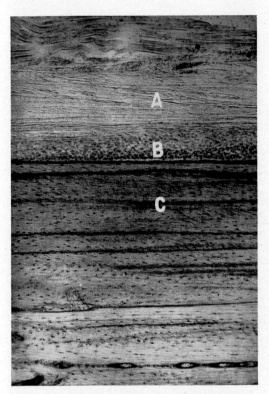

FIGURE 6. Periosteum from the femur of child, age 11. *A.* Fibrous layer. *B.* Cambium layer. *C.* Compact bone.

Bone Marrow

Bone marrow originates from mesenchyme; many of the cells of the mesenchyme differentiate into a reticular type of tissue, which serves as a meshwork to house the amazing variety of cells that constitute red marrow. There are two types of bone marrow: (1) red, or hematopoietic; (2) yellow, or fatty. In the newborn, all of the marrow is red, but with growth more and more of the marrow becomes fatty until, in the adult, red marrow is normally limited to the sternum, ribs, vertebrae, skull and proximal epiphyses of the femur and humerus. In the circulatory system of red marrow, there are numerous large sinus-like vessels called sinusoids. Through the thin walls of the sinusoids, the leukocytes and red blood cells migrate into the blood stream. Yellow or fatty bone marrow is composed almost entirely of fat. In the adult, under physiologic conditions, all of the red blood cells and all of the granulocytes are produced in the red marrow.

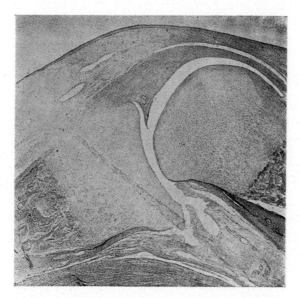

FIGURE 7. A finger interphalangeal joint of a new-born.

Cartilage

Within the human organism there exist three types of cartilage: (1) hyaline, (2) fibrous, (3) elastic. Hyaline cartilage forms the articular surfaces of joints, the anterior ends of ribs, the nasal cartilage, the bronchial rings and parts of the trachea and larynx. Like compact bone, hyaline cartilage contains collagenous bundles which run in a regular and purposeful manner. These collagenous fibers are not visible in the hyaline ground substance since the fibers and their binding material have the same index of refraction. The cells of hyaline cartilage lie in capsule-like lucanae formed in the ground substance, the chondrocytes differing from osteocytes in not possessing processes. Another important difference resides in the capacity of chondrocytes to proliferate within their lacunae. *Cartilage thus possesses the capacity for intrinsic growth, whereas bone does not.* A periochondrium, which is a continuation of the periosteum, covers all hyaline cartilage except for the gliding portions of the articular surfaces.

Articular cartilage presents a noncalcified peripheral layer and a deep calcified layer to be described in detail under the subject Enchondral Ossification. The non-calcified layer may be further divided into a gliding layer and a zone of transmission;

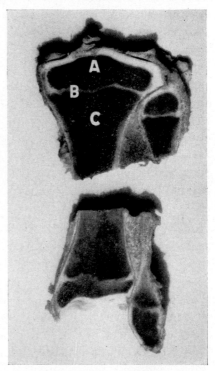

FIGURE 8. Frontal section of the proximal and distal ends of the left tibia of a 11 year old boy. *A.* Epiphysis. *B.* Epiphyseal plate. *C.* Metaphysis.

the gliding layer represents the thin layer of cartilage forming the articular surface, and the zone of transmission, the pure hyaline cartilage which ends at the zone of calcified cartilage. Cells and nuclei of the gliding layer lie in the plane of the surface and are flat and elongated. Due to the fact that collagenous fibers in this layer are frequently visible, the tissue may resemble fibrocartilage more than hyaline cartilage. The lacunae and their chondrocytes in the zone of transmission become larger and somewhat broader as the zone of calcified cartilage is approached. The cells arrange themselves in columns and assume a radial alignment. Collagenous bundles run radially between the columns of cells of the zone of transmission; then, on reaching the gliding layer, turn sharply to run parallel to the surface and anchor at the periphery of the joint.

Fribrocartilage

This form of cartilage is found normally in such locations as the intervertebral disks, symphysis pubis, sternoclavicular joints, glenoidal labrum, ligamentum teres and menisci. Fibrocartilage is a less highly differentiated type of cartilage than is hyaline cartilage, and represents a modified fibrous tissue. Unlike hyaline cartilage, the collagenous bundles are visible in the ground substance and form an unoriented network or lie in uniform waves. Following an arthroplasty, fibrocartilage may develop to cover the adjacent ends of the bones, and this phenomenon is based on the fact that fibrous tissue, subjected to the stimulation of pressure and gliding motion, is transformed into fibrocartilage. Hyaline cartilage may also develop under similar circumstances, but it never attains the high and orderly differentiation of normal hyaline cartilage.

Elastic Cartilage

This type of cartilage is a modified hyaline cartilage; its principal modification is the incluson of networks and strands of yellow elastic fibers, which give elastic cartilage its pale yellow color and elasticity. Elastic cartilage is found in the ligamentum nuchae, the ligamentum flavum, the external auditory canal and the external ear. The origin of the elastic fibers is not settled. Like hyaline cartilage, it undergoes calcification and typical degenerative changes following trauma and during senility.

Joint Capsule

The joint capsules represent membranous tubes or sleeves which enclose articular surfaces, epiphyses and in a few instances metaphases. The capsule is divided into two layers or strata: (1) The fibrous layer *(stratum fibrosum); * (2) The synovial layer *(stratum synoviale).*

(1) Synovial Membrane

This layer represents the joint lining and is the source of the fluid (synovial fluid) that so effectively lubricates the joint surfaces. This

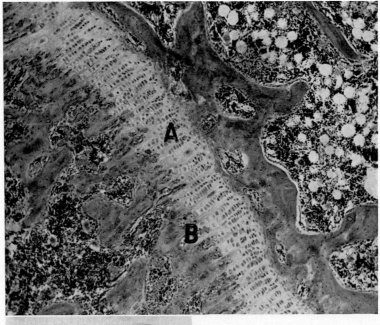

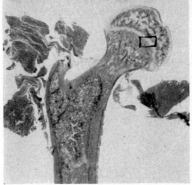

FIGURE 9. Enchondral ossification in an upper femoral epiphyseal plate (insert). *A.* Zone of columns. *B.* Zone of calcified cartilage.

layer does not cover the hyaline articular surfaces as was long erroneously taught, but always attaches and terminates at the margins of the articular surfaces. The synovial membrane is lined, not by endothelial cells, but by an incomplete layer of connective tissue cells. Beneath the lining cells there is considerable variation in different parts of the joint. Key has divided the synovialis into three types according to the character of the tissue beneath the lining cells:

A. Fibrous
B. Adipose
C. Areolar

Fibrous

Fibrous tissue lies beneath the synovial cells where the synovial membrane covers the intra-articular ligaments and tendons, and at points where the capsule is subjected to stress.

Adipose

The best example of this type is seen where the synovial cells lie directly upon the fat layers of the infrapatellar fat pad.

Areolar

Where there is little stress and a demand for considerable mobility, the synovial cells lie on loose areolar tissue. The villi that are seen in the synovial membrane are projections of areolar tissue, enveloped in synovial cells. Villous projections vary from single villi of a few microns to villous clusters many millimeters long. More villi are found along the joint line than elsewhere, and they tend to increase in number and size with advanced age.

The synovial membrane, particularly the areolar type, has a rich blood supply; however, no vessels lie directly on the surface of the membrane. There is also a rich network of lymphatics, and an innervation by both medullated and nonmedullated nerve fibers. After destruction by disease or trauma, the synovial membrane can readily regenerate by direct metaplasia of connective tissue, regeneration being stimulated by joint motion and retarded by immobilization.

(2) The Fibrous Layer (stratum fibrosum)

The synovial membrane is covered peripherally in much of its extent by a dense fibrous tissue layer of varying thickness. Proximal and distal to the joint, the stratum fibrosum of the joint capsule continues as the fibrous layer of the periosteum.

Synovial Fluid

Synovial fluid is secreted by the cells lining the synovial membrane, and lubricates by virtue of its mucin content. The fluid is clear, pale yellow, and is alkalin (Ph. 8.2-8.4). It has a specific gravity of 1.040, total solids 4 to 4.4 percent and has a viscosity of 10.7 to 20 (Kling). Joint motion stimulates secretion of the fluid. In hypertrophic arthritis, there is increased mucin formation, and in atrophic arthritis, decreased mucin.

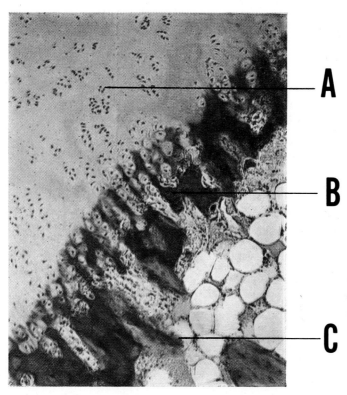

FIGURE 10. Active enchondral ossification at an epiphyseal-metaphyseal junction. *A*. Zone of non-calcified cartilage. *B*. Zone of calcified cartilage. *C*. New bony trabeculum in metaphysis.

HISTOGENESIS OF BONE

Ossification of the skeleton takes place by two strikingly different processes: (1) intramembranous ossification and (2) enchondral ossification.

INTRAMEMBRANOUS OSSIFICATION

The membrane bones are protective, bear no weight and are said to represent the remains of what was once a dermal bone armor

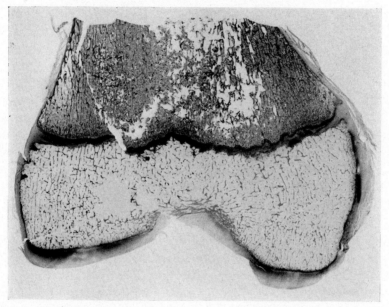

FIGURE 11. Normal lower femur of a 12 year old. Marrow is fatty in the epiphysis and hematogenous in the metaphysis.

(Phemister). In embyronic life the future membrane bones are formed of a fibrous membrane. Intramembranous ossification, a relatively simple process, ossifies these bones. Osteoid trabeculae in the form of a multitude of minute islands are laid down directly in the collagenous meshes of the fibrous tissue, the trabeculae promptly calcify, and eventually join to form primitive cancellous bone. The bone thus formed is steadily replaced by mature lamellar bone, which becomes molded and aligned to the static requirements of the part by a substitution process of bone resorption and new bone formation. Certain conditions alter the membrane bones, one in particular being dysostosis cleidocranialis in which membrane bones incompletely ossify.

Osteomas are limited to membrane bones, while osteochondromas are limited to bones formed by enchondral ossification. Bone formation in and directly beneath the periosteum represents intramembranous ossification. This type of ossification is seen in the embryo in the ossification of parts of the mandible and the diaphyses. Ossification of the mandible is unique in that in the embryo a cartilaginous model forms, but for the major portion of this structure there is no enchondral ossification. The periosteal bone that forms on the surface of the mandible gradually extends, replacing the cartilaginous model layer on layer until much of the mandible has been replaced by bone forming on the basis of intramembranous ossification. In forming diaphyseal bony sleeves in the embryo, the periosteum lays down the bone on the periphery of the cartilaginous model.

Enchondral (Endochondral) Ossification

This is the process of ossification that most concerns us in orthopedic pathology. The entire skeleton, except for the membrane bones and a portion of the mandible, is ossified by this method. This is a cartilaginous replacement process in which hyaline cartilage forms a model, becomes calcified, and is then absorbed and replaced by bony trabeculae. Enchondral ossification never occurs by direct metaplasia of cartilage to bone, as was long presumed until Johannes Müller, in 1836, described the process and clarified the picture. In the discussion of embryology of long bones at the beginning of this chapter, it was pointed out that the first site of cartilaginous replacement by enchondral ossification is in the center of the diaphyses. After the diaphysis is ossified by the proximal and distal extension of the central ossification and by the sleeve of periosteal new bone, an epiphyseal line develops at the junction of the epiphysis and metaphysis. Increased length growth then takes place on the metaphyseal side of the epiphyseal line by the process of enchondral ossification (Fig. 10). Ossification of the epiphysis itself occurs by the cartilage replacement process. A nucleus of ossification forms in the center of the epiphysis and extends peripherally until the entire epiphysis is ossified (Fig. 12). A very slow growth in the epiphysis continues until full growth of bone is attained, at which time the epiphyseal line disappears. For descriptive purposes the process of enchondral ossification will be divided into three steps:

I. At the outset there is a proliferation of chondrocytes in the mother cells which lie near the middle of the epiphyseal plate. The exact site of the mother cells is not often clearly visible microscopically, but their presence is essential to the continuation of the epiphyseal plate. It is held in place above and below by cartilaginous plates. The nucleus pulposus has the task of absorbing and transmitting pressure from one vertebra to the next, like a "hydrodynamic ball bearing." With advancing age it tends to lose some of its resiliency through diminution of its fluid content. This results in narrowing of the disk and loss of height so frequently a part of senility. A comprehensive study of the intervertebral disk and the nucleus pulposus was made by Schmorl.

He found that 38 percent of spines, routinely sectioned at autopsies, showed a prolapse of the nucleus pulposus into adjacent vertebral bodies. He also observed rupture of the nucleus pulposus into the spinal canal. Extrusion of the nucleus pulposus posterolaterally into the vertebral canal frequently impinges a nerve root. Extrusion of the nucleus pulposus through the annulus fibrosus or through the hyaline cartilagenous plates adjacent to the vertebral bodies (Fig. 19) usually results from traumatic rupture at a focus of degeneration or necrosis.

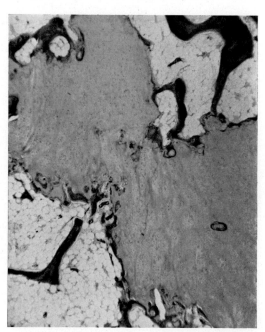

FIGURE 16. Section of a congenitally defective, non-growing epiphyseal plate. The cause of the arrested function is not reflected histologically.

After extrusion of the nucleus, fibrous tissue grows in at the site of the perforation and replaces the center of the disk with scar tissue. Maturity of the scar tissue involves contraction of the tissue which often leaves the disk materially narrowed. Such narrowing of the disk produces a malalignment of the intervertebral articular facets and, in time, creates a traumatic degenerative arthritis in the intervertebral joints.

Occasionally there is calcification in the annulus fibrosus, but only rarely of the nucleus pulposus. The disk may be destroyed by chronic infection, pyogenic infection, or tuberculosis; it may also be destroyed by a malignant neoplasm, but there is considerable resistance to this type of invasion.

CHEMISTRY OF BONE

COMPOSITION OF BONE

Bone is composed of 25% water, 30% organic substances, and 45% inorganic substances. Strength and rigidity of bone depend upon the relative proportions of organic and inorganic constituents. The water content of bone gradually decreases from fetal life to old age, the bones becoming harder and more brittle as the water content diminishes with age. The organic content of bone consists of protein, mainly ossein; there is also osseomucoid and albuminoid. The inorganic content of bone is 85% calcium phosphate, 1.5% magnesium phosphate, 10.5% calcium carbonate. The carbonates, phosphates, and calcium are in the relationship of 1-6-10, this holds only for adult bone.

Analysis of bone ash by Hari:

Calcium	37%	Phosphorus	17.6%
Magnesium	.7%	Carbonate	5.0%
Sodium	.7%	Fluoride	1.0%
Potassium	.2%	Chloride	1.0%

Even in profound deossification (osteoporosis) of the skeleton, the composition of bone remains unaltered. In regard to the structure of bone, it is the organic element, fibers and cells, that determines the structure, rather than the inorganic content.

CALCIUM METABOLISM

Metabolism of calcium is governed by the level of the serum calcium and phosphorus, the absorption of calcium and phosphorus from the intestinal canal, a proper relationship between parathormone and Vitamin D, and kidney function.

A. Absorption of Calcium From the Intestinal Tract

All absorption occurs in the proximal one-third of the ileum. Absorption is favored by an acid chyme and adequate Vitamin D, and conversely, its absorption is impaired by an alkaline chyme and excessive phosphates, fatty acids, and carbonates in the intestinal tract. Excessive fatty acids cause a loss of calcium by combining with it to form soap. Excessive carbonates produce calcium carbonate which is not absorbable. An acid reaction in the stomach is also essential; in senility, when there frequently is an achlorhydria, the impairment of calcium absorption can lead to deossification of the skeleton. In the excretion of calcium, approximately 10% is excreted from the lower one-third of the ileum and the colon, and 90%+ is excreted from the urine. In the adult, 2% of the body weight is calcium, and 99% of the body calcium is in the skeleton, only 1% existing in the blood stream, in muscles, and in other soft tissues. The calcium stored in the skeleton is readily available for use elsewhere, but in order to mobilize it, both the organic and inorganic elements of the bone must be absorbed. Much of the resorption for mobilization of calcium takes place in metaphases because of the facts that the bone in these areas is cancellous and the blood supply is rich.

B. Negative and Positive Calcium Balance

Normally the calcium intake and the calcium output balance each other. In childhood, more calcium is absorbed than is excreted; therefore, during the growing period, the calcium balance is positive. A positive balance also exists during pregnancy. During senility there usually is a negative calcium balance in that more calcium is excreted than is absorbed. One hundred to two hundred milligrams of calcium may be lost each day by the senile individual but this is such a small amount that it is difficult to detect. However, over a period of years such a loss may amount to enough calcium to produce advanced osteoporosis. There is approximately two pounds of calcium in the normal skeleton. In an individual weighing one hundred and fifty pounds, the weight of the skeleton is aproximately 23 pounds. During pregnancy an ounce or more of calcium is transferred from the mother's skeleton to the fetus.

C. Calcium Fractions

Three calcium fractions reside in the blood serum:

1. *Colloid:* This is calcium combined with protein of the serum and represents 4 mg.% of the total serum calcium. It is physiologically inactive, non-ionized and nondiffusible.

2. *Calcium Phosphate:* This calcium salt is in solution in the serum, is dialyzable but is non-ionized. It constitutes 4 mg.%, is physiologically active, and its level is maintained by the parathyroids.

3. *Ionized Calcium:* This calcium fraction is combined with phosphorus, is physiologically active and is ionized. It equals 2.5 mg.%.

Calcium of the second and third types is diffusible and forms 40% to 60% of the total calcium. It is the diffusible form of calcium that reaches the spinal fluid. In hyperarathyroidism the diffusible calcium may be increased and yet the total calcium in the blood serum remain normal.

Heterotopic Calcification

Most of the body tissues have a neutral reaction and this, plus their protein content, prevents precipitation of calcium. In the presence of necrosis, degeneration, chronic inflammation, scars or infarcts, the CO_2 production is low or nil, and an alkaline medium may follow which invites calcium deposits.

Phosphatase

Robinson, in 1923, observed a substance in hypertrophic epiphyseal cartilage and in osteoblasts at sites of active osteogenesis, which proved to be the enzyme phosphatase. It is consistently found at sites of new bone formation and makes its appearance at the time the osteoid and callus begin to calcify. Phosphatase appears to break down organic phosphoric esters, liberating phosphorus (PO_4) ions which upset the local calcium-phosphorus balance, and precipitate calcium salts. The high phosphatase content of the blood during generalized osteitis fibrosa, Paget's disease and some of the malignancies is due to the wide-spread stimulation of osteoblastic new bone formation in these conditions. It must be pointed out, however, that the presence of phosphatase is not the only mechanism essential to calcification and, although phosphatase probably does play an important part definite proof has not yet been established that it is essential in the calcification of bone.

F. Vitamin D

Vitamin D has two essential rôles in calcium metabolism: first, it aids in the absorption of calcium from the intestinal tract, and second, it aids in the deposition of calcium in bone formation. In physiologic doses, vitamin D produces calcification of osteoid directly after the formation of the osteoid. In very large doses Vitamin D causes degeneration and necrosis of certain of the soft tissues, particularly those in the viscera and in the vascular system. It may also create conditions that lead to generalized osteoporosis of the skeleton. Familiar changes develop from inadequate vitamin D, and these will be discussed in the chapter on rickets and osteomalacia.

G. Parathormone

Parathormone and vitamin D work together in the metabolism of calcium. Whereas vitamin D is essential to the assimilation of calcium, parathormone functions in the mobilization of calcium. Parathormone acts principally on ionizable calcium, and functions in the maintenance of a proper level of calcium in the blood. In calcium deficiency diseases and in adenoma of the parathyroid gland, there is increased calcium mobilization from the skeleton; in the first instance to maintain the blood level of calcium above the tetany stage and, in the latter, because the increased parathormone secretion from the adenoma keeps the blood calcium at a pathologically high level.

THEORIES OF BONE FORMATION

For two centuries the subject of bone formation has been the center of much interest and extensive investigation (Ham). Several famous polemics have developed around the subject, but in spite of the numerous investigations and the addition of much new information, some fundamental problems remain unsolved and the controversy carries on. Accounts of the numerous investigations abound in conflicting experimental results and data. Two theories of bone formation have been widely discussed. These theories are the cellular theory, also known as the osteoblastic theory, and the humoral, or physico-chemical, theory.

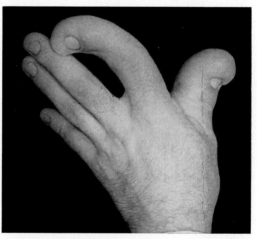

FIGURE 17. Congenital anomaly (localized gigantism) of the thumb and index finger associated with distorted epiphyseal plates, and overgrowth of the soft tissues.

THE CELLULAR THEORY

Proponents of this theory see the osteoblast as a highly differentiated cell created for the specific purpose of producing bone. Just how the osteoblast accomplishes this predestined function is not a point on which there is agreement. It has been contended that the osteoblast actually secretes osseomucin and calcium in the process of building bone. Others believe these cells secrete the osseomucin but not the calcium, while still others view the osteoblast as secreting neither osseomucin nor calcium, but rather secreting substances which precipitate the bone forming materials from the intercellular fluid.

That there are osteoblasts with a predestined capacity to form bone appears indicated by the metastases of osteoblastic osteogenic sarcoma (Brunschwig and Harmon). A group of malignant osteoblasts can be delivered to a lung by the blood stream, and there in an environment as unadapted to bone formation as lung pharenchyma, successfully build tumor bone.

Convincing experimental evidence to support the cellular theory was observed by Fell and Robinson when they cultured cartilage explants from chick embryos. Growth continued in the explants and the cartilage was gradually replaced by bone, which proceeded to differentiate into well formed parts of the skeleton. This observation warranted the conclusion that certain cells of the anlage are predestined to differentiate into osteogenic cells.

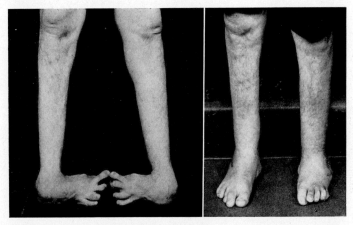

FIGURE 18. Congenital club foot (before and after surgery). Congenital anomaly manifested by abnormal position and alignment of bones and joints.

Lichwitz states that osteoid is a colloid and is the product of the osteoblast. Whether the osseo-mucin of the osteoid and the collagen of the collagenous fibers is actually secreted by the osteoblasts, or whether these substances are precipitated as a result of something the osteoblast brings to the environment, is a point of little practical significance. An increasing number of investigators who support the cellular theory believe that the osteoblast secretes neither the osseomucin nor the calcium, but by some method yet unknown, causes the precipitation of both of these substances from the intercellular fluid. That the factors which govern the osteogenic environment are as yet little known was emphasized by Shipley: "The actual precipitation of calcium phosphate (Ca_3PO_4) is probably covered by simple laws of chemistry but the mechanism by which the environment is controlled which makes the operation of these laws possible, is most complex and many apparently remote forces enter into it." The sex hormones and kidney function represent two of these "remote forces."

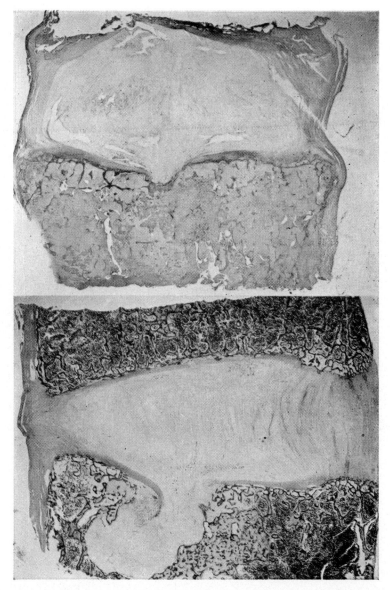

FIGURE 19. Pathologic intervertebral discs. A. *(Above)* Protrusion of the intervertebral disc into the inferior cartilaginous plate. B. *(Below)* Rupture of an intervertebral disc with extrusion of the nucleus pulposis into the vertebral body.

The Humoral Theory

Periodically during the past century the cellular theory has been challenged as giving specific cells too much credit, and the physico-chemical phenomena too little credit in bone production. As the name suggests, the humoral theory gives the tissue fluids, or humors, the principal responsibility for forming bone. The outstanding ex-

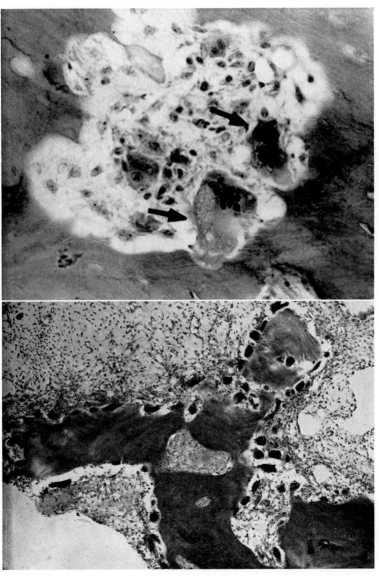

FIGURE 20. Multinucleated osteoclasts lying in Howship's lacunae.

ponents of this theory were Leriche and Policard. In the preface of their book, *Normal and Pathological Physiology of Bone,* they stated, "The problem of osteogenesis has passed through many phases. It has been histological and surgical and the present time it is above all chemical." It is claimed that, given the primitive tissue mesenchyme, bone will form whenever differentiation of the mesenchyme takes place in the presence of abundant calcium and a good blood supply. Bone is simply metaplastic connective tissue. The osteoblasts

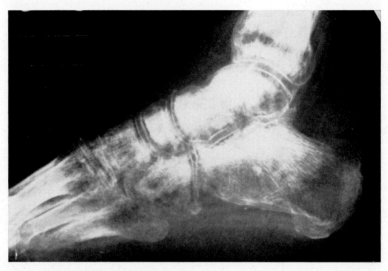

FIGURE 21. Osteoporosis. Roentgenogram of a foot after a prolonged period of immobilization for a fractured femur.

seen during ossification are said to represent connective tissue cells, altered in appearance due to swelling and hypertrophy associated with activity. Secretory functions of the osteoblast, described by a few exponents of the cellular theory, are said not to exist.

Metaplasia of connective tissue to form bone is divided by Leriche and Policard into four stages: (1) Edematous infiltration, (2) Multiplication of the connecting fibrils, (3) Deposition of a preosseous substance, and (4) Calcereous hardening of the pre-osseous substance to form bone.

In order to attain the primitive state of the connective tissue in which bone is to form, it is claimed that adult cells "dedifferentiate," and subsequently redifferentiate during the bone forming process. This aspect of the cellular theory is untenable to McLean, Bloom, Maxinow, and others.

FACTORS INFLUENCING BONE DENSITY

Greig has given us a good summary of the changes in bone density that occur when the blood supply is increased, decreased or obliterated: "(1) Maintain circulation within certain limits and bone remains unchanged; (2) Produce a definite hyperemia and bone undergoes rarefaction, decalcification, osteoporosis; (3) Restrict the blood supply and bone undergoes consolidation, increased density, osteosclerosis; (4) Cut off the blood supply and bone undergoes necrosis."

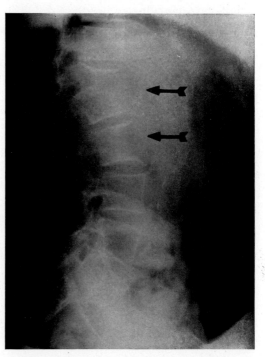

FIGURE 22. Massive bone absorption in response to the pressure of a large aortic aneurysm.

It appears illogical that bone should develop an increased circulation during immobilization, but nevertheless it is true that with disuse, the blood supply steadily increases. Likewise, areas of trauma, such as fracture sites, incur bone atrophy and the associated increased circulation. Part of traumatic atrophy is from disuse and part from traumatic inflammation.

In spite of a certain degree of overlapping of the various causative factors it is useful to outline the numerous sources of diminished bone density.

ETIOLOGIC FACTORS IN THE REDUCTION OF BONE DENSITY

1. Dissuse
2. Inflammation
   a. Infection
   b. Trauma
3. Metabolic disturbances
   a. Vitamin C and D deficiency
   b. Calcium deficiency
   c. Protein deficiency
   d. Senile osteoporosis

4. Glandular unbalance
    a. Hyperparathyroidism
    b. Hyperthyroidism
    c. Basophilism
    d. Hypogonadism (particularly hypoestrinism)
    e. Acromegaly
    f. Adaption syndrome of Selye
5. Nephritis
    a. Renal rickets
    b. Renal acidosis
6. Congenitally defective bone formation
    a. Osteogenesis imperfecta
7. Neurotrophic disturbances
    a. Sudeck's atrophy
8. Chemical ingestion
    a. Strontium
    b. Magnesium
9. Gastro-intestinal disturbances
    a. Biliary and pancreatic fistulas
    b. Sprue
    c. Streatorrhea (idiopathic)
10. Idiopathic diseases
    a. Paget's disease

Reduction in bone density takes place by *osteoporosis* and by *osteomalacia*. First and most important clinically is osteoporosis or deossification. In this condition there is loss of bone tissue, a quantitative loss. Through either diminished osteoblastic activity or excessive osteoclasia the cortices are reduced in thickness, and the cancellous trabeculae become thinner and the marrow spaces are widened. Histologically there are relatively few osteoblasts and little new bone apposition. In most instances, osteoporosis is the symptom of a disturbance of anabolism, which may involve all tissues, as in Cushing's syndrome, or be limited to the skeletal system as in osteogenesis imperfecta. While osteoporosis very often causes a negative calcium balance during its evolution, the disturbance is not due either to insufficient calcium available to the bone or to a disturbance in the character of the calcium. Protein deficiencies of malnutrition cause osteoporosis simply because the bone matrix is protein and if insufficient protein is available to the body, skeletal anabolism (new bone formation) is diminished. When osseous anabolism is disturbed and osseous catabolism carries on a normal rate there is eventually generalized osteoporosis; this is an etiologic factor in senile osteoporosis. While the process is definitely generalized from a histologic viewpoint, there are certain bones and parts of bones that become porotic more rapidly than others. Cancellous bone becomes porotic more rapidly than does compact bone. And the spine and pelvis frequently reflect the porosis to a more advanced degree than do the long bones; this is particularly well illustrated in postmenopausal osteoporosis (Albright).

Albright and his group have written comprehensively on the part that an excessive secretion of the adrenal cortex can play in the etiology of osteoporosis. The adrenal cortex secretes so called sugar or "S" harmones which are essential to the transformation of proteins to sugars (glycogenesis). Either a tumor or hyperplasia of the adrenal cortex may cause an excess of the "S" harmones and thereby, through excessive proteolysis and suppressed anabolism, lead to atrophy of all tissues, including the skeleton. This is Albright's explanation of the principal changes in Cushing's syndrome (basophilism). The

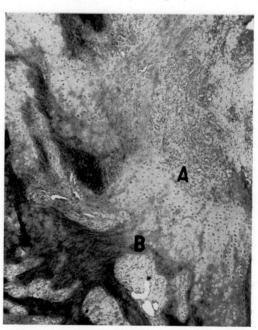

FIGURE 23. Bone formation by direct metaplasia. A. Pre-cartilage differentiating to cartilage. B. Cartilage transforming to bone.

osteoporosis associated with the general adaptation syndrome or so called "alarm reaction" of Selye is explained by Albright on the same basis. Selye observed, as a consistent part of the syndrome of adaptation, a hypertrophy of the adrenal cortex. Selye defines the "alarm reaction" as, "The sum of all biological phenomena elicited by sudden exposure to stimuli to which the organism is quantitatively or qualitatively not adapted." Three stages can be identified: 1. Shock; 2. Counter-shock; and, 3. Exhaustion. It is the second stage that is characterized by the "general adaptation syndrome." Disuse often enters into the picture as an additional cause of the osteoporosis in that the patient frequently is bed-fast.

The other source of diminished bone density, skeletal malacia (osteomalacia), is caused by a disturbance in calcium metabolism. For one or more of several reasons the bones do not have available to them the calcium necessary for the transformation of the newly formed osteoid to bone. Osteoblasts are unhampered and are present in normal numbers; they procede in a normal manner with their part in the formation of bone matrix. Since calcium is not available the osteoid remains and, as new layers are applied, becomes increasingly thicker, reducing the relative proportions of the previously existing bone to the newly formed osteoid. Since osteoid is soft the bones are reduced in density. This process may advance to the point where the bones can be cut with a knife. Chapter VIII, *Metabolic Diseases* presents numerous illustrations of the malacic diseases. Vitamin D deficiency rickets and osteomalacia are the outstanding examples of skeletal malacia. Calcium deficiency, either dietary or from gastro-intestinal disturbances, also causes malacia of the bones. It is common for more than one factor to exist in a given case, just as it is in osteoporosis. Osteoporosis and

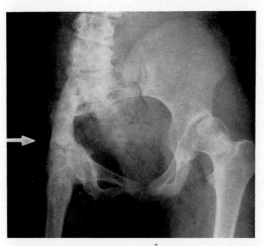

FIGURE 24. Bone hyperplasia in lines of stress (Wolff's law). Roentgenogram taken many months after total resection of the ilium for chronic pyogenic osteomyelitis.

osteomalacia may exist in the same case, particularly in advanced stages. Renal rickets (renal osteodystrophy) causes skeletal malacia with osteoid seams by eliciting a secondary hyperparathyroidism (Albright). Additional parathormone is demanded to cause a withdrawal of extra calcium from the skeleton for use in neutralizing the excessive acid ions (sulfate and chloride) created by the diminished ability of the kidney to excrete the phosphates necessary for the production of urinary ammonia.

Primary hyperparathyroidism deserves to be included in the group of malacic diseases. Generalized osteitis fibrosa is characterized by osteoid distributed throughout the skeleton. The continuous and often rapid mobilization of calcium from the skeleton prompted by excessive parathormone does not permit the newly forming osteoid to have calcium for its change into bone. Of course, there is, in hyperparathyroidism, a destructive aspect, seen as pathologically active osteoclasia, which is not present to the same degree in the other malacic diseases.

In all of the malacic diseases there is some degree of hyperparathyroidism. In primary hyperparathyroidism the adenoma is usually responsible; in all of the other malacic diseases of the skeleton there is secondary hyperparathyroidism brought about by the need for an additional calcium mobilization to maintain the serum calcium at a physiologic level.

The following classification divides the conditions that produce a generalized decrease in skeletal density into two groups; (1) Osteoporosis; and, (2) Skeletal malacia. Etiologic factors causing a localized osteoporosis are not included. There are no conditions that cause localized osteomalacia.

Osteoporosis (Deossification)

(Disturbances of protein metabolism and osteoblastic function)

1. Disuse (bed-fast)
2. Protein deficiency (Malnutrition)
3. Basophilism (Cushing's syndrome)
4. Hyperthyroidism
5. Post-menopausal syndrome
6. Acromegaly
7. "Alarm reaction" of Selye
8. Osteogenesis imperfecta
9. Chemical ingestion (Strontium, Magnesium)
10. Senility
11. Vitamin C deficiency (Scurvy)

Skeletal Malacia (Osteomalacia)

(Disturbances of calcium metabolism)

1. Vitamin D deficiency rickets and osteomalacia
2. Calcium deficiency rickets and osteomalacia
3. Renal rickets and renal acidosis (Albright)
4. Primary hyperparathyroidism

BONE RESORPTION

The exact mechanism by which bone is absorbed remains a mystery. However, several of the factors that enter into the process are known, and have practical significance. Bone is absorbed, both physiologically and pathologically, for a wide variety of reasons. There is anabolism and catabolism in bone as in all living tissues, and in bone this means a never ending process of bone apposition and bone resorption.

During the growing years this process is particularly active. The manner in which the bones serve as a storehouse of calcium and how the parathyroid glands preserve and protect the blood calcium level has already been described. One feature of bone resorption appears clear of controversy: that is the fact that to mobilize calcium in a given area of bone, the organic as well as the inorganic elements of the bone must be absorbed. This may seem uneconomical, but nevertheless, it is a fact. At times there have been claims that the osteoid layers in rickets and osteomalacia represent sites from which calcium has been "leached" or absorbed. These osteoid seams represent sites of osteoid apposition, which have remained in the osteoid stage due to lack of proper calcium.

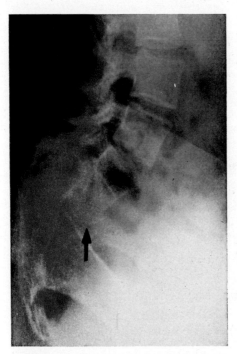

FIGURE 25. Spondylolisthesis, 3rd degree. A strong curved exostosis has grown out from the sacrum in response to the need for support beneath the 5th lumbar vertebral body.

THEORIES OF BONE RESORPTION

Bone appears to be resorbed by cellular action and by a physico-chemical mechanism. *The cellular theory* credits multinucleated and mononuclear osteoclasts with matrix resorption either by their direct apposition to bone or by contributing a substance to the tissue fluids, which causes the resorption. Radasch found osteoclastic resorption particularly active in senile bone atrophy. Bony lacunae (Howship's lacunae), in which multinucleated osteoclasts are so often moored, are such a consistent finding at sites of bone resorption that it is difficult to escape the conviction that the bony notch was somehow related to the presence of the osteoclast. However, McLean and Bloom have shown conclusively that the osteoclast does not take up the calcium by phagocytosis. Multinucleated osteoclasts produce lacunar resorption; smooth resorption when related to cells is associated with mononuclear osteoclasts, cells about the size of osteoblasts, and likely a close relative, or the same cells acting in a different role. Arey believes the multinucleated osteoclast represents several fused osteoblasts.

PHYSICO-CHEMICAL RESORPTION of bone was described first by von Recklinghausen. It was his belief that the tissue fluids adjacent to bone became acid in reaction and "washed out" the calcium, very much as hydrochloric acid will dissolve calcium salts out of bone. The physico-chemical process of bone resorption has been given the name halisteresis. All who have studied bone sections have seen areas of bone which are undergoing resorption but which fail to disclose an adequate cellular

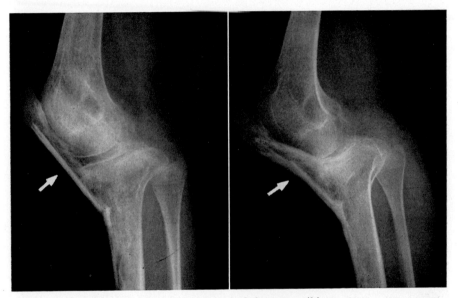

FIGURE 26. Bone graft between the patella and the upper tibia to prevent genu recurvatum. A. *(Left)* Three months post-operative. Graft has united to the tibia and patella. B. *(Right)* Two years post-operative. Hyperplasia is pronounced; the bony bridge now has a tubular cortical wall and a well-formed medullary canal.

pattern to explain the disappearance of the bone. In such instances it is tempting to resort to the "halisteresis" concept. So far as the resorption of the inorganic component of bone is concerned, it is not difficult to visualize the process as related to tissue fluids, but removal of the cells, collagen and osseo-mucin by tissue fluids requires more imagination. However, the physico-chemical theory of bone formation and resorption has gained considerable ground in recent decades. Leriche and Policard state that, "The disappearance of bone generally takes place without the intervention of cellular elements, and under the influence of a purely humoral process. Osteolysis is a rupture of the chemical balance of the phospho-carbonates of lime and a reversal of the precipitation or apposition process."

VASCULAR RESORPTION is associated with the ingrowth of blood vessels, particularly capillaries, into bone. Bone is resorbed ahead of the advancing vessels, but the exact mechanism is unknown. Pressure of the vessels against the bone may be a factor. Jaffe believes bone resorption to be much more a vascular and chemical than an osteoclastic phenomenon.

Osteosclerosis

Whereas a multitude of factors produce generalized osteoporosis, there is only hypoparathyroidism and fluorosis create a generalized increase in bone density. Albers-Schönberg's disease, erroneously called marble bones, may involve all, or nearly all of the skeleton formed by enchondral ossification, but this disease gives the impression of generalized osteosclerosis only in the roentgenogram. Pathologic examination discloses that the bone is more like chalk than marble, and that the increase in density is due to innumerable intratrabecular islands of calcified cartilage, the entity being the result of defective and incompleted enchondral ossification.

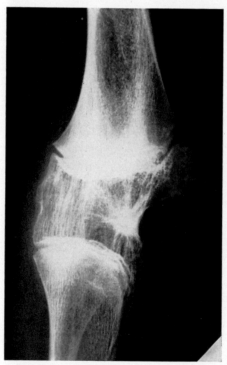

FIGURE 27. Lines of stress transmitted through this ankylosed knee joint are reflected by the trabecular systems (Wolff's law).

Localized osteosclerosis is a familiar part of chronic osteomyelitis, degenerative arthritis, certain abnormal mechanical stresses, and in bones whose circulation has been diminished by vascular disease. Details of the histogenesis of osteosclerosis are included under the several entities characterized by areas of osteosclerosis.

PHYSICAL PROPERTIES OF BONE

Steindler, in a classical treatise on kinesiology stated that "of all the factors influencing bone, mechanical factors are the most potent in determining its form and architecture . . . it is permissible (in normal adult bone) to reason deductively from the form and architecture to mechanical external forces."

As has been pointed out, the skeleton develops embryonically without mechanical stresses dictating form and internal architecture. Throughout life biologic factors exert important influences upon bone structure, many of which defy mathematical calculation. But mechanical factors often reflect themselves in a conspicuous manner, and much has been learned from the mechanical analyses given to us by such pioneers in this field as Meyer, Wolff, Jansen and Steindler.

Julius Wolff, in 1870, pointed out that whenever a bone is subjected to a change in function and stresses, the trabeculae align themselves with the new lines of stress. In 1892 this observation was formulated into the "law of functional adaptation of bone," known since as Wolff's law. It states that; "every change in form of a bone, or of its function, is followed by certain definite changes in the internal architecture and equally definite secondary alterations in external form in accordance with mathematical laws." It was Wolff's opinion that mechanical factors "absolutely dominated" bone development and architecture. Wolff did not take biologic factors into full account; we now know that infections, metabolic disturbances, growth and senility all alter the physical properties and architecture of bone.

Trabecular Systems (Trajectories)

The trabecular systems in the upper femur (Fig. 28) have been compared to the structure of a crane, and it was Wolff's opinion that the systems crossed at right angles. There is disagreement on this point and on the exact distribution of pressure and tension stresses, but the clear reflection of mechanical forces is impressive. Steindler has described the trabecular system in bones of the foot. One system runs from the astragalus posteriorly through the os calcis, and a second runs distally from the astragalus through the metatarsals and phalanges. Both systems cross in the astragalus at right angles and this point represents "the mechanical center of the systems."

Types of Stresses

Stresses which bones must resist are tension, pressure, shear, bending, and torsion. Combinations of these extrinsic stresses are the rule, and in a given bone at a given time all of the above stresses may be represented in various areas of the bone. In the femur, for example, during the standing position the femoral head is subjected to pressure (compression) stresses; the neck, to bending and shear stresses, and the diaphysis, to torsion and compression stresses. To analyze the femoral

neck stresses further, there are tension stresses in the superior aspect
and compression on the inferior aspect. Bending and shear stresses on
rod-like structures showing some degree of bend, reveal tension stresses
on the convex side of the bend and compression on the concave side.

The direction of the forces at work in creating the various stresses
deserve mention. Pressure stresses are exerted on an object when two
forces in a direct line point toward each other. When these same forces

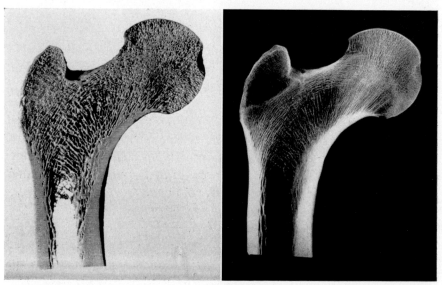

Figure 28. Trabecular systems of the upper femur. A. *(Left)* Specimen. B. *(Right)*
Roentgenogram.

pull away from each other a tension stress results. Shear and bending
stresses occur from the same application of forces, i.e.: two parallel
forces directed toward each other, but offset from each other (not in
a straight line as with pressure stress). Torsion stress results when two
forces in parallel planes occur opposite each other and at right angles
to the axis of the object acted upon. A force exerted parallel to the
longitudinal axis of a long bone is compression; if exerted at a right
angle it is shear; if exerted at a 45 degree angle it is one-half compression and one-half shear.

Response of bones to excessive stresses: Pressure stresses stimulate
bone formation up to a certain point, whereas they produce osteoresorption when excessive. Examples of this are seen where tumors or
aneurysms create prolonged excessive pressures (Fig. 22). Shear and
bend, when excessive, may be poorly tolerated. Bone grafts, placed in

scoliotic or kyphotic spines, not uncommonly develop a transverse defect or fracture at the site of maximum shear and bend; the defect or fracture is the result of a localized area of resorption inflicted by the overload.

Changes in Bone Architecture

The architecture of bone undergoes profound changes through growth, the postmenopausal state, during senility, and from such diseases as rickets and osteomalacia. In bone atrophy there may be endosteal absorption, as in excentric atrophy, or subperiosteal absorption, leading to the narrowed shafts of concentric atrophy. Advanced osteoporosis may reduce the long bones to membranous tubes. Paget's disease and hyperparathyroidism in advanced stages completely disrupt the internal architecture of involved bones.

REFERENCES

Articular Cartilage

Clark, E. R. and Clark, E. L.: Microscopic observations on new formation of cartilage in the living mammal. *Am. J. Anat., 70*:167, 1942.

Efskind, L.: Experimental investigations on anatomy and physiology of the joints and synovia. *Acta orth. Scandinav., 12*:1, 1941.

Fell, H. B.: Histogenesis of cartilage and bone in the long bones of the embryonic fowl. *J. Morphol. & Physiol., 40*:417, 1925.

Freund, E.: Active and passive pleat formation of joint cartilage. *Arch. Path., 18*:168-198, 1934.

Haas, G. M.: Studies of cartilage: A morphologic and chemical analysis of aging human cartilage. *Am. J. Path., 35*:275, 1943.

Ham, A. W.: Cartilage and bone. *In Cowdry: Special Cytology*, Vol. II, New York, 1932.

Hunter, W.: On the structure and diseases of articulating cartilages. *Philosophical Trans. London, 42*:514, 1742.

Ogston, A.: On articular cartilage. *J. Anat. & Physiol.*, London, *10*:49, 1876; *12*:503, 1878.

Phemister, D. B.: Causes of and changes in loose bodies arising from articular surface of joint. *J. Bone & Joint Surg., 6*:278, 1924.

Phemister, D. B.: Changes in articular surfaces in tuberculous and pyogenic infections of joints. *Am. J. Roentgenol., 12*:144, 1924.

Phemister, D. B.: Effect of pressure on articular surfaces. *Ann. Surg., 80*:481, 1924.

Santos, J. V.: Changes which the articular cartilage of the hip joint may undergo. *Surg. Gynec. & Obst., 45*:650, 1932.

Shands, A. R., Jr.: Regeneration of hyaline cartilage. *Arch. Surg., 22*:137-178, 1931.

Silberberg, M. R.: Response of cartilage and bone of new-born guinea pig to stimulation by various hormones. *Anat. Rec., 78*:549, 1940.

Synovial Membrane

Ghormley, R. and Deacon: Synovial membranes in various types of arthritis: A study of differential stains. *Am. J. Roentgenol., 35*: June 1936.

Key, J. A.: Cytology of the synovial fluid of normal joints. *Anat. Rec., 40*:193, 1928.

Key, J. A.: The reformation of synovial membrane in the knees of rabbits after synovectomy. *J. Bone & Joint Surg., 7*:793, 1925.

KLING, D. H.: *The Synovial Membrane and the Synovial Fluid*. Medical Press, Los Angeles 1938.

SIGURDSON, L. A.: The structure and function of the articular synovial membrane. *J. Bone & Joint Surg., 12*:603, 1930.

VAUBEL, E.: The form and function of synovial cells in tissue culture. *J. Exper. Med., 58*:63, 1938.

BONE

ALBRIGHT, F.: Cushing's Syndrome. *The Harvard Lecture Series, 38*:123, 1942-43.

AREY, L. B.: The origin, growth and fate of osteoclasts and their relation to bone resorption. *Am. J. Anat., 26*:315, 1920.

ARIES, L. J.: Experimental analysis of growth pattern and rates of appositional and longitudinal growth in rat femur. *Surg. Gynec. & Obst., 72*:679, April 1941.

BANKS, S. W., AND COMPERE, E. L.: Regeneration of epiphyseal cartilage. *Ann. Surg., 114*:1076, 1941.

BAST, T. H., SULLIVAN, W. E., and GERST, F. D.: The repair of bone. *Anat. Rec., 31*: 255, 1925.

BAST, T. H.: Studies on the structure and multiplication of bone cells facilitated by a new technique. *Am. J. Anat., 29*:139, 1921.

BATTS, M.: Rupture of the nucleus pulposis, anatomical study. *J. Bone & Joint Surg., 21*:121, 1939.

BAUER, W. and AUB, J. C., and ALBRIGHT, F.: Studies in calcium and phosphorous metabolism. *J. Exper. Med., 49*:145, 1929.

BELL, G. H. and CUTHBERTSON, D. P.: Effect of various hormones on the physical properties of bone. *J. Endocrinol., 3*:302, 1943.

BELL, G. H., CUTHBERTSON, D. P., and ORR, J.: Strength of bone in relation to calcium intake. *Am. J. Physiol., 134*:299, 1941.

BISGARD, J. D.: Osteogenesis; An experimental study. *Arch. Surg., 30*:748, 1935.

BISGARD, J. D.: Ossification. *Arch. Surg., 33*:926, 1936.

BLOOM, W. and BLOOM, M. A.: Calcification and ossification of developing bone in embryonic and new-born rats. *Anat. Rec., 78*:497, 1940.

BLOOM, W., BLOOM, M. A. and McLEAN, F. C.: Calcification and ossification. Medullary bone changes in reproductive cycle of female pigeons. *Anat. Rec., 81*:443, 1941.

BOGERT, L. J. and HASTINGS, A. B.: The calcium salts of bone. *J. Biol. Chem., 94*:473, 1931.

BRASH, J. C.: Some problems in growth and developmental mechanics of bone. *Edinburgh M. J., 41*:305, 1934.

BRUNSCHWIG, A. and HARMON, P. H.: Studies in bone sarcoma. Malignant osteoblastoma as evidence for existence of true osteoblasts. *Surg. Gynec. & Obst. 57*:711, 1933.

CORBIN, K. B. and HINSEY, J. C.: Influence of the nervous system on bone and joints. *Anat. Rec., 75*:307, 1939.

COWDRY, E. V.: *Special Cytology*. Vol. II, Paul B. Hoeber, New York 1932.

CRETIN, A.: Histogenesis of bone tissue in the light of study of delayed consolidation. *La Presse Med., 48*:996, Dec. 11, 1940.

DAWSON, A. B.: Histologic study of the persisting cartilage plates in retarded or lapsed epiphyseal union in the albino rat. *Anat. Rec., 43*:109, 1929.

DEAKINS, M.: Bone composition, correlation between density and ash, organic and water content. *Proc. Soc. Exper. Biol. & Med., 46*:62, 1941.

DODDS, G. S.: Row formation and other types of cartilage cells in endochondral ossification. *Anat. Rec., 46*:385, 1930.

DODDS, G. S.: Osteoclasts and cartilage removal in endochondral ossification of certain mammals. *Am. J. Anat., 50*:97, 1932.

DOWNS, W. G. and McKEOWN, R. M.: Histology of healing of fractures in rats on diets low in total salt, calcium, and phosphorus. *Arch. Surg., 25*:108, 1932; 25:94, 1932.

DRAGSTEDT, C. A.: Some aspects of the physiology of bone. *Nebraska M. J., 17*:93, 1932.

DRAGSTEDT, C. A. and KEARNS, T. E.: Bone formation in thyroparathyroidectomized dogs. *Am. J. Physiol., 100*:262, 1932.

EHRENHAFT, H. L.: Development of the vertebral column as related to certain congenital and pathological changes. *Surg. Gynec. & Obst., 76*:282, March 1943.

FELL, H. B.: Osteogenic capacity in vitro and periosteum and endosteum isolated from the limb skeleton of fowl embryos and young chicks. *J. Anat., 66*:157, 1932.

FELL, H. B.: Osteogenesis in vitro. *Arch. f. exper. Zellforsch., 11*:245, 1931.

FELL, H. B. and ROBINSON, R.: Embryonic bone development. *Biochem. J. 23*:767 and 860, 1929.

FRANSEEN, C. C., SIMONS, C. C. and McLEAN, R.: The phosphatase determination in the differential diagnosis of bone lesions. *Surg. Gynec. & Obst., 68*:1038, 1939.

GALLI, W. E. and ROBERTSON, D. E.: The repair of bones. *Brit. J. Surg., 7*:211, 1919.

GEDDES, A. C.: The origin of the osteoblast and of the osteoclast. *J. Anat. and Physiol., 47*:159, 1912.

GILL, A. B.: Bone metabolism. Its principles and its relation to orthopedic surgery. *J. Bone & Joint Surg., 18*:4, 1941, 1936.

GLUCKMANN, A.: Studies on bone mechanics in vitro. *Anat. Rec., 72*:97, 1938; *73*:39, 1939.

GLUCKMANN, A.: The role of mechanical stresses in bone formation in vitro. *J. Anat., 76*:231, 1942.

HAAS, S.: Experimental transplant of the epiphyses with observation on the longitudinal growth of bone. *J. A. M. A., 65*:1965, 1915; *Surg. Gynec. & Obst. 52*:958, 1931.

HAAS, S.: The relation of blood supply to the longitudinal growth of bone. *Am. J. Ortho. Surg., 15*:305, 1917.

HAM, A.: The last hundred years in the study of bone. *J. Am. Dent. A., 21*:3, 1934.

HARBIN, M.: Overgrowth of the long bones of the lower extremity. *Arch. Surg., 14*:142, 1927.

HARI, P.: *Physiologische Chemie*, p. 226, Berlin 1922.

HARREL, D. J.: The nerve supply of bone. *J. Anat., 72*:54, 1938.

HARRIS, H. A.: Bone formation and the osteoblast. *Lancet, 2*:489, 1928.

HARRIS, H. A.: Lines of arrested growth in long bones in childhood. *Brit. J. Radiol., 4*:561, 1931.

HARRIS, H. A.: *Bone Growth in Health and Disease*. Oxford Press, 1933.

HOWSHIP, J.: Experiments and observations in order to ascertain the means employed by the animal economy in the formation of bone. *Tr. Med.-Chir. Soc., London, 6*:263, 1817.

HUGGINS, C. B.: Composition of bone and the function of the bone cell. *Physiol. Rev., 17*:119, 1937.

HUGGINS, C. B., McCARROL, H. R. and BLOCKSOM, B. H.: Experiments on the theory of osteogenesis. *Arch. Surg., 32*:915, 1936.

HUNTER, D.: Studies in calcium and phosphorus metabolism in generalized diseases of bone. *Proc. Roy. Soc. Med., 28*:1619, 1935.

HYNDMAN, O. R.: Pathologic intervertebral disc and its consequences. *Arch. Surg., 53*:247, 1946.

INGALLS, T. H.: Epiphyseal growth. Normal sequence of events at epiphyseal plate. *Endocrinology, 29*:710, 1941.

JAFFE, H. L.: Methods for the histologic study of normal and diseased bone. *Arch. Path., 8*:817, 1929.

JAFFE, H. L.: The resorption of bone. *Arch. Surg., 20*:355, 1930.

JOHNSON, R. W., JR.: A physiological study of the blood supply of the diaphysis. *J. Bone & Joint Surg., 9*:153, 1927.

JORDAN, H. E.: Varieties and significance of giant cells. *Anat. Rec., 31*:51, 1925.

KAY, H. D.: Phosphatase in growth and diseases of bone. *Physiol. Rev., 12*:384, 1932.

KEITH, SIR A.: Bone growth and bone repair. *Brit. J. Surg., 6*:19, 1918-19.

KEITH, SIR A.: Wolff's Law of bone transformation. *Lancet, 1*:250, 1918.

KEY, J. A.: Factors in atrophy of bone. *J. Am. Dent. A., 17*:1660, 1930.

KOCH, J. C.: Laws of bone architecture. *Am. J. Anat., 21*:177, 1917.

LERICHE, R. and POLICARD, A.: *The Normal and Pathological psysiology of bone*. C. V. Mosby Co., St. Louis, 1928 (Trans. by. S. Moore and J. A. Key).

LICHTWITZ, L.: *Functional Pathology*. Grune and Stratton, New York, 1941.

McEWEN, W.: *The Growth of Bone*. Glasgow, Maclehose, Jackson and Co. 1912.

McLean, F. C. and Bloom, W.: Calcification and ossification. *Arch. Path., 32*:315, 1941.

McLean, F. C. and Bloom, W.: Calcification and ossification. Calcification in normal growing bone. *Anat. Rec., 78*:333, 1940.

McMaster, P. E.: Bone atrophy and absorption. *J. Bone & Joint Surg., 19*:74, 1937.

Maximow, A. U. and Bloom, W.: *Textbook of Histology.* W. B. Saunders Co., Philadelphia, 1942.

Munnemacher, R. F.: Experimental studies on the cartilage plates in the long bones of the rat. *Am. J. Anat., 65*:253, 1939.

Murray, P. D. F.: *Bones.* A Study of the Development and Structure of the Vertebrate Skeleton. Cambridge Univ. Press, London, 1936.

Ollier, L.: Traité experimental et clinique de la régenération des os et de la production artificielle du tissue osseux, Paris, 1867, 1. *Arch. Klin. Chir., 22*:343, 1878.

Peters: Chemistry and physiology of calcification. *Am. J. Surg., 10*:550, 1930.

Phemister, D. B.: Repair of bone in presence of asceptic necrosis resulting from fractures, transplantation and vascular obstruction. *J. Bone & Joint Surg., 12*:769, 1930.

Phemister, D. B.: Studies in reduction of bone density. *Am. J. Roentgenol., 8*:355, 1921.

Phemister, D. B.: Bone growth and repair. *Ann. Surg., 102*:261, 1935.

Pollock, G. A. and Ghormley, R. K.: Early repair of bone. *J. Bone & Joint Surg., 23*:273, 1941.

Pommer, G.: Ueber osteoporose, ihren Ursprung und ihren differential diagnostische Bedentung. *Deutsche Klin. Chir., 136*:1, 1925.

Radasch, H. E.: Senility of bone and its relationship to bone rapair. *Surg. Gynec. & Obst., 51*:42, 1930.

Robinson, R.: The possible significance of phosphoric esthers in metabolism. *J. Biochem., 17*:286, 1923; *24*:1922, 1930.

Selye, H.: On the mechanism of controlling the growth in length of the long bones. *J. Anat., 68*:289, 1934.

Selye, H.: The general adaptation syndrome. *J. Clin. Endocrinol., 6*:117, 1946.

Shands, A. R., Jr.: Studies in bone formation. The effects of the local presence of calcium salts on osteogenesis. *J. Bone & Joint Surg., 19*:1065, 1937.

Shear, M. J. and Kramer, B.: Composition of bone. *J. Biol. Chem., 83*:697, 1929.

Shipley, P. G. and Macklin, C. C.: Some features of osteogenesis in the light of vital staining. *Am. J. Physiol., 42*:117, 1916.

Siegling, J. A.: Growth of the epiphyses. *J. Bone & Joint Surg., 23*:23, 1941.

Siegling, J. A. and Fahey, J.: The fate of transplanted cow's horn. *J. Bone & Joint Surg., 18*:439, 1936.

Steindler, A.: Physical properties of bone. *Arch. Phys. Therapy, 17*:336, 345.

Steindler, A.: *Mechanics of normal and pathological locomotion in man.* Charles C Thomas, Springfield, 1935.

Stump, C. W.: Histogenesis of bone. *J. Anat., 59*:136, 1925.

Todd, W.: The development and growth of bone. *J. Anat. & Physiol., 47*:177, 1913.

Urist, M. R. and McLean, F. C.: Calcification and ossification. I. *J. Bone and Joint Surg., 23*:1, 1941. II. *J. Bone & Joint Surg., 23*:283, 1941. III. *J. Bone & Joint Surg., 24*:47, 1942.

Watson-Jones, R. and Roberts, R.: Calcification, decalcification and ossification. *Brit. J. Surg., 21*:30, 1934.

Watt, J. C.: Development of bone. *Arch. Surg., 17*:1017, 1928.

Wenger, H. L.: Transplantation of epiphyseal cartilage. *Arch. Surg., 50*:148, 1945.

Willis, R. A.: The growth of embryo bones transplanted whole in the rat's brain. *Proc. Roy. Soc., London, 120*:496, July 1, 1936.

CHAPTER II

Acute Infections of Bones and Joints

Contents

Acute infections of the skeletal system are the pyogenic infections. In the majority of cases the pyogenic organisms are carried to a bone or joint via the blood stream. An exception exists under battle conditions in that the greater number of cases develop from direct innoculation in compound fractures and traumatic arthrotomies. The account of the reactions of bones and joints to the presence of pyogenic organisms is one of the most important chapters in any dissertation on skeletal pathology. This is true both because of the relative frequency of these diseases, and the insight to be gained into pathologic and physiologic mechanisms, as they apply to skeletal reactions. An understanding of the pathogenesis of these entities is indispensable to the proper direction of their therapy.

Bones, even when extensively involved, generally are capable of retaining their continuity and, with proper treatment, achieve a near-normal restoration. Joints, on the other hand, once seriously involved in an acute pyogenic infection, are incapable of a complete recovery, and indeed there are many instances when the joint is utterly destroyed.

Antibiotics have reduced the tragedy of acute osteomyelitis and of suppurative arthritis, but have by no means eradicated these diseases.

PYOGENIC ARTHRITIS

Pyogenic arthritis, commonly called suppurative arthritis, is the outcome of a successful invasion of a joint by pyogenic organisms. While it may occur at any age, it occurs most frequently during the first and second decades and is the most common of the joint infections created by micro-organisms (Campbell).

Although several types will be described, based upon the mode of entry and causative organisms, the morbid anatomy is essentially similar in all instances.

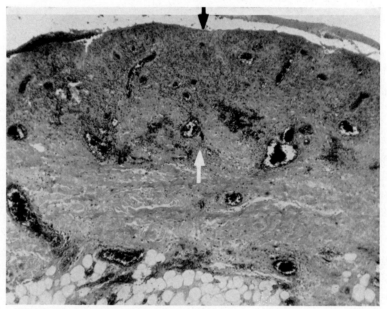

FIGURE 29. Acute pyogenic synovitis. Neutrophils thickly infiltrate the granulation tissue that has replaced the stratum snyoviale.

ETIOLOGY

All of the pyogenic organisms have been identified with pyogenic arthritis; the most frequent are staphylococci, streptococci, gonococci, pneumococci and the meningococci. A combination of organisms is not unusual: for example, tuberculous arthritis with secondary staphylococci; staphylococci with Vincents infection, which may occur when metacarpo-phalangeal joints strike human teeth in fist fights.

Pyogenic arthritis may make its appearance as a complication of osteomyelitis, measles, scarlet fever, meningitis, pneumococcic pneumonia, septicemias or gonorrhea. It may also complicate traumatic joint perforations. In some instances no definite source of the organism can be identified. Periodically, foci of infection are claimed as sources of pyogenic arthritis.

Mode of entry into joint: (1) *Hematogenous:* Blood borne infections deposit the organisms directly into the joint capsule, presumably into the synovial membrane. (2) *Direct extention:* Organisms may advance from a nearby bone or soft tissue infection directly into the joint. When there is direct extention from an osteomyelitic focus, one of several routes may be taken. A metaphyseal osteomyelitis may deposit pus beneath overlying periosteum, and since the periosteum is continuous with the joint capsule, entry of pus into the joint becomes possible. Less commonly an organizing exudate may make its way from a metaphysis directly through an epiphyseal plate and epiphysis to perforate the articular surface. Rarely in children, more frequently in adults, a primary epiphysitis occurs in which organisms enter the joint through erosion of articular cortex and cartilage. An osteomyelitis of the patella may empty its exudate directly into the knee joint. (3) *Perforation of a joint by trauma or surgery:* Pyogenic organisms, once carried into a joint on foreign bodies, often set up suppuration. In rare instances a pyogenic joint infection represents a post-operative complication.

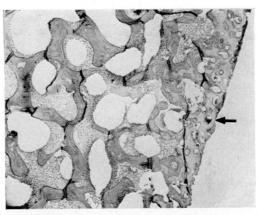

FIGURE 30. Pyogenic arthritis of the hip. Photomicrograph of a section from the femoral head. All of the non-calcified cartilage has been destroyed by the proteolytic enzyme released from necrotic neutrophils, leaving only the calcified cartilage (arrow). The infection has extended into the epiphysis, and pus fills many of the marrow spaces.

Once inside the joint, the extent of the infection depends upon the usual factors that control pyogenic infections, i.e., number and virulence of the organisms, and the resistance of the host.

PATHOGENESIS

Acute Stage

The earliest changes in the joint appear in the synovial membrane as active hyperemia, edema, and accelerated secretion of synovial fluid. Neutrophils are concentrated at the site of the invading pyogenic organisms, and soon leucocytes and organisms overflow into the joint fluid. This is the seropurulent stage, and fortunately, many cases do not advance further. Healing is prompt and permanent damage only slight.

If the invading organisms continue to hold the upper hand, the synovial fluid steadily thickens with exudate, frank pus ultimately filling the joint. During this, the purulent stage, intra-articular pressure may steadily rise until the joint capsule either ruptures at a site of necrosis or is drained surgically. With a rupture into adjacent soft tissues, large areas of muscle and fascia may become shot through with a multitude of minute abscesses or destroyed en masse by large abscesses.

Cartilage Changes

Most interesting of the joint responses to pyogenic infections are the striking changes that take place in the articular cartilages. Phemister's classical experiments have done much to elucidate cartilage reactions to the exudates. When hyaline cartilage was incubated at 55 degrees C. in organism suspensions or in exudates of non-pyogenic infections, such as tuberculosis, no changes occurred in the cartilage. But when incubated in pus from a pyogenic infection, the cartilage was completely digested, in from three to 24 hours. From the dead neutrophilis a proteolytic ferment (protease) is released which produces the chondrolysis characteristic of

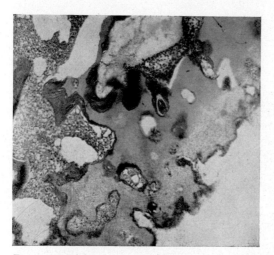

FIGURE 31. High power magnification of the zone of calcified cartilage, Figure 30.

suppurative arthritis. At the outset the superficial layers of the articular surfaces become involved through loss of matricial substance, exposing the collagenous fibers. The normal, hyaline, wet, glistening surface gives away to a dull, granular, opaque surface. If the infection subsides early, the chondrolytic process may end here, the superficial layers flake off from friction, and a new gliding surface forms.

If the suppurative process advances and the articular cartilage is bathed in frank pus, chondrolysis progresses until the cartilage is entirely lost. Destruction is most rapid at sites of contact of the articular surfaces. An extension of the pus through the thin zone of calcified cartilage that lies between the articular cortex and articular cartilage is not readily accomplished until granulation tissue forms. The proteolytic enzyme readily digests uncalcified cartilage and most soft tissues, but is unable to destroy calcified cartilage and bone.

Bone Involvement

In older children and adults the epiphyses are ossified; therefore, only a protracted and severe pyogenic arthritis can advance through the articular cortex to fill subchondral marrow spaces with pus. Only rarely do deep extensions or sequestration develop.

In children, suppuration in the hip joint may interrupt the blood supply to the capital epiphysis of the femur by compression or thrombosis, creating an aseptic necrosis. Dislocations, and epiphyseal separa-

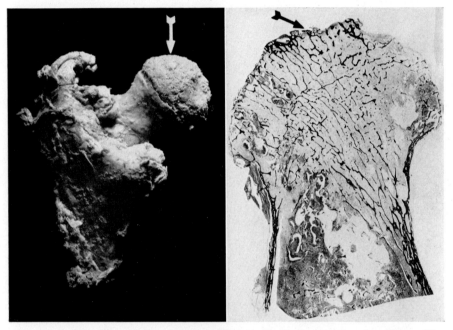

FIGURE 32. Pyogenic arthritis of the hip joint. A. *(Left)* Photographs of specimen. The articular cartilage and most of the articular cortex (arrow) have been destroyed. Infection of the joint was secondary to an acute osteomyelitis of the femoral neck. B. *(Right)* Histologic section of femoral head and neck. A large abscess occupies much of the neck. Nothing remains of the articular surface.

tions are not uncommon complications of the more severe pyogenic joints.

Chronic Stage: As the acute stage subsides, the exudate organizes and part or all of the synovial membrane is replaced by granulation tissue. Granulation tissue then grows over peripheral portions of the articular cartilage as a pannus. A thin tongue-like projection of the pannus may extend between articular surfaces, creeping only part way, or advancing to join its fellow from the opposite side. In the microscopic picture the neutrophiles steadily diminish in numbers. Fibroblasts increase, and soon the granulation tissue is transformed to young fibrous tissue. When the synovial membrane is damaged, the secretion of synovial fluid is diminished or lost; the cartilage is deprived of its nutrition and dies.

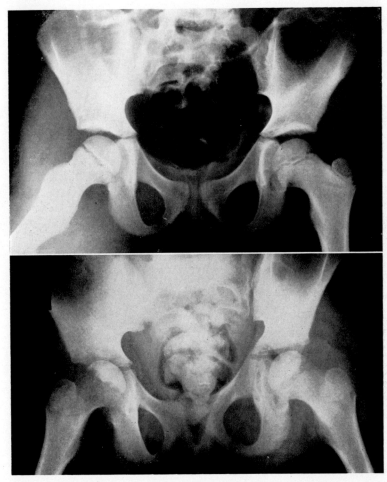

FIGURE 33. Bilateral streptococcus hemolyticus arthritis of the hip joints of an eight year old girl. Involvement of the hip joints occurred following an acute pyogenic middle-ear abscess. Left hip incised (Ober incision), right hip aspirated. A. *(Above)* 4-26-38. Three days after onset. B. *(Below)* 6-13-38. Necrosis of capital epiphyses, presumably from vascular occlusion.

In the chronic stage, any articular cartilage surviving the action of protease, may forthwith be destroyed by the granulation and fibrous tissue pannus on the surface, and by granulation and fibrous tissue growing through the articular cortex into the deep side of the articular cartilage. Osteoclasts and chondroclasts are numerous during this period. Dense fibrous adhesions develop within the synovial sac as the exudate disappears or organizes. If the joint ruptures or is drained surgically, sinuses with their scar tissue walls and epithelialized openings in the skin may persist for many months. Rarely a small sequestrum

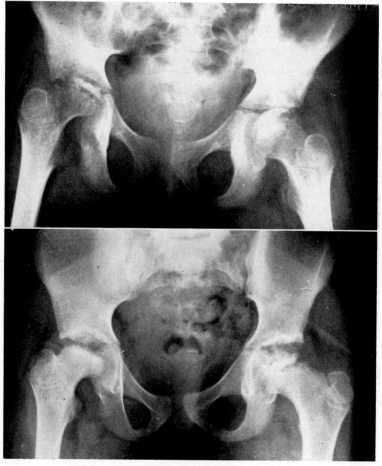

FIGURE 33. *(Continued)* C. *(Above)* 8-1-38. Left capital epiphysis is regenerating, right is absorbing. D. *(Below)* In excellent health. Flexion right hip, 150 to 140 degrees; flexion left hip, 180 to 100 degrees.

develops around and adjacent to the articular cortex. Occasionally an untreated pyogenic arthritis in childhood extends into an epiphysis, rapidly spreads throughout and may invade the epiphyseal plate and stop its growth.

If the blood supply of the femoral head has been cut off by a suppurative arthritis of the hip, the resulting aseptic necrosis of the capital epiphysis must pass through the long process of creeping substitution.

Healing Stage: During the healing process granulation tissue, displacing involved areas of synovialis, undergoes fibrous condensation. If function in the joint is re-established, the areas of synovial membrane that were replaced by fibrous tissue become transformed into a synovial-like tissue that secretes joint fluid. If the joint undergoes anklylosis during the healing process, no functional transformation of the fibrous areas takes place. If pannus formations are present, they also undergo condensation and often play an important role in ankylosis.

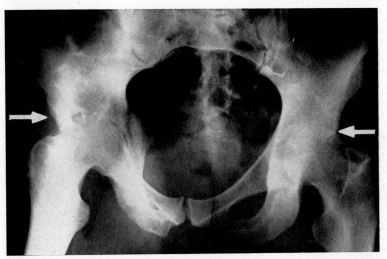

FIGURE 34. Pneumococcic arthritis hip, bilateral. Male age 37. Hips became involved following a pneumococcic pneumonia. Pneumococcus type II cultured from pus obtained during arthrotomy right hip joint. Result was bilateral ankylosis of the hips.

Ankylosis

Suppurative arthritis is one of the leading causes of ankylosis. During the healing stage one of three types of ankylosis may be established: (1) fibrous; (2) cartilaginous; or, (3) bony. *Fibrous ankylosis* occurs when the articular surfaces fuse to an interposed fibrous tissue pannus. When the pannus is young and the joint infection is in the chronic stage, active absorption of articular cartilage by the pannus takes place, but when the healing stage appears, the pannus cells mature, cease their invasion of the cartilage, and may bind adjacent cartilage surfaces together. *Cartilage ankylosis* occurs in one of two ways. Following the acute stage of a pyogenic infection, the softened articular surfaces may fuse without the advent of an interposed pannus. Another type of cartilaginous ankylosis may develop if a fibrous ankylosis permits a few degrees of mobility. The friction plus pressure gradually transforms the interposed fibrous tissue to fibrocartilage. Transverse fissures in such a zone of fibrocartilage are the rule. *Bony ankylosis* may result in older children or adults if there has been complete destruction of the articular cartilage, particularly so if the joint is immobilized during the healing stage. Fibrous tissue unites the adjacent bone ends at the outset; then, with bony trabecularization of the fibrous tissue, the bony ankylosis is established. In time mature lamellar bone replaces the original fibrous bone, the mature trabeculae extending across the

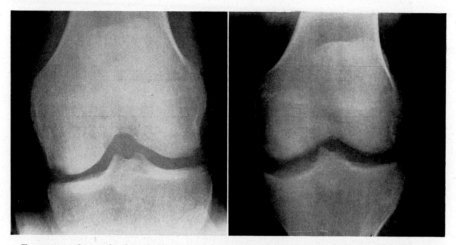

FIGURE 35. Gonorrheal arthritis left knee. A. *(Left)* Four weeks after onset. Note marginal notching of femoral condyles similar to tuberculosis arthritis. B. *(Right)* Nine weeks after onset. X-ray taken with knee in traction.

former joint aligning themselves in the directions of functional stresses.

If joint motion is preserved in spite of thinned cartilaginous surfaces, degenerative arthritis with its marginal osteophytes and subchondral sclerosis slowly develops through the years.

Clinical Correlation

Since joint damage occurs rapidly in the more severe cases of suppuration, it is important to make the diagnosis early. Early aspiration facilitates diagnosis and at the same time relieves the intraarticular tension. Unheeded distention of a joint by pus destroys the synovial membrane, stretches ligaments, and produces chondrolysis. Adequate drainage is mandatory if antibiotic therapy fails to control the infection.

With early and proper treatment, the joint will reveal a remarkable capacity for retrieving its function. The synovial membrane shows fairly substantial resistance to infection in early stages, and also in later stages, if effective treatment is instituted and the synovial membrane protected from becoming overwhelmed by the invading organisms.

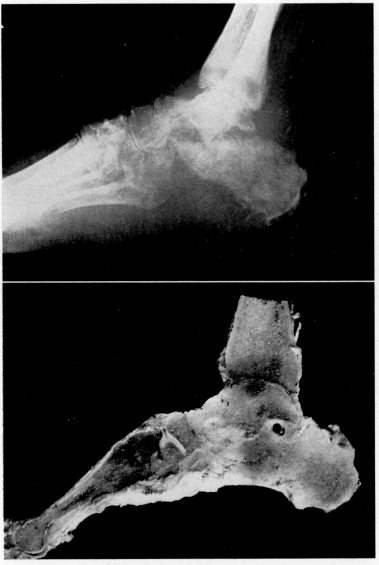

FIGURE 36. Pyogenic arthritis of all tarsal joints. Female age 50. Acute onset five months previously. Hemolytic staphlococcus aureus cultured from drainage. A. *(Above)* Lateral roentgenogram. B. *(Below)* Amputation specimen. The round subastragaloid perforation is a sinus tract.

When ankylosis is inevitable, every effort should be made to secure a bony ankylosis, and to achieve it with the joint in the best possible position for function. This usually requires protracted immobilization. In the majority of cases mobility can be preserved, and early joint motion is employed to attain this end. If dense adhesions are permitted to form between folds of synovial membrane and between articular surfaces, only a few degrees of motion will be possible. Such a joint gives the patient a useless range of motion and a distressing amount of pain.

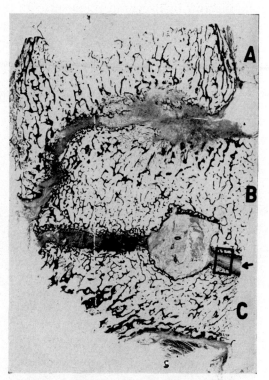

Formerly, after several years of quiescence of the infection, elective surgery to correct alignment, to transform a painful fibrous ankylosis to a bony ankylosis, or to perform an anthroplasty was hazardous because of the existence of minute hidden nests of granulation tissue and organisms. Post-operative infections on this basis are less feared now that antibiotics are in our armamentarium.

Differential diagnosis is not often a problem if aspirations are employed and cultures and smears are made. Pyogenic arthritis may need to be differentiated from acute traumatic arthritis, particularly when associated with hemarthrosis; and rheumatoid arthritis, when it involves only one joint; and rarely from tuberculous arthritis.

FIGURE 37. Fibrous and cartilaginous ankylosis of ankle and subastragaloid joints. Residual of pyogenic arthritis in a 20 year old male. A. Lower tibia. B. Astragalus. C. Os calcis.

Roentgenographic Correlation

Early in the process the roentgenogram shows only the joint distention. Later a narrowed cartilage space and bone atrophy are visualized. One of the most significant points to be noted relates to the articular cortices. In pyogenic arthritis, the articular cortex remains intact until there is pronounced narrowing of the cartilage space. In the chronic granulomata, particularly tuberculosis, the articular cortex loses its definition and integrity early while the cartilage space is yet preserved.

ACUTE OSTEOMYELITIS

Acute osteomyelitis is a destructive invasion of bone, periosteum, and marrow by pyogenic organisms. On the basis of gross and roentgenological examinations, inflammation of the skeleton is termed osteitis, periostitis, or osteomyelitis. Microscopic examination does not support this classification since such localization of the inflammatory process rarely occurs, there being some degree of involvement of all anatomical components. Actually, the acute infection holds forth in the marrow spaces, in the haversian canals, and beneath the periosteum. The bone proper plays a passive role: in early stages it is actively resorbed; later it is actively reconstructed; or it may succumb to the infection or to vascular thrombosis and sequestrate.

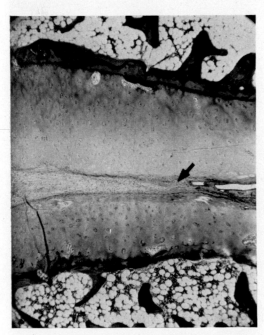

FIGURE 38. Photomicrograph of the segment of the subastragaloid joint in square drawn on Figure 37. Ankylosis was achieved through a fibrous tissue pannus (arrow).

ETIOLOGY

It is estimated that 90 percent of all cases of acute hematogenous osteomyelitis are due to staphylococci. Streptococcic infections, gonorrhea, pneumonia, typhoid, and colon bacillus infections account for approximately ten percent of the cases.

AGE INCIDENCE

Acute osteomyelitis occurs most frequently during the growing years, the highest incidence being reached during the first decade. As would be expected, trauma is held responsible for the greater number of cases in males.

DISTRIBUTION

Wilensky and Kulowski have emphasized that hematogenous pyogenic osteomyelitis is a septicemia at the outset, the skeletal lesions representing only one of many potential manifestations of the disease. No part of the skeleton is immune from becoming a focus, but the usual location is in a long bone metaphysis. The following reasons are given for the pronounced susceptibility of metaphyses: metaphyses are the site of the most rapid skeletal growth; metaphyses receive many terminal branches (end arteries) from the nutrient arteries; and, it is claimed, metaphyses have within them less active phagocytosis. Phemister has pointed out that the incidence of osteomyelitic involvement in a given long bone metaphysis is in direct proportion both to the rate of growth at that metaphysis, and to the size of the bone. The longer and larger the bone, the more susceptible it is to acute osteomyelitis, the more rapidly growing end being the more susceptible. Thus the lower femur has a higher incidence than does the upper femur; and the upper tibia and upper humerus have a higher incidence than the lower metaphyses of these bones.

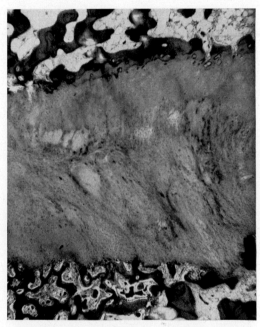

FIGURE 39. Fibrocartilaginous ankylosis. Fibrocartilage has replaced most of the normal hyaline cartilage.

Pathogenesis: Potential sequences of events in acute hematogenous osteomyelitis will be portrayed step by step, beginning with the pyogenic organisms being swept along in the blood stream. The organisms reach a metaphysis via a nutrient artery. To be able to establish a suppurative infection in the bone, the organisms must arrive in rather large numbers and possess a fairly high virulence. At the site where the organisms lodge, a minute area of bone is killed. An active hyperemia promptly develops, and mature neutrophilic leucocytes move into the area to defend the bone against the invading organisms. The result is an exudate, which is thin and serous at first, but soon becomes purulent if the organisms survive and multiply. With the enforced immobilization of the bone by pain, and the hyperemia from the infection, active osteoabsorption takes place which is reflected in the roentgenogram in one to three weeks as bone atrophy. In the process of bone absorp-

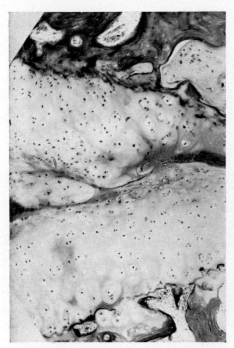

FIGURE 40. Cartilaginous ankylosis. An uncommon type of ankylosis in which the contacting articular surfaces fuse to each other. Probably the result of a mild pyogenic arthritis.

tion, the cortical Volkmann and haversian canals enlarge and serve as channels to carry the newly formed exudate to the surface where it is deposited beneath the periosteum. With vast numbers of microscopic channels to the surface, it should not be surprising when a subperiosteal abscess forms at an early manifestation of the disease. If the organisms are less virulent and nature's defenses more effective, infection may subside before an abscess forms. Since the advent of penicillin and the sulfonamides, this has been frequently observed. When frank pus forms, it may localize and encapsulate to become a Brodies' abscess. Details of the pathogenesis of this type of abscess will be presented in the discussion of chronic osteomyelitis. When pus flows to the surface or in any other manner accumulates beneath the periosteum, extension distally and proximally may be rapid, since in children the periosteum is only loosely anchored to the cortex. The exudate may so extensively elevate the periosteum as to form a veritable "cloak of pus" about the diaphysis.

Extension of pus down the medullary canal may occur, the normal marrow elements being destroyed as they are displaced by myriad neutrophils. In this process the cancellous bony trabeculae and the inner aspect of the cortex are deprived of their blood supply and therefore must sequestrate. When so advanced a stage is reached that the periosteum is elevated and much of the medullary canal filled with pus, the entire diaphysis may become a sequestrum. It is possible for an extensive sequestrum to form in the presence of only a small amount

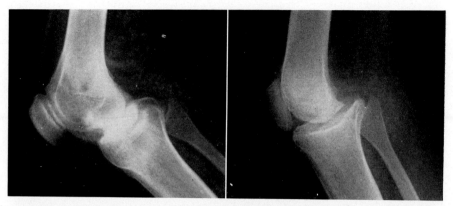

FIGURE 41. Bony ankylosis of right knee in a female, age 17. Result of a Neisserian infection. A. *(Left)* Lateral roentgenogram showing bony ankylosis and flexion contracture. B. *(Right)* Post-arthroplasty. Motion 175 to 90 degrees. No pain.

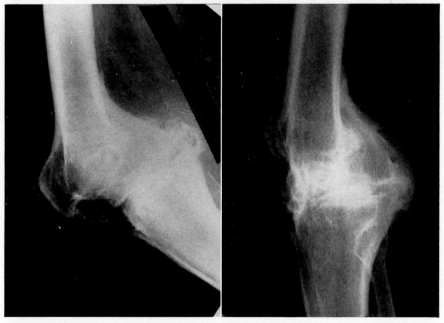

FIGURE 42. Fibrous ankylosis of the right knee in a 67 year old man. Result of a pyogenic arthritis that followed a laceration into knee by an axe in 1895. Knee was in a flexed position and was painful. A. *(Left)* Pre-operative. B. *(Right)* After wedge resection. Bony ankylosis. No pain.

of pus if the nutrient vessels become involved in a thrombosing phlebitis and arthritis. Obliteration may occur in the nutrient foramen of the cortex, since the bone is unyielding to edema and little extra space exists around the vessels. Large areas of diaphysis undergo aseptic necrosis when death of the bone occurs by obliteration of the nutrient

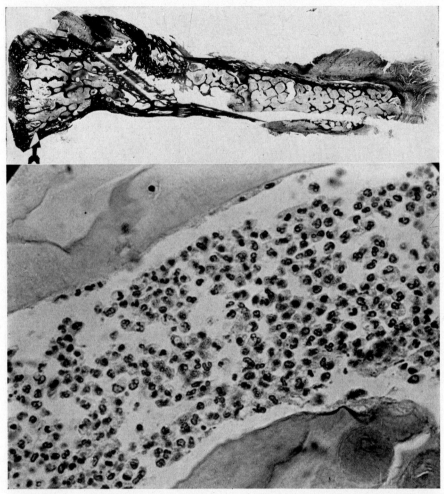

FIGURE 43. Acute osteomyelitis, left transverse process, 4th lumbar vertebra. The bone is necrotic. Marrow spaces are filled with pus. Male, age 39. Fulminating acute infection. Left lumbar abscess drained, but patient expired in ten days from a staphylococcus meningitis. A. *(Above)* Transverse process. B. *(Below)* Photomicrograph of field at arrow point showing acute inflammatory cells.

vessels. Larsen infused medullary canals of dogs with salt solution under pressures up to 180 cm. of water. The extent of necrosis in marrow and diaphyseal cortex depended on the duration of the pressure. At 180 cm. of water for 12 hours, the entire diaphysis was killed. These experiments emphasize the necessity for early and adequate drainage in acute osteomyelitis associated with mounting intramedullary pressure.

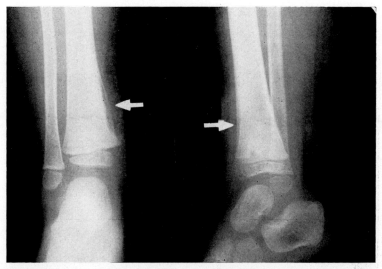

FIGURE 44. Acte osteomyelitis localized in the lower tibia. Note the layers of immature periosteal bone (arrows).

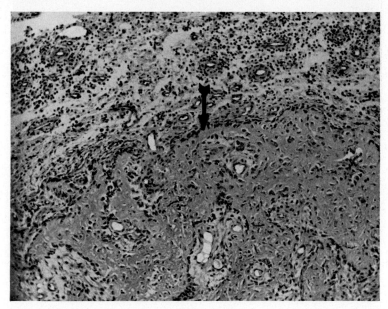

FIGURE 45. Periosteal bone (arrow) forming adjacent to and in spite of subacute and chronic inflammation.

Extensive destruction of the periosteum is uncommon. When pressure in a subperiosteal abscess becomes great, the periosteum usually decompressess itself by perforating. Pus may escape into adjacent muscles and cause serious damage; or the pus may travel far via fascial planes, eventually coming to the surface.

Compound Fractures

Osteomyelitis, complicating a compound fracture, usually develops insidiously, but occasionally begins as an acute osteomyelitis with all

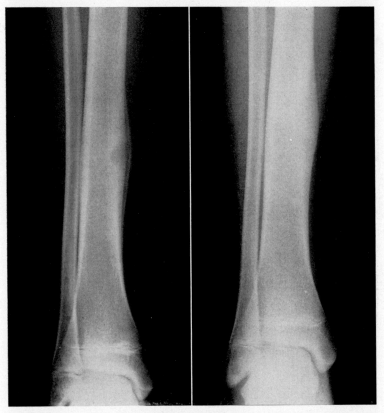

FIGURE 46. Acute osteomyletis of the tibia. A *(Left)* One month from onset. B. *(Right)* Five and one-half months from onset. Completely healed.

of the local and systemic symptoms of the hematogenous type. If adequate drainage of the pus is attained through the compound wound or a surgical wound, spread of the infection is unlikely. On the other hand, a tightly sutured compound wound, upon becoming infected by pyogenic organisms, can have a fulminating course with extensive bone involvement. Aseptic necrosis of a segment of bone at a fracture site has been mistaken for an osteomyelitis. During the long period of creeping substitution, a superficial resemblance to a chronic bone infection arises from the numerous areas of decreased density that form while the dense necrotic bone is being replaced.

Clinical Correlation

Severe pain and alarming systemic symptoms are a characteristic reflection of acute hematogenous osteomyelitis. Pus forming under the sensitive periosteum is the principal source of pain. Once the periosteum perforates or is drained adequately there is at least temporary relief from pain. The bone proper, the marrow, and even the endosteum, have little pain sensation. On numerous occasions the author has sawed out segments of bone, using only local infiltration of procaine over the periosteum. No pain was mentioned by these pa-

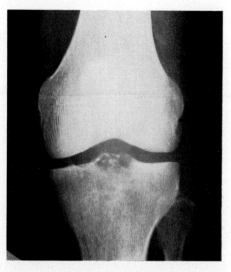

FIGURE 47. Acute osteomyelitis in the region of the tibial spines. Male, age 19. Soon after onset the knee joint became involved requiring an arthrotomy.

tients when the bone and endosteum were cut.

The proper time for drainage of an acute osteomyelitis has been the center of numerous polemics. Unquestionably many patients have been lost by the institution of drainage before the patient was physically prepared for the surgery. Wilensky, and Wilson and Mc Keever have waged protests against indiscriminate immediate surgery. It is now recognized that in most cases antibiotics, fluids, and transfusions are mandatory prior to surgical intervention. Recent reports in the literature indicate that surgery has been unnecessary in many in-

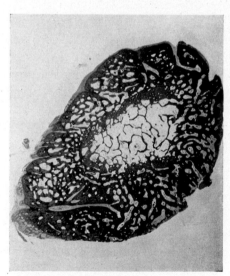

FIGURE 48. Transverse section of porotic cortex from a tubular bone to show that with osteoporosis there are many channels by which pus can travel from the medullary canal to beneath the periosteum.

stances when adequate conservative measures have been utilized.

Acute osteomyelitis must be differentiated from a cellulitis, trauma, acute rheumatoid arthritis, and rheumatic fever.

Roentgenologic Correlation

Seldom does the roentgenogram offer any help in the very early diagnosis of acute osteomyelitis. Soft tissue films occasionally show a thickened or elevated periosteum soon after the onset but ordinarily it is eight to 20 days before areas of osteoporosis, destruction or repair become visualized.

REFERENCES

Acute Pyogenic Arthritis

Bisgard, J. D.: Relation of pyogenic arthritis to osteomyelitis. *Surg., Gynec. & Obst.,* 55:74, 1932.

Blaisdell, J. and Harmon, P. H.: Suppurative joint disease and its relation to pyogenic arthritis. *Surg. Gynec. & Obst.,* :796, 1942.

Cooperman, M. B.: Acute pyogenic arthritis of the hip joint in infancy and childhood. *Am. J. Dis. Child., 31:*183, 1926.

L'Episcopo, J. B.: Suppurative arthritis of the sacro-iliac joint. *Ann. Surg.,* Aug. 1936.

Phemister, D. B.: Pathology and treatment of pyogenic arthritis. *Pennsylvania M. J., 32:*52, 1928.

Reich, R. S.: Purulent arthritis. *J. Bone & Joint Surg., 10:*554, 1928.

Russo, P.: Acute suppurative arthritis of the hip in childhood. *Am. J. Roentgenol., 51:*447, 1944.

Veal, J. R.: Acute suppurative arthritis. *New Orleans M. & S. J.,* 87:549, 1935.

Willems: Treatment of purulent arthritis by wide arthrotomy followed by immediate active immobilization. *Surg. Gynec. & Obst.,* 28:546, 1919.

Acute Osteomyelitis

Atsatt, R. F.: Acute osteomyelitis of a vertebral body following compression fracture. *J. Bone & Joint Surg.,* April 1939.

Key, J. A.: The rational treatment of acute hematogenous osteomyelitis. *J. A. M. A.,* June 17, 1938.

Maxfield, J. E. and Mitchell, C. L.: Acute hematogenous osteomyelitis in the adult. *J. Bone & Joint Surg.,* July 1942.

Moore, T.: Acute osteomyelitis of the patella. *Lancet,* March 5, 1938.

Robertson, D. C.: Acute hematogenous osteomyelitis. *J. Bone & Joint Surg., 9:*8, 1927.

Simpson, D. B.: Studies on the pathogenesis of acute hematogenous osteomyelitis. *Mil. Surgeon,* Jan. 1943.

Starr, C. L.: Acute hematogenous osteomyelitis. *Arch. Surg., 4:*567, 1922.

Wilensky, A. O.: *Osteomyelitis; Its pathogenesis, symptomatology and treatment.* The Macmillan Co., New York, 1934.

Williams, S.: Source of staphlococcus infection in acute osteomyelitis. *M. J. Australia,* :717, Oct. 29, 1938.

Wilson, J. C. and McKeever, F. M.: Hematogenous acute osteomyelitis in children. *J. Bone & Joint Surg., 18:*323, 1936.

Zadek, I.: Acute osteomyelitis of the long bones of adults. *Arch. Surg.,* Oct. 1938.

CHAPTER III

Chronic Osteomyelitis

Contents

Tuberculous Osteomyelitis
Tuberculous Arthritis
Sarcoid
Syphilis of Bones and Joints
Actinomycosis
Blastomycosis
Coccidioides

Sporotrichosis
Streptothricosis
Histoplasmosis
Torula
Leprosy
Yaws
Echinococcus

Once an infection has taken a firm hold on a bone or joint, the character and architecture of the skeleton invite chronicity. Replacement of an area of dead bone is a long slow process and usually must be conducted in the face of persisting infection. To maintain continuity and strength in a long bone and at the same time replace as much as an entire diaphysis is by no means a simple task. That such can be accomplished at all is a tribute to natural processes.

Even with antibiotics many acute infections of bone become chronic infections. The chronic granulomata pursue a chronic course from the beginning. A wide variation exists in the rate of aggression and the rate of healing in the chronic exudative infections, but all have important features in common. All present both bone destruction and bone proliferation. As complex as certain pathological reactions in the skeleton appear, it is still a fact, and one we must not lose sight of, that skeletal tissues when disturbed from their usual "severe tranquility," possess only a narrow group of rather stereotyped responses.

Three great forces mold the alterations in an infected bone or joint: (1) The invading organisms and their toxins; (2) The defense reaction to the invader; and, (3) The reparative processes of the healing phase. The changes wrought by these forces will be described in detail for each of the entities in this important group.

CHRONIC PYOGENIC OSTEOMYELITIS

A discussion of the chronic stage of pyogenic osteomyelitis must include a description of involucrum formation, sequestration, Brodie's abscesses, nonsuppurative osteomyelitis, and the factors that perpetuate a chronic bone infection.

INVOLUCRUM FORMATION

As the acute stage of the infection subsides, round cells become infiltrated among the neutrophils of the pus, and, if an exacerbation does not supervene, lymphocytes, monocytes, and wandering cells soon become as numerous at neutrophils. This is sometimes designated as the subacute stage. With organization of the exudate by the ingrowth

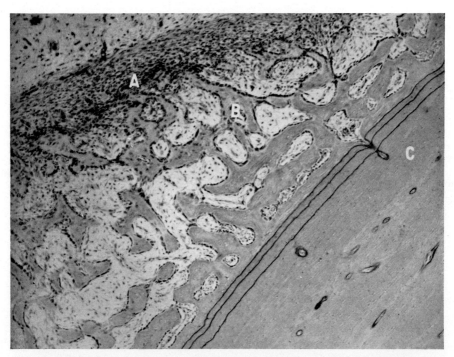

FIGURE 49. Involucrum formation, early stage. *A*. Cambium layer actively forming new trabeculae. Note the numerous osteoblasts. *B*. Periosteal fibrous bone. *C*. Tibial cortex (not yet involved at this site by the infection).

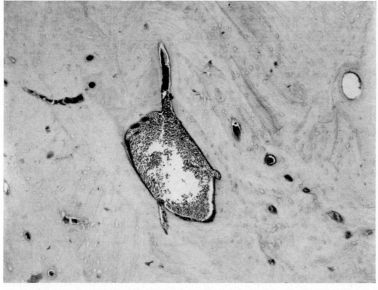

FIGURE 50. Histologic section through a cortical sequestrum. The Haversian marrow space in the center is filled with neutrophils (pus). Haversian canals are filled with necrotic debris. Lacunae of cortex are "empty tombs" of dead osteocytes.

of granulation tissue, the neutrophils steadily decrease in number until they disappear from the picture. Once the acute stage of the infection is under control, considerable activity begins in the periosteum through cellular proliferation in its cambium layer, provided of course that this structure has not been destroyed. Within the proliferating young fibrous tissue a multitude of bony trabeculae make their appearance to transform the tissue into a layer of fibrous bone, often referred to

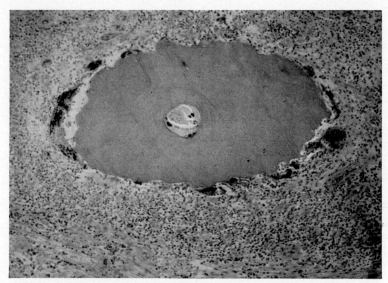

FIGURE 51A. Sequestrum lying in granulation tissue and being absorbed by giant cell osteoclasts.

as a periosteal osteophyte (Fig. 49). In children the periosteal osteophyte stops at epiphyseal plates because of the secure fixation of the periosteum to the periphery of the epiphyseal cartilage.

Layers of periosteal bone may form one on top of the other to give a lamellated appearance, resembling the "onion peel" character of periosteal bone in Ewing's tumor. But usually the bone of the involucrum is bulky and flamboyant, and microscopically shows no tendency to align its trabeculae with the lines of stress. An involucrum may have one to several crater-like openings, which represent either sites of sinus tracks, communicating with the sequestrum or localized areas of periosteal destruction. If the infection is controlled and sequestra absorbed or removed, the massive involucrum rapidly narrows down, becomes smooth, and is gradually replaced by mature lamellar bone. With complete reconstruction of the involved area, the trabeculae and haversian systems again align themselves with the lines of func-

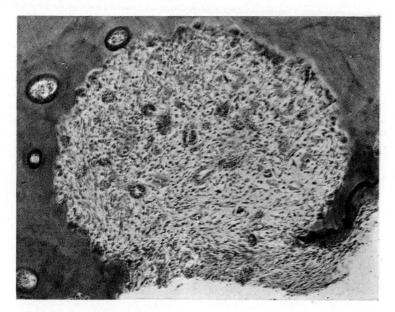

FIGURE 51B. Granulation tissue and osteoclasts invading a sequestrum.

tional stresses passing through the bone. In long bones a well defined medullary canal with normal marrow elements is the last portion of the bone to be resorbed.

SEQUESTRATION

Sequestra vary in size from a microscopic spicule (Fig. 51A) to an entire diaphysis (Figs. 52, 53, & 54). In pyogenic infections sequestra are largely cortical while in tuberculous and leutic osteomyelitis sequestra generally are cancellous.

The Fate of a Sequestrum

If a sequestrum is small and particularly if composed of cancellous bone, it may be absorbed and gradually replaced by viable bone. A larger sequestrum is slowly severed at its periphery by a border of granulation tissue with its vast numbers of osteoclasts and foreign body giant cells. If the area of dead bone is large, it is not severed from its junction with viable bone until the overlying involucrum has grown strong enough to assume the mechanical function formerly invested in the sequestrum. All necrotic bone to which the

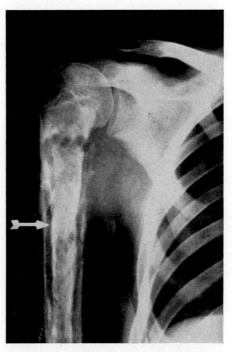

FIGURE 52. Sequestration of the humeral diaphysis (arrow).

granulation tissue has access becomes deeply pitted through osteoclastic action. This action goes below the surface through granulation tissue growing into haversian canals and marrow spaces of the sequestrum (Fig. 51B). Necrotic debris and pus is replaced by osteoclastic granulation tissue. Histologically, numerous osteoclasts are seen lying in their Howship's lacunae. This type of osteoclasis is referred to as lacunar absorption. Numerous mononuclear cells also appear to take part in the absorption process, but their site of absorption is smooth and not characterized by the row of notches so conspicuous in lacunar absorption. Any surface of the sequestrum not acted upon by granulation tissue remains white, hard, and smooth.

Cortical sequestra may be broken up into small pieces, and extruded with astonishing skill through sinus tracts. But a large sequestrum is trapped in its involucrum and requires surgical removal once it is completely separated from its attachment to viable portions of the host bone. When an entire diaphysis sequestrates a long window in the involucrum and morcellation of the dead bone become necessary to facilitate its removal.

Separation of a large area of necrotic bone requires many months, and even years. The sequestrating process may be interrupted at any time by an acute exacerbation of the infection. Granulation tissue is destroyed, and the sequestrum lies in a field of pus. Pyogenic pus does not appreciably alter the bone, so until granulation tissue returns, no progress is made toward separating necrotic bone from the viable. Another cause for retarded absorption is observed when a sequestrum becomes encapsulated in fibrous tissue. Over a period of years there may be only microscopic evidence of alteration in the sequestrum. Exacerbations after long periods of quiescence are sometimes due to an encapsulated sequestrum.

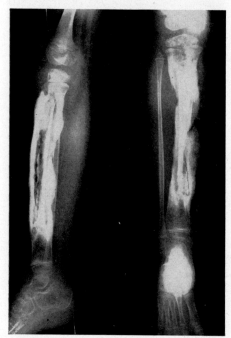

FIGURE 53. Sequestration of the tibial diaphysis.

Axhausen requested that we use the term sequestrum to apply only to necrotic bone in an exudative process. An area of bone that is necrotic from vascular embarrassment is not a sequestrum. Such bone is dealt with by the process of "creeping substitution" and not by sequestration.

BRODIE'S ABSCESS

Sir Benjamin Brodie, in 1830, reported a series of chronic bone abscesses. The lesion he described was chronic from the onset, but the majority of bone abscesses now termed Brodie's abscesses, have an acute onset. Both types are fairly common, but the type with an acute beginning has the higher incidence. Although they are referred to as bone abscesses throughout their course, the contents of the abscess cavity frequently becomes sterile after the early stages. Ordinarily metaphyseal in location, a Brodie's abscess may represent either a primary acute hematogenous osteomyelitis or a metastasis from a pyogenic osteomyelitis. Systemic symptoms may or may not accompany the abscess. The classical case is a metaphyseal osteomyelitis caused by staphylococci of low virulence. The infection is rapidly localized and solidly walled off. Absorption of bone in a sharply circumscribed round or oval area makes space for the pus. A pyogenic membrane forms a sack enclosing the pus. Peripheral to this granulation tissue wall, the normal bone marrow elements are replaced by fibrous tissue for as much as a centimeter or more.

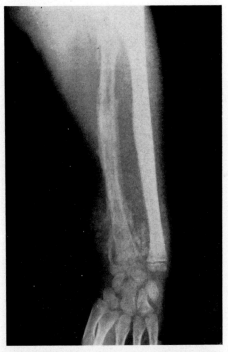

FIGURE 54A. Staphylococcic osteomyelitis of the radius with sequestrated diaphysis.

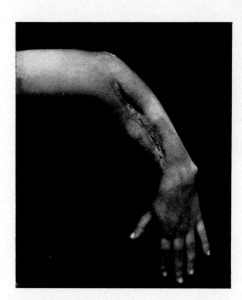

FIGURE 54B. Appearance of forearm following early diaphysectomy.

Bony trabeculae in this zone show increasing dimensions from repeated layers of new bone (Fig. 59). In time this process leads to the osteosclerosis so well visualized in the roentgenogram. A complex pattern of blue cement lines testifies to the periodicity of bone apposition.

The pus becomes sterile and either persists as such, or becomes organized and replaced by granulation tissue. If the infection flares up, all granulation tissue present is reduced to debris, and the cavity again fills with pus. But if the granulation tissue is not disturbed, it gradually matures to fibrous tissue which either persists as such or is trabecularized by bone. If ossification occurs, the fibrous bone is replaced by lamellar bone, completing the healing process. Frequently these abscesses are drained surgically. After surgery they can be depended upon to heal uneventfully.

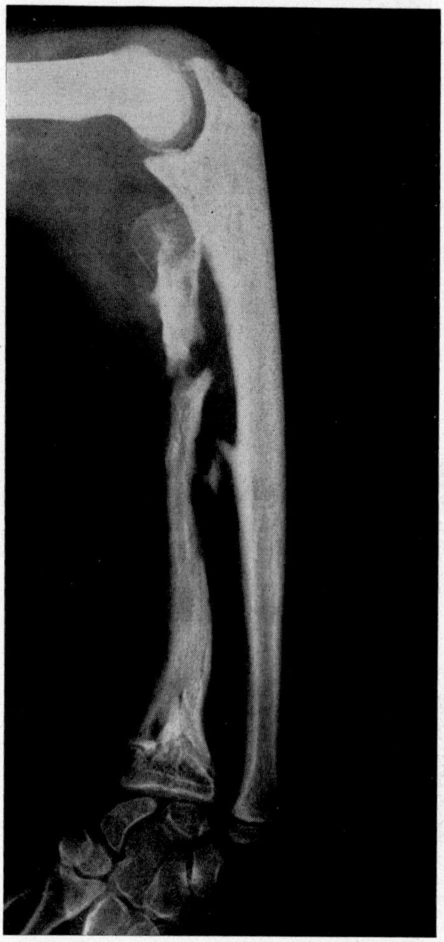

NON-SUPPURATIVE CHRONIC OSTEOMYELITIS

Types of non-suppurative osteomyelitis, which have a chronic course from the beginning and are seldom associated with frank pus, will be included here. These types include: (1) Sclerosing osteomyelitis; (2) Fibrous osteomyelitis; (3) Osteomyelitis variolosa; (4) Typhoid osteomyelitis; and, (5) Undulant fever osteomyelitis.

(1) SCLEROSING OSTEOMYELITIS has a protracted course, leads to fusiform thickening of a long bone, and does not form sequestra, or abscesses. Inflammatory cells are not a prominent part of the picture microscopically. Bone apposition is active, leading to osteosclerosis, and a complex pattern of blue cement lines indicate remissions and exacerabations.

FIGURE 54C. A defect in regeneration persists at the junction of the middle and upper one-thirds, epiphyses are premature fused. These defects are the reason why early diaphysectomy is no longer popular.

In reviewing medical literature it is evident that osteoid osteomas occasionally have been mistaken for sclerosing osteomyelitis.

(2) FIBROUS OSTEOMYELITIS, described by Phemister, is not so much an entity as it is a stage of osteomyelitis. Almost any pyogenic osteomyelitic lesion may long remain in a state of fibrosis during its healing stage and during that period be called a fibrous osteomyelitis. However, there are cases that have an extensive fibroblastic response from the outset, never suppurate, and never repair spontaneously by bony trabecularization of the fibrous tissue. That

pyogenic organisms definitely cause these lesions is not established. A streptococcus, particularly streptococcus viridans, has been suspected.

(3) OSTEOMYELITIS VARIOLOSA: This extremely rare entity was reviewed by Brown and Brown in 1924. Most cases appear as a form of

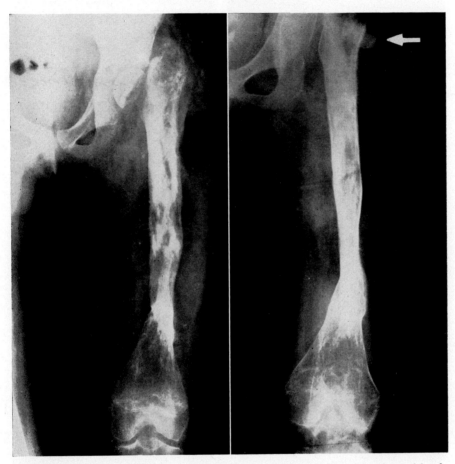

FIGURE 55. A. *(Left)* Chronic osteomyelitis of the femur with sequestration femoral head, and absorption of the neck. B. *(Right)* Nine months after A. The sequestrated head has moved through a sinus tract from the acetabulum to just below the skin (arrow).

necrosing, non-suppurative osteomyelitis, involving metaphyses and epiphyses of long bones. Since the majority of cases occur during childhood, epiphyseal plates frequently are destroyed, leading to disabling late deformation. Extension into joints has occurred and resulted in ankylosis. The smallpox virus is considered to be the cause of this type of osteomyelitis.

(4) In years gone by, typhoid fever accounted for an occasional

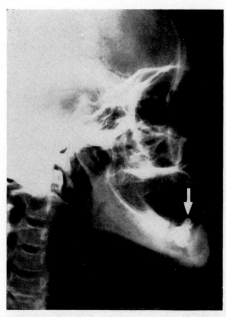

FIGURE 56. Sequestrum of mandible from an osteomyelitis associated with a compound fracture.

case of low grade, usually non-suppurative, chronic osteomyelitis. There was a predelection for the spine; hence the term "typhoid spine." Collapse of a vertebra was common. Onset was generally during convalescence.

(5) UNDULENT FEVER *(Brucellosis)* produces a rare non-suppurative osteomyelitis similar to typhoid, and tends to involve the vertebra (Fig. 65). Brucellosis spondylitis generally occurs one month to one year after the onset of systemic symptoms. Spontaneous bony fusion is the rule, particularly if the spine is immobilized. Only rarely is there suppuration and a paravertebral abscess.

CAUSES OF CHRONICITY IN PYOGENIC OSTEOMYELITIS

The most frequent cause of chronicity in pyogenic osteomyelitis is the presence of sequestra. Other causes are: (1) Extension of the infection to adjacent or remote soft tissues; (2) Extension of the suppurative process into a joint; (3) Persistence of soft tissue sinus tracts; and, (4) Ephithelization of soft tissue and bony sinuses with and without malignant degeneration.

Sequestra and suppurative arthritis have been discussed. Soft tissue abscesses need no elaboration. Sinus tracts with walls of dense scar tissue can persist long after the underlying bone lesions have healed. Metabolism of the tissue is low, the walls relatively impervious, and the stimulus for healing is weak.

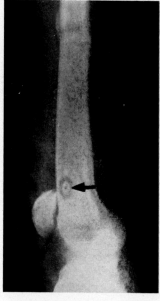

FIGURE 57. Sequestrum from an infection following the insertion of a Steinman pin.

Epithelization of a sinus can become a serious aspect of protracted cases. Stratified squamous epithelium of the skin enters the sinus at the skin orifice and grows slowly down into the sinus to form a lining membrane. Milgram reported a case in which there had been a draining sinus for 62 years. Stratified squamous epithelium had lined the sinus tract as well as a considerable area in the marrow cavity, displacing much of the original pyogenic membrane. In this case malignant changes had not occurred.

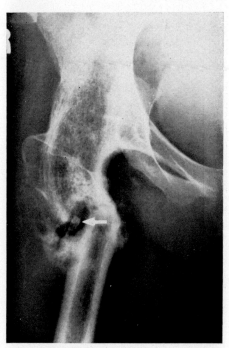

In a small percentage of cases epithelial sinuses of long standing become malignant by transforming to a squamous cell epithelioma. The incidence is highest in sinuses over the antero-medial aspect of the leg. Two types are recognized: the superficial type, often associated with fungation that makes the diagnosis obvious, and the deep type, in which the carcinoma originates deep in the sinus and in walls of bone cavities. Although the degree of invasiveness varies widely, growth is slow as a rule, and metastases uncommon. Most cases have occurred during middle or old age in sinuses of many years standing. A foul odor and hemorrhages are

FIGURE 58. Osteomyelitis and sequestrum from post-operative infection of a subtrochanteric osteotomy.

significant symptoms, but the diagnosis should be confirmed by biopsy. Once the diagnosis is established, radical excision is not attempted where amputation is feasible.

Regarding the incidence of epitheliomata in foci of chronic osteomyelitis, Benedict (1931) found 12 malignancies out of 2400 cases of chronic osteomyelitis at the Massachusetts General Hospital. Henderson and Swart of the Mayo Clinic reported five epitheliomas in 2,396 cases of osteomyelitis. In one case a fibrosarcoma was associated with the epithelioma.

Roentgenologic Correlation

Sequestra appear relatively more dense than neighboring bone for the reason that they long retain the density possessed at the time the bone was killed by the infection or by vascular obliteration. Having no circulation, the sequestrum cannot share in the osteoporosis taking place in the adjoining live bone. This phenomenon is a great help in radiographically visualizing both septic and aseptic necrosis of bone. In long standing cases, the involucrum may become so dense that small sequestra are hidden from view. Using more penetration and taking films at several angles frequently visualizes previously unseen sequestra, and deep seated smaller cavities.

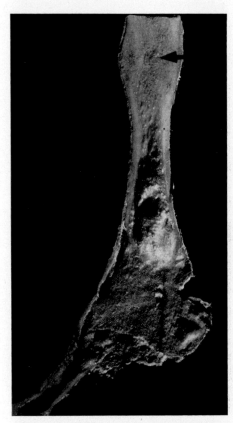

FIGURE 59. Circumscribed bone abscess (at arrow). Pyogenic osteomyelitis and suppurative arthritis had destroyed all of the tarsal joints and some of the tarsals. Amputation was the treatment of choice.

Soft tissue films give a sharper view of newly formed periosteal bone, as seen in acute osteomyelitis.

The zone of osteosclerosis, surrounding the cavity of a localized osteomyelitis, helps differentiate these lesions from bone cysts and tuberculous bone abscesses since these seldom have a reactive margin.

Sequestra of pyogenic osteomyelitis generally are cortical. Sequestra of tuberculosis and syphilis are predominately cancellous and are located near joints.

Tuberculous osteomyelitis of long bone diaphyses, a rare entity, closely resembles pyogenic osteomyelitis on the roentgenogram. Luetic osteomyelitis may also resemble pyogenic osteomyelitis with the exception that it frequently has multiple areas of destruction and proliferation.

Sooner or later most of us mistake a Ewing's tumor or an osteogenic sarcoma for an osteomyelitis; or an osteomyelitis for a tumor. A cavity is not often associated with bone sarcoma; whereas, it frequently is associated with an osteomyelitis. In early stages of bone sarcoma the differentiation may be impossible either roentgenographically or clinically. A biopsy must be the last tribunal.

Clinical Correlation

In chronic osteomyelitis radical excision of necrotic bone offers the best assurance against an exacerbation. A Brodie's abscess needs only to be unroofed. In acute osteomyelitis requiring surgery good drainage is the objective, not radical excision. Diaphysectomy in a major bone is rarely indicated, because of the danger of incomplete regeneration (Fig. 54C). Draining sinuses should not be permitted to persist through the years in view of the potential malignant changes, and the protracted distress to the patient.

TUBERCULOUS OSTEOMYELITIS AND ARTHRITIS

Tuberculosis of bones and joints, a predominantly destructive infection, practically always develops secondary to a primary infection in such locations as the respiratory or alimentary systems. Both human and bovine tubercle bacilli invade the skeleton. Since both produce similar lesions, and since the prognosis is the same, it is not necessary clinically to differentiate the two types. Pasteurization of milk has profoundly reduced the prevalence of the bovine type.

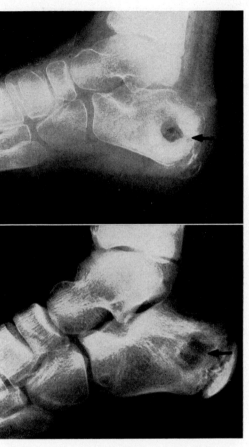

FIGURE 60. A. *(Above)* Pyogenic localized osteomyelitis of the os calcis. Note the characteristic reactive marginal osteosclerosis. B. *(Below)* Tuberculous osteomyelitis of the os calcis for comparison. Note the characteristic absence of marginal sclerosis.

The disease is most common during the first decade, but occurs at all ages. Since tuberculous lesions of bones and joints are so intimately related in most instances, both lesions will be discussed together. Lesions of vertebral bodies are the most frequent in skeletal tuberculosis. In the order of their frequency, as given by Knaggs, other skeletal sites are the hip, knee, ankle, elbow, wrist, and skull. As in tuberculosis else-where in the body the tubercle is the characteristic pathologic unit, and is associated with tuberculous granulation tissue, caseation ne-crosis, exudation, and fibrosis. Typical epithelioid and Langhan giant

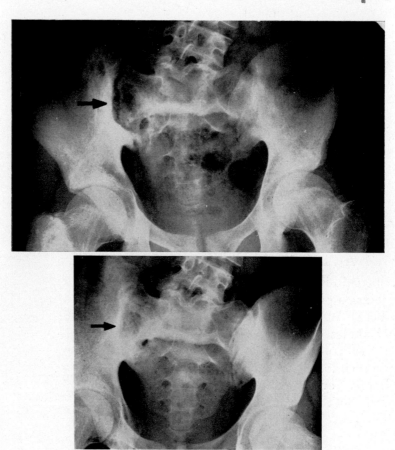

FIGURE 61. A. *(Above)* Chronic osteomyelitis of the right sacro-iliac region, and pyogenic arthritis of the sacro-iliac joint. B. *(Below)* After healing of the osteomyelitis and bony ankylosis of the sacro-iliac joint.

cell tubercules occur in the bone marrow and synovial membrane (Figs. 66 & 67). Epitheloid cells are considered of more diagnostic significance than are Langhan giant cells. The giant cells are believed to be derived from epithelioid cells. Although the exact origin of epithelioid cells is uncertain, it is generally agreed that they are fixed tissue cells and are phagocytic for tubercle bacilli. The lymphocytes, lying in the periphery of most tubercles, are delivered by the blood circulation.

Pathogenesis

Tubercle bacilli are carried from remote foci to the skeleton via the blood stream. Except for vertebral lesions the majority of cases of skeletal tuberculosis involve a joint. A controversy developed regarding the incidence of tuberculous arthritis of synovial origin as compared to the incidence of primary metaphyseal and epiphyseal lesions that had innoculated the joint by direct extension. The exact ratio of occurrence of these two mechanisms of joint invasion is unknown. Smith, after a thorough examination of pathological material from 23 tuberculous joints, concluded that in 17 there had been a primary synovial infection. To quote Allison and Ghormley, "...we feel that it is of the least importance where the infection begins." After an extensive clinical and pathological survey, these authors state further: "The question of the existence of pure synovial tuberculosis is to our minds a futile one. Theoretically its existence is no doubt possible. Practically, the early invasion of

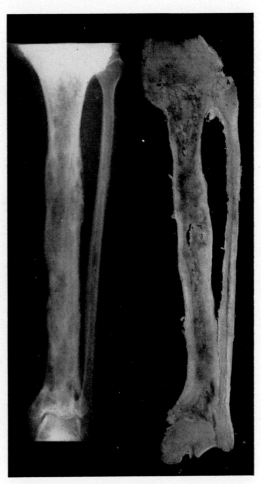

Figure 62. A pyogenic infection of the knee joint spread through the entire tibia and into the ankle, male age 55. A. *(Left)* A.P. roentgenogram. B. *(Right)* Amputation specimen.

the subchondral region by tuberculous granulations has been seen to accompany the synovial disease in all of our sections."

Virtually all metaphyseal and epiphyseal foci sooner or later involve the adjacent joint. A metaphyseal focus accomplishes this by extention subperiosteally and subcapsularly, or less commonly, and only in older children, by a direct advance through the epiphyseal plate and epiphysis.

An epiphyseal focus generally extends into the adjacent joint at a margin near the synovial-cartilage junction. Metaphyseal foci are common in children, and epiphyseal foci are uncommon. During adult life the reverse is true, with primary epiphyseal lesions becoming the more frequent. A primary bony focus may be large and extensively

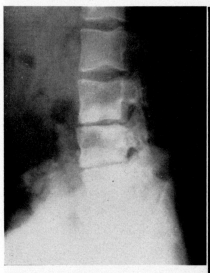

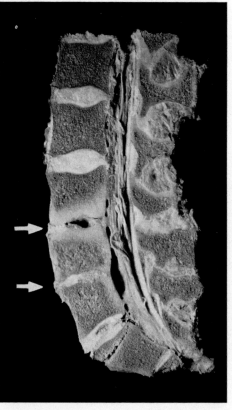

FIGURE 63. Chronic pyogenic osteo-myelitis of the 3rd and 4th lumbar vertebral bodies of a male age 25 who expired after a vertebral abscess perforated into the peritoneal cavity. A. *(Left)* Lateral roentgenogram lumbar spine. B. *(Right)* Sagital section lumbar vertebrae. Note the reactive sclerosis and destruction of two discs.

destructive, or so minute and of such short duration that it is never seen roentgenographically or pathologically.

With invasion of the joint, whether it be primary in the synovial membrane from a blood stream innoculation, or secondary to an adjacent bony focus, all of the joint components become involved. It is the reaction of the capsule, cartilage, and subchondral bone and marrow to the disease that is responsible for the numerous pathological and clinical manifestations.

SYNOVIAL MEMBRANE

Although the attack by the tubercle bacilli involves the cartilage and bone very early in the disease, it appears likely that in many cases the initial lesion is in the capsule. The earliest defensive response to the organisms is not a mobilization of lymphocytes and monocytes but a local concentration of polymorphonuclear neutrophils. Within a few days the neutrophils are replaced by lymphocytes, plasma cells and monocytes. Where the defensive response is at least partially successful, capillary buds from the synovial membrane sprout into the newly formed exudate. Granulation tissue thus formed frequently spreads to cover most of the surface of the syno-vial membrane. Numerous Langhan giant cell and cpi thelioid cell tubercles, to-gether with areas of casea-tion necrosis, are character-istically scattered through the granulation tissue. The pattern of the alterations varies from one part of the synovialis to another. Whereas one area may be in a florid exudative stage, another may be fibrotic and healing. This is the reason that most of the older classi-fications of the process, based as they were upon spe-cific stages of the disease, are untenable.

Perforation of a tubercu-lous joint with the forma-tion of a sinus tract is not infrequent. Secondary pyo-

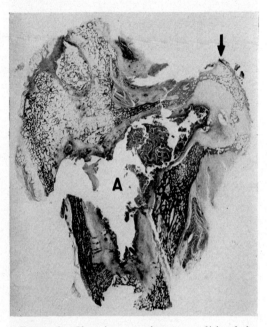

FIGURE 64. Chronic pyogenic osteomyelitis of the upper femur with destruction of head (arrow). In-fection was of many years' duration and a sinus tract leading to the large cavity, A, was epithelial-ized. Dense fibrous tissue lined the cavity. Amyloi-dosis was far advanced at death.

genic infection can then enter at the skin opening of the sinus to complicate the clinical course and the pathological changes.

The capsule becomes edematous, and often greatly thickened, but it does not develop the hyperplastic villosity seen in proliferative arthritis. *Rice bodies* in large numbers do not form as frequently in tuberculosis as they do in proliferative arthritis. Rice bodies in tubercu-losis appear to form principally from fibrin which is deposited on villi layer on layer, the villus ultimately severs to drop free into the joint as a rice body. When there is joint motion, rice bodies may form from the fibrin rolling up into small oval or round bodies.

Articular Cortex and Subchondral Marrow

The early invasion of the articular cortex is a striking feature of tuberculous arthritis. At the joint margins where cartilage and synovialis meet tuberculous granulation tissue erodes through the edge of the cartilage to create a notch of destruction in the articular cortex (Fig. 68). When the epiphysis has not yet ossified to the periphery, such marginal notches are not to be expected. A second source of articular cortex disintegration is the non-specific subchondral granulation and fibrous tissue (Fig. 69). When there is tuberculous involvement of the capsule, a non-specific granulation tissue appears in the subchondral marrow spaces. Only rarely has a tubercle been seen in this tissue, and there is never caseation necrosis. It is therefore agreed that this is a non-specific tissue growing in response to the presence of the tuberculous joint infection, but not as a local response to tubercle bacilli. Lymphocytes and plasma cells are often richly infiltrated among the fibroblasts and

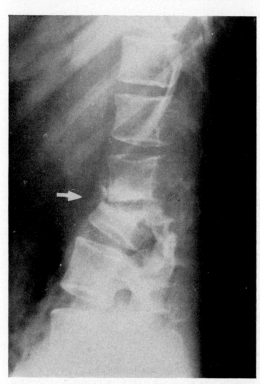

FIGURE 65. Brucelosis (Malta fever) osteomyelitis 2nd and 3rd lumbar vertebrae. Male age 22; symptoms 6 months. Subsequently underwent spontaneous bony fusion.

capillaries. Contact with the articular cortex is soon followed by absorption of the trabeculae that make up the cortex. At first the articular cortex continuity is interrupted at numerous points by tongue-like inroads. At a later stage only scattered fragments of the subchondral trabeculae remain. The process of absorption does not stop with the articular cortex but procedes against the zone of calcified cartilage and then absorbes the non-calcified articular cartilage. It is a common experience to see an extensive area of articular cartilage so undermined by subchondral erosion that it lies free in the joint.

Just what calls forth this active subchondral response is not known.

It has been suggested that endotoxins, released by dead tubercle bacilli, filter through the cartilage to the subchondral region. Another theory

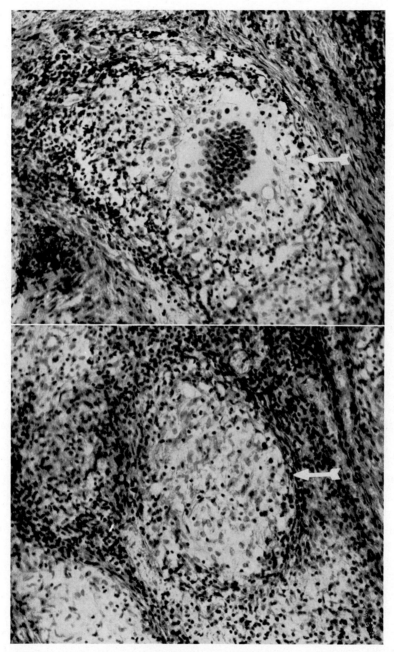

FIGURE 66. Typical tubercles (in synovial membrane) High power. A. *(Above)* Langhan giant cell tubercle. B. *(Below)* Epitheloid cell tubercle.

attributes the response to the death of the articular cartilage, the sub-chondral reaction being established to help absorb the dead cartilage which acts as a foreign body. The latter theory would be more convincing if the articular cartilage were consistently found to be necrotic. In many of the cases disclosing an active subchondral reaction, the articular cartilage is quite alive. To add a philosophical touch: Perhaps

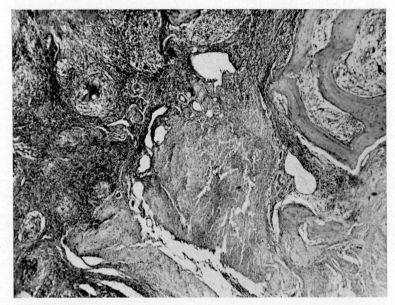

FIGURE 67. Tubercles and tuberculous granulation tissue filling marrow spaces.

nature, faced with a joint infection that can heal only after bony ankylosis, strives to remove the articular cartilage as a step toward facilitating the needed ankylosis.

Subchondral marrow fibrosis occurs also in proliferative and in suppurative arthritis; in fact, in these conditions, the zone of fibrous and granulation tissue is considerably wider than the narrow zone in tuberculosis. However, the subchondral reaction in proliferative and suppurative arthritis is not nearly so destructive, and forms only after the disease is moderately or far advanced. In proliferative arthritis the numerous lymphocytes tend to concentrate into follicles; in tuberculosis the lymphocytes are diffuse and less numerous.

ARTICULAR CARTILAGE

Surface erosion of the articular cartilage occurs beneath a tongue-like projection of granulation tissue extending out from the synovial membrane at the joint margin. As would be anticipated, the cartilage at the periphery is the first destroyed. Once a given area of cartilage is absorbed, the tuberculous granulation tissue has access to underlying articular cortex. When subchondral marrow spaces are reached, the specific and non-specific granulation tissues meet. As Phemister has so well described, contacting articular surfaces are a temporary barrier to the advance of the creeping pannus. Therefore, absorption occurs first at the margins, and at other parts of the joint where the opposing articular surfaces are not in contact. In the hip joint, the fovea centralis offers space for the ingrowth of granulations; in the olecranon, there is a narrow transverse zone near its center (Fig. 70); in the knee and shoulder, only a relatively small part of the articular surfaces are in contact with each other at any given time. Marginally located specific granulation tissue rarely undermines the articular cartilage to any extent unless the subchondral granulation

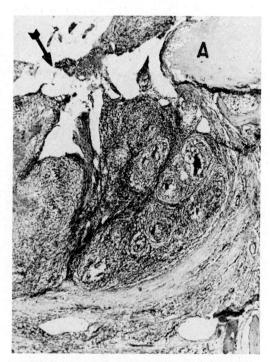

FIGURE 68. Photomicrograph of a "marginal notch" (arrow) showing that the eroded notch is filled with tuberculous tissue which is destroying articular cartilage, *A*, and subchondral bony trabeculae.

tissue should sever the cartilage from its bed. In this instance there is rapid spread of the tuberculous granulations over the end of the bone.

In far advanced cases all of the articular cortex and cartilage may be destroyed. Fragments of cartilage may persist, enclosed in fibrous tissue created by a condensation of tuberculous granulation tissue (Fig. 83).

As described in Chapter II, the exudate from tuberculous abscesses does not usually possess a proteolytic enzyme capable of dissolving cartilage, as does neutrophilic pus from a pyogenic infection. This explains why the cartilage space is so long preserved in tuberculous arthritis.

In the knee joint a sagitally placed curtain of fibrous tissue may form to screen off an advance of the infection from one side of the joint to the other. As shown in Figure 82, the articular cartilage is normal in the lateral one-half of the joint, and completely destroyed in the medial one-half. A fibrous tissue partition protected the lateral one-half of the joint.

Tuberculous Sequestra

Cancellous sequestra are rather commonly associated with tuberculous arthritis, particularly in adults. Primary sequestra form at the

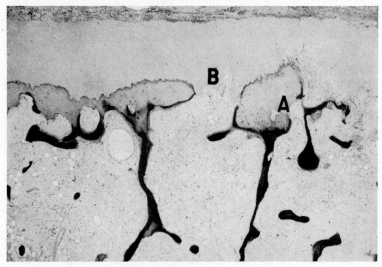

Figure 69. Subchondral non-specific granulation and fibrous tissue. Articular cortex has been absorbed at *A,* and zone of calcified cartilage destroyed at *B.*

site of a primary bony focus in the epiphysis or rarely, in the metaphysis (Figs. 71, 79, & 84); secondary sequestra are traceable to a direct extention of a joint infection through the articular cartilage and into the epiphysis, making all secondary sequestra epiphyseal. Sequestra may be small and rapidly absorbed, or they may be large and exist for many years. Regeneration of the necrotic bone is accomplished much more readily in children than in adults. All sequestra retain the density existing at the time the necrosis occurs, although occasionally a slight increase in density can be attributed to calcium deposited in caseated granulation tissue.

PRIMARY SEQUESTRA, because they form at the beginning of the infection, possess trabeculae of normal size and contour. After the disease has been present for several months and neighboring bone has undergone atrophy, there is a striking contrast between the full sized trabeculae of the sequestrum and the thin atrophic trabeculae of the adjacent viable bone.

SECONDARY SEQUESTRA, form long after the onset of the tuberculous

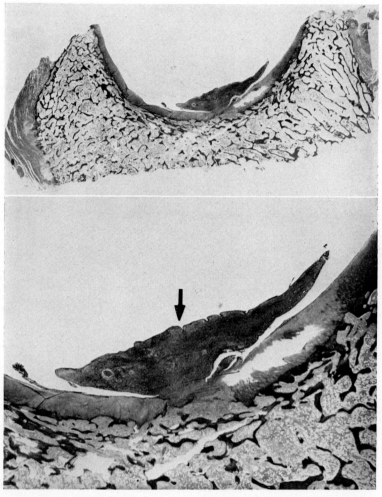

FIGURE 70. Sagital section of olecranon. A tuberculous granulation tissue pannus (arrow) with numerous tubercles gained access to the olecranon articular cartilage by way of the transverse groove at center of sulcus.

arthritis and therefore possess atrophied trabeculae. Little contrast exists roentgenographically unless demineralization in the epiphysis increases further after formation of the sequestrum, or unless calcium is deposited in the necrotic granulation tissue, or unless a zone of absorption encircles the sequestrum as a result of granulation tissue growing in to absorb or to sequestrate the sequestrum.

"Kissing" sequestra represent twin secondary sequestra and form directly opposite each other in opposing epiphyses (Fig. 72). They occur at sites of maximum pressure stress and it is Phemister's opinion that pressure plays an important part in their etiology. It was Koenig's teaching at the turn of the century that secondary sequestra were infarcts forming as a consequence of emboli composed of tuberculous material. Since the sequestra are usually cone or wedge shaped, this theory appeared reasonable until Nussbaum and others demonstrated that no end arteries exist in the epiphyses.

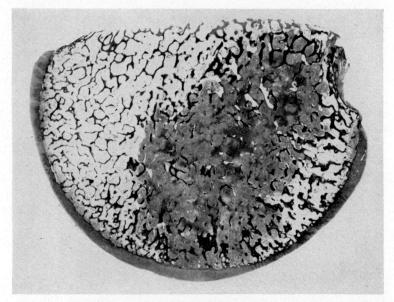

Figure 71. Large primary sequestrum of capitellum humeri. Articular cartilage intact.

The healing process: The healing process in skeletal tuberculosis is slow and faltering. In children, under optimum conditions, tuberculous arthritis frequently is self-limited and tends toward spontaneous healing. After the first decade the capacity to heal diminishes with the years. Complete spontaneous healing in an adult seldom occurs.

The state of the granulation tissue, forming in the bone or joint, holds the key to the status of healing. In the beginning the granulation tissue sets up a defence against the tubercle bacilli by bringing in leucocytes and nutrition. In a later stage when an exudate and necrotic debris have to be dealt with, the granulation tissue displays an absorptive function; in the final stage the granulation tissue undergoes fibrous condensation to heal damaged areas by fibrous tissue. At any time the infection may fulminate and destroy areas of granulation tissue.

Only in rare instances do tuberculous joints heal with the preservation of a useful range of motion. And even when this does occur, the contours of the joint are so extensively altered (Fig. 80) that disabling degenerative arthritis can be expected.

Healing in a tuberculous joint occurs first by a fibrous ankylosis which may subsequently change to a bony ankylosis, particularly in childhood. By the time most of the articular cartilage has been destroyed, so also has the synovial membrane. The healing joint becomes a mass of dense fibrous adhesions. As the scar tissue contracts, the fixation becomes increasingly rigid. In children the fibrous tissue tends to ossify, but this tendency is not striking in the adult. If the articular surfaces are completely destroyed, either by granulation tissue or by surgery, the epiphyses may lie in sufficiently close proximity to unite by bone in very much the same manner that fracture fragments become bridged. The surgical operation of intraarticular arthrodesis

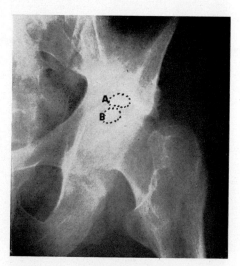

FIGURE 72. "Kissing sequestra" in far advanced tuberculosis of the hip. *A.* Acetabular sequestrum. *B.* Femoral head sequestrum.

facilitates bony bridging by removing remaining cartilage, scar, and granulation tissue lying between the bone ends. An autogenous bone graft or bone chips may be inserted to bring about further bony contact. In an extraarticular bone graft, there usually is bony union of the graft above and below the joint long before the joint itself bridges across by bone. But with the effective internal splinting of a good bone graft, bony ankylosis eventually develops inside the joint. Intervertebral and hip joints are the joints best adapted to extraarticular arthrodesis.

TUBERCULOUS SPONDYLITIS

In children, tuberculosis of the spine commences as an osteomyelitis and in adults, as a periostitis. In children the process ordinarily begins in the vertebral body near its anterior aspect. This characteristic has an anatomical basis; in the young the major artery, a branch of the posterior spinal, enters the central area of the vertebral body coming in by way of the posterior wall. In the adult, the major vessels to vertebral bodies are from the intercostal and lumbar arteries, and enter anteriorly, branching out subperiosteally. This explains the high incidence in adult tuberculosis of lesions occurring at the anterior aspect of vertebral bodies and discs beneath the periosteum and anterior longitudinal ligament.

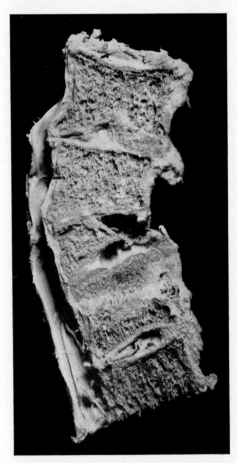

FIGURE 73. Tuberculosis of the spine at the dorso-lumbar junction, involving three vertebra and two discs.

In children, central destruction of the vertebral body may lead to collapse, perforation, and extension of the infection to adjacent vertebral bodies. In adults, the lesion long remains localized to a single vertebra or disc, or else spreads proximally and distally beneath the periosteum and anterior longitudinal ligaments.

Involvement of more than one vertebra, particularly in the dorsal region, is relatively common in tuberculous spondylitis. Multiple involvement with normal vertebra separating sites of involvement is not rare. Spread of the infection in these cases is hematogenous.

Vertebral collapse may cause spinal cord pressure. More frequent causes of cord pressure are: (1) Abscesses; (2) Tuberculous granulation tissue growing epidurally to encircle and constrict the cord; and, (3) Edema associated with vertebral compression and proximity of the infection.

On the basis of pathologic studies, cold abscesses are found in practically all cases of tuberculous spondylitis. Widely variable in size and distribution, these abscesses become filled with an exudate composed of serum, leucocytes, bone sand, caseated debris, and tubercle bacilli.

Healing of psoas abscesses by a massive deposition of calcium occurs occasionally in children. These large, impressive masses form conspicuous shadows in the roentgenogram (Fig. 75).

Finder studied a specimen of healed tuberculous spondylitis and observed that osteoclerosis was a prominent part of the healing response; its presence was not dependent upon secondary pyogenic infection or mechanical irritation. Evidence was presented to support the contention that bone marrow is stimulated to fibrosis and osteogen-

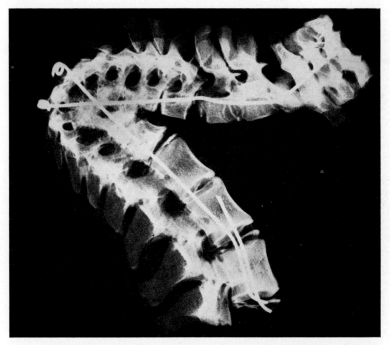

FIGURE 74. Tuberculosis of the lower dorsal spine. A 148° kyphotic angulation led to fusion of the lower dorsal vertebral bodies across the apex of the angle.

esis by irritating toxic substances liberated at the death of tubercle bacilli. Marrow fibrosis developing under this circumstance showed signs of having acquired resistance to tubercle bacilli.

DIAPHYSEAL TUBERCULOUS OSTEOMYELITIS

Except for spina ventosa, diaphyseal tuberculosis is very rare. It is associated with pronounced proliferation of periosteal bone, and the death of an area of diaphysis. Sequestra seldom separate; the necrotic bone is regenerated gradually without a fragment becoming freed and surrounded by exudate or granulation tissue. Abscess formation is exceptional in diaphyseal tuberculosis. The tendency is toward spontaneous healing whenever the general condition of the patient improves.

Spina Ventosa

Spina ventosa is a term given to diaphyseal tuberculosis that involves phalanges, metacarpals or metatarsals (Figs. 92, 93, & 94). The process is low grade as a rule and seldom occurs except in small children. Emboli, containing tubercle bacilli, lodge in the medullary canal of the diaphysis, presumably because the major nutrient artery, upon entering the diaphysis, immediately breaks up into numerous minute vessels. Granulation tissue forms inside the diaphysis, then advances through the cortex to the surface, prompting the formation of periosteal bone. Typical tubercles, and areas of caseation necrosis are seen. Lamellation of the periosteal bone occurs when tuberculous granulation tissue penetrates the initial periosteal osteophyte. During healing, the periosteal bone gradually disappears and, grossly, the bone returns to normal.

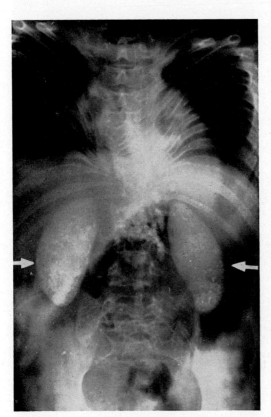

FIGURE 75. Calcified psoas abscesses.

CARIES SICA

Caries sica (dry decay) is an obsolete term applied to a low grade type of tuberculous involvement of the shoulder joint and humeral head. An advanced degree of osteoporosis and multiple small foci of tuberculous granulation tissue are characteristic. Through a long slow process, granulation tissue destroys the articulation, undergoes fibrous condensation, and creates a fibrous ankylosis. The old name caries sica grew out of observations that this form of tuberculosis is not associated with grossly evident caseation necrosis and exudation.

Roentgenologic Correlation

In young children the roentgenogram may not show a tuberculous arthritis for a considerable period of time. If the epiphysis has only a small core of ossification, the characteristic marginal notches, impaired definition of the articular cortex, and even narrowing of the cartilage space, are not visualized. Joint distention, osteoporosis, and metaphyseal lesions will be reflected in the roentgenogram. A roentgen ray study at regular intervals may be necessary to identify even reasonably

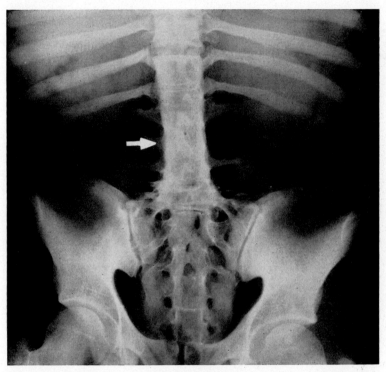

FIGURE 76. Healed tuberculosis of the 4th and 5th lumbar vertebrae. A spinal fusion was performed 15 years previously when the patient was age nine. Lumbar vertebral bodies (arrow) have fused, and the discs have disappeared.

early, the changes that develop. Substantial narrowing of the cartilage space does not take place until the disease is well advanced (Fig. 85).

After ossification of the epiphyses, the marginal changes and loss of the articular cortex become evident. As was described under the discussion of pyogenic arthritis, the articular cortex definition is lost early in tuberculous arthritis while the cartilage space remains intact, whereas, in pyogenic arthritis, the cartilage space is narrowed before the articular cortex is damaged.

Marginal notching is not pathognomonic of tuberculous arthritis; it is also seen in proliferative arthritis and gout. A superficial resemblance to a marginal osteophyte of the type associated with degenerative arthritis may be achieved by the marginal notching, but there is little reason to make this error in interpretation.

Sequestra are not usually visualized in the roentgenogram for at least ten weeks (Finder), and frequently not at all in secondary sequestra possessing advanced deossification.

Collapse of a vertebral body in the presence of intact disks is not uncommon in tuberculous spondylitis of children, but, when the roentgenogram reveals such a picture in an adult, the chances are good that the collapse is due to a malignancy and not to tuberculosis.

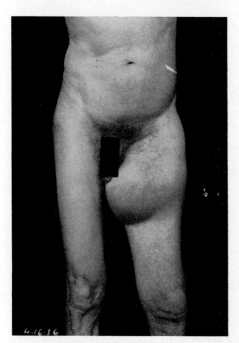

FIGURE 77. Tuberculosis of the left hip, with a large abscess, in a 56 year old man. A. Photo of patient.

Clinical Correlation

The clinical diagnosis of skeletal tuberculosis is not a simple matter, and, according to published statistics, a substantial percentage of error occurs even in the best of our orthopedic clinics. In 39 cases of tuberculous arthritis, Smith reported that 14 were erroneously diagnosed on admission. Milgram reported 38.7 percent erroneous diagnoses in 142 cases.

Diagnosis by histological sections stained by ordinary methods is also subject to error. In a strict sense the only way in which a positive diagnosis can be made is by identifying the tubercle bacilli. This can be accomplished through special cultures, guinea pig innoculation, or by special staining of histological sections.

The treatment of tuberculous arthritis is directed toward developing a sound bony ankylosis. Synovectomy, no longer employed, failed because of the early associated bone involvement. Referring to the possibility of curing tuberculous arthritis by synovectomy, Allison and Ghormley state, "Its possibility seems so remote to us that we feel that all cases should be regarded as having both bone and synovia as well as cartilage involved." Streptomycin is a welcome adjunct in the treatment of skeletal tuberculosis.

SARCOID

Although sarcoid was described by Hutchison in 1898, credit goes to Boeck for the first complete description. Impressed by the microscopic similarity to sarcoma, Boeck named the entity benign sarcoid.

The etiology is unknown, but numerous investigators have expressed a strong conviction that the disease is somehow caused by the tubercle bacillus, even though no organisms can be recovered from the diseased tissues. In order to explain the negative tuberculin reaction, and the absence of an exudate, caseation necrosis, and tubercle bacilli the claim is made that the disease occurs only in cases where there is a high resistance to the tubercle bacillus. The organisms are said to be killed by the host defense mechanisms, and the tubercles of epithelioid cells are said to represent a response to products released by the dead organisms.

Schauman saw a resemblance and relationship, not to tuberculosis, but to Hodgkin's disease, and named the entity benign lymphogranuloma.

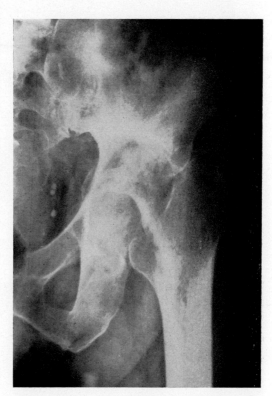

FIGURE 77. *(Continued)* B. Roentgenogram of left hip.

In the majority of instances skin lesions are a prominent feature of the disease, a fact which explains why so many cases have been reported by dermatologists. Systemic symptoms are astonishingly mild and do not reflect the widespread lesions seen in so many cases. Any organ in the body may show typical lesions, but involvement may be particularly extensive in the lungs, lymph nodes and spleen. In the lungs, the lesions tend to involve the hilus region and show no caseation and cavitation.

BONE LESIONS

Bone lesions are neither frequent nor prominent, but do present a characteristic pattern in typical cases, upon which a roentgenological diagnosis can be made.

Sites of bone lesions approximately in order of frequency are phalanges of hands and feet, metacarpals, metatarsals, wrist, elbow, ankle

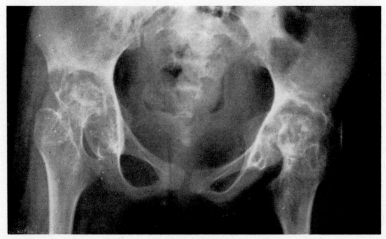

FIGURE 78. Bilateral tuberculosis of the hips.

and the long bones. The earliest changes are seen most often in terminal phalanges, and are characterized by an increased coarseness of the

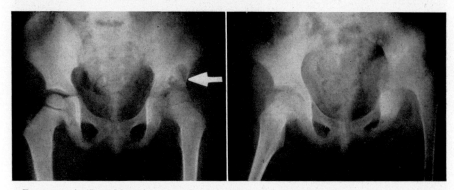

FIGURE 79. A. *(Left)* Metaphyseal and epiphyseal acetabular primary tuberculous osteomyelitis with a large primary sequestrum. B. *(Right)* Acetabular focus finally ruptured into hip joint, and the femoral head telescoped into the abscess cavity. Healing followed an arthrodesis.

trabecular pattern. Multiple, small, punched-out, cystic-like areas of rarefaction appear later and represent a consistent feature. The areas of rarefaction are not cysts but are circumscribed deposits of sarcoid tissue varying from 1 mm to 1 cm in diameter. Only a minimal degree of local bone atrophy, and no generalized atrophy is seen.

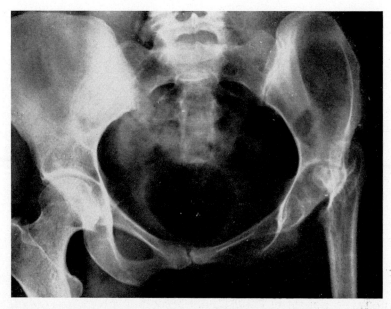

FIGURE 80. Healed tuberculosis of the left hip. Female age 24. Hip symptoms began at age 10. Abscess aspirated, pus contained tubercle bacilli. At the time the above roentgenogram was taken there was 50% of a normal range of motion and no pain. Patient also had pulmonary tuberculosis.

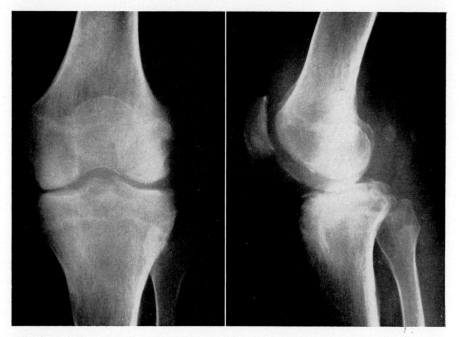

FIGURE 81. Tuberculosis of the knee. (Antero-posterior and lateral X-rays). Cartilage space is narrowed and areas of the articular cortex are losing their definition.

Since there is no significant inflammatory element in the tissue, there is little or no reactive sclerosis peripheral to the zones of rarefaction.

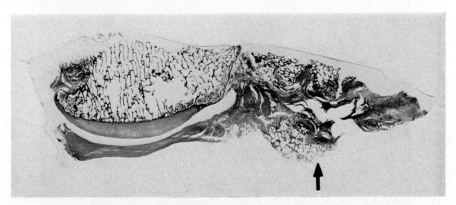

FIGURE 82. Tuberculosis of knee. Frontal section. An inter-condylar fibrous curtain localized the infection to the medial one-half of the joint (arrow).

Sequestra do not form, joints do not become involved, and only seldom is there an interruption, or expansion of the cortex. Fingers with involved phalanges may present pronounced thickening or none.

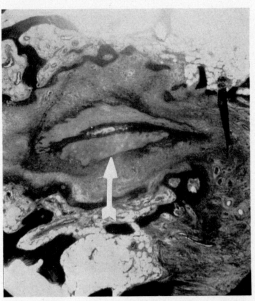

FIGURE 83. Necrotic fragments of articular cartilage (arrow) inclosed in fibrous tissue. Specimen removed from an area of fibrous ankylosis in a tuberculous knee.

Histopathology

The characteristic microscopic lesion is the so-called "hard tubercle," or sarcoid. A sarcoid is a collection of epithelioid cells with characteristic large polygonal, pale staining nuclei. The cells may not be concentrically arranged but "fitted together like tiles in a floor" (Longcope). Except for scattered lymphocytes there is no peripheral zone of inflammatory cells. Tubercles have no central necrosis, but occasionally have degeneration of central cells. Giant cells are fairly common, but

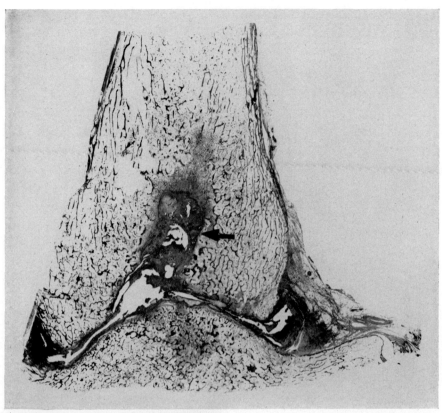

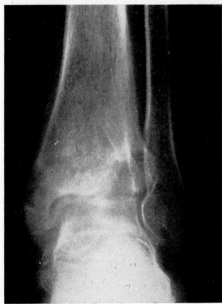

FIGURE 84. Tuberculosis of the ankle, advanced, in a 20 year old male. A *(Above)* Sagital section. A tibial primary epiphyseal abscess (arrow) extended into the ankle joint. Only scattered small fragments of articular cartilage remain. B. *(Below)* Antero-posterior roentgenogram.

typical Langhan giant cells with their peripherally placed nuclei are exceptional. Solitary tubercles, which are about the size of miliary tuberculous tubercles, increase in numbers, but not in size. Sarcoids frequently coalesce to form large tumor-like masses.

Clinical Features

Cases are seen in all age groups, but the incidence is highest in the second and third decades. Masses of sarcoid tissue may interfere with function of an organ, but serious disability is exceptional. The disease may be protracted, extending over a period of many years, with relapses and remissions, but spontaneous recovery eventually occurs in most instances. A positive diagnosis may be made by histologic study of an involved lymph node. Lung lesions, far advanced as indicated by the roentgenogram, have been occasionally discovered after routine chest films. Seeing the lesions as they are portrayed in the roentgenograms, one is impressed that the clinical symptoms could be so slight. This feature helps differentiate sarcoidosis from exudative pulmonary tuberculosis.

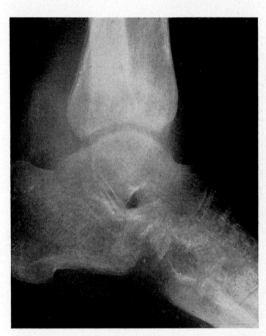

FIGURE 85. Tuberculosis of the ankle (lateral roentgenogram). Articular cortex has been destroyed, but cartilage space is preserved.

Osteitis Tuberculosa Multiplex

In 1920 Jungling reported what he termed osteitis tuberculosa multiplex or cystic tuberculosis of bone. It was his belief that the lesions represented a form of tuberculosis; it is now evident that the lesions described were those of sarcoid. Most of the cases were in younger adults and were not associated with significant systemic symptoms at any time. The bone lesions were described roentgenologically as small, round or oval, cystic-like areas of rarefaction, having no appreciable peripheral or periosteal reactive ossification. Although most of Jungling's cases involved only bones of the hands and feet, there are reports in the literature of long bone involvement. Boeck's Sarcoid skin lesions were present in many of the cases. Tissue from the bone lesions showed

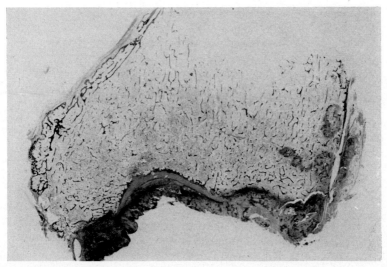

FIGURE 86. Tuberculosis of the ankle joint. Section of lower tibia shows only central area of cartilage remaining, a thick pannus over entire joint area, extensive destruction of the articular cortex, and profound osteoporosis.

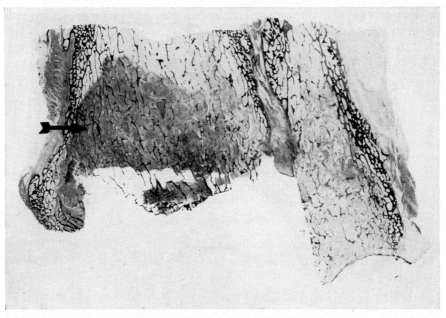

FIGURE 87. Tuberculous osteomyelitis (arrow) resulting from secondary extension after complete destruction of the ankle joint.

numerous epithelioid cells, but few inflammatory cells, and no caseation necrosis. Tubercle bacilli were never identified.

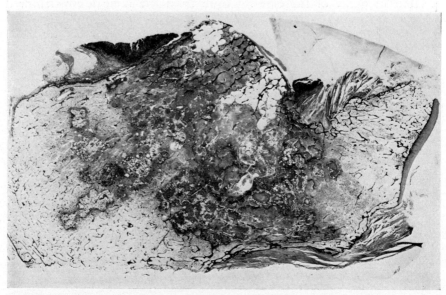

FIGURE 88. Tuberculous osteomyelitis of the os calcis. There were numerous areas of caseation necrosis. The process was gradually extending throughout the os calcis; no reactive osteosclerosis.

The group of investigators that considered Boeck's sarcoid to be a form of low virulence tuberculosis would no doubt class the Jungling

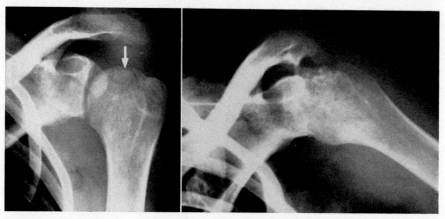

FIGURE 89. Tuberculosis of the shoulder joint. A. *(Left)* Arrow points to a sequestrum. B. *(Right) Steindler arthrodesis.*

cases with tuberculosis. But all must agree that there is a profound difference between the typical response of bone and other tissues to the exudative type of tuberculous infection and the response seen in sarcoid.

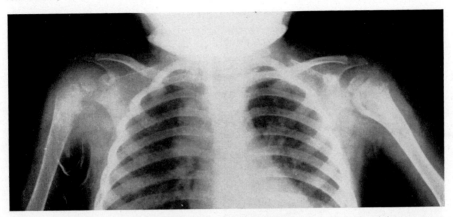

FIGURE 90. Bilateral tuberculosis of the shoulders; metaphyseal origin.

Bone lesions tend to heal with reossification of the sites of rarefaction.

Differentiation from chondromas, and spina ventosa usually is not difficult; chondromas are larger and expand the cortex, spina ventosa has more periosteal reaction and frequent sinuses.

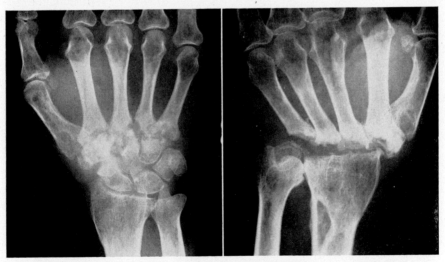

FIGURE 91. A. *(Left)* Tuberculosis of the carpals and the metacarpal bases. B. *(Right)* After surgical resection.

SYPHILIS OF THE SKELETAL SYSTEM

The roentgen-ray has shown us that syphilis of bone is more widespread than was previously presumed. Pathological studies on this subject have greatly increased in the past three decades in spite of the fact that effective therapy has created a paucity of pathological material.

The organism responsible for syphilis was identified by Fritz Schaudinn in 1905 and given the name spirochaeta pallida. The revised name, treponema pallidum, is widely used in laboratories but seldom by clinicians. This organism has been found to bear resemblance to several other spirochaetes: for example, the spirochaetes of yaws, relapsing fever, yellow fever, rat bite fever, and Weil's disease. The Spirochaeta pertenius of yaws so closely resembles the spirochaeta pallida that yaws was once considered tropical syphilis.

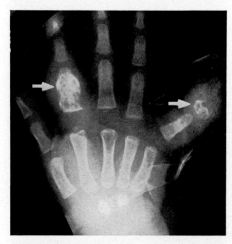

FIGURE 92. Tuberculous dactylitis *(Spina ventosa)* of the index and fifth fingers. The fifth finger developed a sinus. Note the periosteal bone, and the fusiform enlargement of the involved fingers.

Bartarelli, by the use of special staining technique, was able in 1906 to observe spirochaeta pallida in bone marrow and periosteum. Since this time Neisser and others have shown that bone, periosteum, and marrow are favorite sites for the

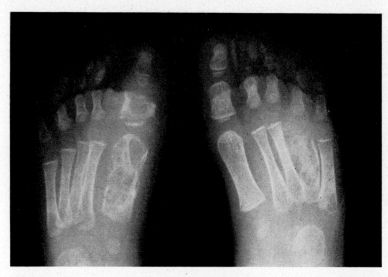

FIGURE 93. Tuberculosis of the left 1st metatarsal, right 4th metatarsal, and proximal phalanx left 1st toe.

organisms. Spirochaetes in the greatest numbers are found in the metaphyses of the syphilitic new born.

CONGENITAL SYPHILIS

Syphilis of the new born is syphilis of the secondary period. The changes characteristic of the primary period presumably occur in utero, but they have never been observed. Secondary changes, on the other hand, present a striking and well known picture in the skeletal system. No other changes in congenital syphilis occur more consistently than the bone changes. (This is by pathological examination, not by X-ray.) Thomson found these characteristic osteochondritic changes in 97 per cent of syphilitic foetuses over six months old. In decomposed stillbirths, luetic skeletal changes can be detected when all other signs of syphilis are lost through maceration. The foetus acquires the organisms sometime during the course of its development; therefore, the term hereditary syphilis or heredo-syphilis, is not legitimately used for it erroneously suggests that the disease originates in the germ plasm.

Pathogenesis

Stage of round cell infiltration: We begin the discussion of pathogenesis with the arrival of the spirochaete, apparently via the blood stream, in the foetal bone

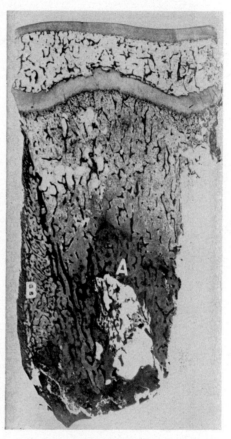

FIGURE 94. Tuberculosis 1st metatarsal in an 11 year old boy. Healing by conservative measures failed. After an abscess and sinus developed, the metatarsal was excised. Note the diaphyseal destruction, *A*, and the thick layer of periosteal bone, *B*. The epiphyseal plate was not disturbed.

marrow. The blood supply is richest in the metaphysis, and this may explain why the most striking pathological alterations occur in the vicinity of the enchondral line. The first visible local defensive response to the presence of the organisms is a mobilization of lymphocytes and plasma cells. Thus, round cell infiltration throughout the marrow spaces becomes a conspicuous early feature of the picture. The spirochaeta pallida have a tendency to remain in the metaphyses and diaphyses, the organisms having no tendency to migrate to joints as do tubercle bacilli.

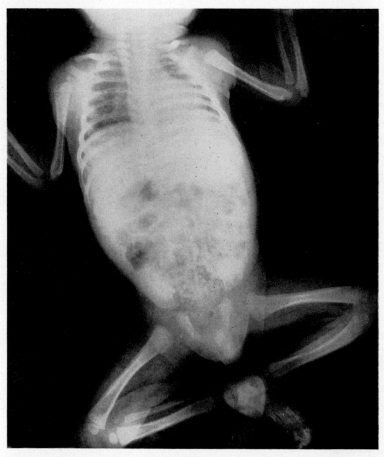

FIGURE 95. Congenital syphilis of the skeleton, secondary stage. Characterized by ossifying periostitis, metaphysitis, and osteochondritis; most pronounced in the long bones.

There is a wide variation in the degree of virulence in luetic osteochondritis, and so, in turn, there is wide variation in the defensive and healing responses. In mild or moderate metaphyseal invasions, enchondral ossification may be accelerated, but, with greater degrees of virulence, there is impairment of growth. Histologic studies disclose that the retarded growth stems from a disturbance of the new trabeculae forming at the enchondral line. The process of osteoclastic resorption is retarded, and, as a result the intratrabecular islands of calcified cartilage, are found at an abnormally great distance from the enchondral line. At the same time the trabeculae are thin, and possess irregular borders. These points are important in the histological diagnosis of this condition. As a consequence of poorly formed trabeculae, together with the inflammatory tissue in the metaphysis, the epiphyseo-metaphyseal junction is greatly weakened (Figs. 96 & 97). This situation explains the frequency with which slipped epiphyses are observed in luetic osteochondritis, both in utero, and after birth.

The osteochondritic changes previously described take place principally in the long bones and the nasal bones. In the periosteum of the long bones, usually the femur, tibia, and humerus, the important pathological alteration, leutic periostitis, consistently develops. Luetic periostitis is most evident in the periosteum covering the metaphyses and the adjacent portion of the diaphysis; it is always bilateral and co-existent with luetic osteochondritis.

Grossly the periosteum becomes thickened and hyperemic, and may be elevated by a thin exudate. Histologically there is a leucocytic response of the same round cells that infiltrate the metaphyses. Periosteal changes generally are most striking in the upper third of the tibia and the lower third of the femur. The formation of subperiosteal granulation tissue, fibrous tissue and reactive bone is essentially the same in syphilis as in other types of chronic inflammation.

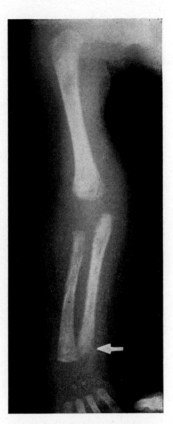

FIGURE 96. Congenital syphilis, secondary stage. Note the advanced metaphyseal changes in the lower end of the ulna (arrow).

Stage of Granulation Tissue: Just as in other types of chronic inflammation, the granulation tissue stage follows the stage of leucocytic round-cell infiltration. A well formed bed of granulation tissue that succeeds in remaining intact represents a successful defense and a broad step toward healing.

Metaphyseal luetic granulation tissue possesses a yellowish tinge during early stages of organization and turns a brighter yellow in later stages. Toward the end of the granulation tissue stage, when fibrosis begins, the yellowish color gradually turns into grey. The budding granulations fill the marrow spaces of the metaphysis in their process of organizing the leucocytic exudate. Granulations erode their way into the zone of provisory calcification and often extend even farther to

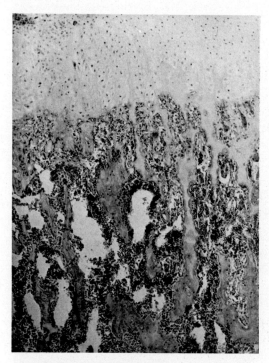

make tongue-like inroads into the zone of non-calcified cartilage. It is this aggressiveness on the part of the granulation tissue that gives rise to the saw-tooth irregularity of the epiphyseo-metaphyseal junction—a diagnostic point in the roentgenogram. Cases are reported in which the granulation tissue ultimately eroded its way to the skin surface, creating a sinus.

Stage of fibrosis: Again, as in other types of chronic inflammation, the granulation tissue, if not destroyed, undergoes fibrous condensation to form fibrous tissue. Variable degrees of leucocytic round cell infiltration are present until healing approaches completion. Fibrous tissue fills the meta-

FIGURE 97. Congenital syphilis, secondary stage. Photomicrograph of epiphyseo-metaphyseal junction. Luetic granulation tissue and round cell infiltration disturb the final stage in the formation of new bony trabeculae.

physeal marrow spaces and also the inroads made into the epiphyseal cartilage.

The fibrous tissue stage may be followed by complete healing with return of normal marrow elements and normal enchondral ossification. Luetic osteochondritis usually is a self-limited process whether treatment is instituted or not. Most cases subside by the sixth months of extra-uterine life, and many subside much earlier.

As previously mentioned, there is a wide variation in the degree of virulence. In mild cases there may be healing by resolution in the stage of leucocytic infiltration. The round cells disappear early and normal marrow promptly reappears. In such cases growth is not re-traded and may even be accelerated.

Late Congenital Syphilis *(Tertiary)*

Tertiary congenital syphilitic bone and joint lesions ordinarily make their appearance toward the end of the first decade. Occasionally such

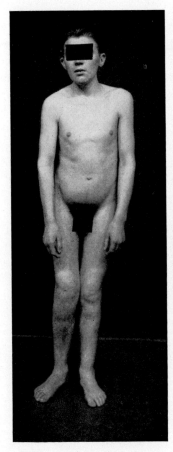
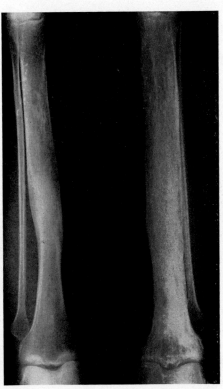

FIGURE 98. Congenital syphilis, tertiary stage. Note, in A *(left)*, enlargement of the right leg from the luetic periostitis and osteomyelitis shown in the roentgenogram, B *(Right)*.

lesions are identified as early as the second and third years of life, and as late as adulthood.

In the secondary stage of congenital syphilis the major lesion is in the metaphyses; in the tertiary stage it is in the diaphyses. At this late stage of the disease the bone lesions, characterized by reparative or osteoplastic changes, are found mainly in the tibia, femur and skull. The commonest bone lesion is the so-called saber shin in which the anterior and antero-medial aspects of the tibia become greatly thick-

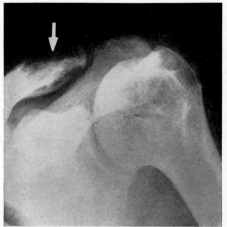

FIGURE 99. Tertiary congenital syphilitic osteomyelitis lateral end of the clavicle (from patient in Figure 98).

ened by an ossifying periostitis (Fig. 100A). Actual bending of the bone does not take place unless there is associated rickets. Periosteal new bone may involve a localized area of the shaft or extend along the entire diaphysis. While it is thickest over the antero-medial aspect, it may form in a thinner layer around the entire circumference of the bone. The fibrous layer of the periosteum is elevated, and the interval between it and the bone fills with granulation tissue thickly infiltrated by round cells. When the granulation tissue becomes fibrous tissue there is a rapid transformation to fibrous bone. As the periosteal bone matures it becomes more and more dense. Eventually there is transformation of the cancellous periosteal bone to compact bone with assimilation to the cortex. If this point is reached, the saber deformity is permanent. In earlier stages, adequate anti-luetic therapy will usually stop the process and even cause resorption of the periosteal bone already formed (Fig. 100B).

Occasionally the luetic inflammatory process does not confine its activities to the periosteum but penetrates the cortex and medullary canal to produce a luetic osteomyelitis. Rarely, an extensive osseous necrosis develops, presenting a picture similar to that of chronic pyogenic osteomyelitis. Luetic osteomyelitis is much more common in acquired

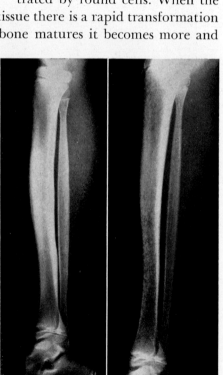

FIGURE 100. Ossifying periostitis of tertiary congenital syphilis. A. *(Left)* Before treatment. B *(Right)* After treatment.

than in congenital syphilis and will be described in detail later.

Skull changes occasionally appear in late untreated congenital syphilis and lead to variable degrees of skull thickening, often with the formation of nodules. In rare instances an osteoclastic process is established in the skull, leading to the formation of numerous small, crater-like defects. Both types of lesions involve both tables of the skull and may extend inward to invade the dura, or outward to ulcerate the skin.

Luetic dactylitis, a lesion of tertiary congenital lues, occasionally involves the small bones of the hands and feet. These lesions are osteoplastic and occur bilaterally in a symmetrical distribution. The symmetrical distribution helps to differentiate luetic from tuberculous dactylitis. The clinical and roentgenological features may be identical.

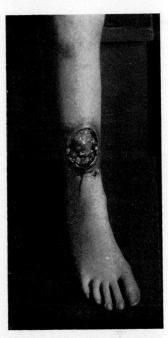

FIGURE 101. Ulcer of tertiary congenital syphilis. There was also a periostitis of the tibia.

Luetic joint involvement rarely advances beyond simple hydrarthrosis, low grade synovitis being responsible for the hydrops. Pathologically the picture is one of simple chronic low-grade inflammation with the usual round-cell infiltration. Gummatous synovitis is rare but it has been described. Joint lesions are usually multiple and occur most frequently in the knees.

DIFFERENTIAL DIAGNOSIS: The osteochondritis and periostitis of early congenital syphilis must be differentiated from the following diseases: (1) rickets, (2) tuberculosis, (3) pyogenic osteomyelitis, (4) scurvy, (5) sarcomata.

There are several characteristics by which rickets may be differentiated: (1) Calcium is diminished or absent at the zone of provisory calcification. In luetic osteochondritis there usually is an increase in calcified cartilage at the enchondral line together with a widening of the line, seen as a white zone in the roentgenogram. The enchondral line in rickets is widened, irregular, and radiolucent. (2) Rickets is rare during the first three or four months of life—the period when true luetic osteochondritis is most manifest. (3) Growth slows or ceases during active rickets. Luetic osteochondritis may even accelerate growth. (4) Metaphyses widen and flare (trumpet) in rickets. (5) Periostitis is less pronounced in rickets than in early congenital lues.

Tuberculosis is rare during the early months of life. **Pyogenic osteomyelitis** has a more acute onset and does not involve several metaphyses simultaneously. **Scurvy** leads to more periosteal changes and less metaphyseal alteration than early congenital lues. **Sarcomas** are very rare in the early months of life and present only a solitary lesion.

The saber shin tibiae of late congenital syphilis are easily differentiated roentgenographically from the anterior bowing of rickets. In leutic periostitis there is no actual bowing, merely a thickening of the bone

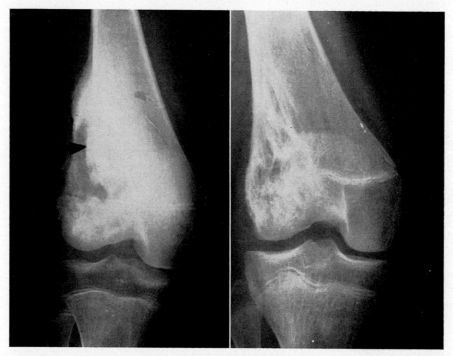

FIGURE 102. Tertiary congenital syphilitic osteomyelitis. A. *(Left)* Before treatment. Arrow points to a large sequestrum. B. *(Right)* After treatment. Sequestrum absorbed.

anteriorly and antero-medially, to form an anterior curve. In rickets the anterior curve is the result of a tibial bend. Tibial thickening, if present in rickets, is on the concave aspect of the curve and represents a static reinforcement.

Acquired Syphilis

Practically all bone and joint lesions of acquired syphilis occur during the tertiary stage, and rarely appear sooner than two years after the disease is acquired. The incidence of these lesions has never been accurately determined, but is considerably higher than earlier observers believed. In the examination of twenty-seven syphilitic cadavers, Chiari found gummatous lesions of the long bones in nine. From a study of 165 syphilitics, Wile and Senear found bone or joint lesions in 60 percent. Clinicians are becoming more and more conscious of luetic bone lesions; so the future should bring forth more information on this subject. The roentgenogram of bone syphilis is not often specific. There are certain distinctive features which are helpful but not infallible. According to Stokes, the outright diagnosis of bone syphilis could not be made by the roentgenogram or any other one method in a higher proportion than 50 per cent.

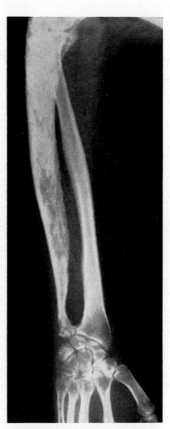

Pathogenesis

Invasion of a bone by spirochaeta pallida and its toxins precipitates an immediate defensive response which attempts to destroy or wall off the invader. The leucocytes which are mobilized in the area are predominately lymphocytes and plasma cells. Granulation tissue forming from organization of the exudate may, as Knaggs has pointed out, undergo the same fates as does granulation tissue in tuberculosis: (1) resolution, (2) fibrosis, or, (3) necrosis.

(1) Resolution during the granulation tissue stage is usually the result of antiluetic therapy. The granulations simply are absorbed and disappear.

(2) Fibrosis occurs when the granulation tissue remains viable and unresorbed long enough to undergo fibrous condensation. Fibrous tissue thus formed may ossify or later be absorbed.

FIGURE 103. Tertiary congenital syphilitic osteomyelitis of the ulna.

(3) Necrosis of localized areas of granulation tissues together with the adjacent tissue responses create the interesting syphilitic lesion—the gumma. Gummata vary in size from a fraction of one centimeter to several centimeters in diameter. The core of these lesions is filled with a yellowish gum-like material which represents the caseated necrotic debris of luetic granulation tissue (Fig. 104). Two factors appear responsible for the death of the granulation tissue: first, the spirochaetes

or their toxins; and second, the endarteritis and periarteritis in the arteries leading to the involved area. The vessels are obliterated mainly by a proliferation of their endothelial lining. Peripheral to the necrotic area are the foreign body giant cells, round cells, and a zone of fibrosis. Beyond the fibrous zone there may be normal tissue. Unlike tubercles, gummata may sit solitarily in a field of otherwise normal tissue. Gummata may be absorbed or replaced by fibrous tissue; occasionally they become the site of an abscess; when close to the skin surface they may perforate the skin and discharge a mucinous or even cheesy material. Secondary infection usually follows perforation, the discharge then becoming purulent.

In both early and late acquired syphilis, periostitis is the predominating skeletal lesion (Fig. 105). Probably the most frequent sites of involvement are the tibial diaphysis and the inner one-third of the clavicle. The skull is next in frequency, and in some statistics skull involvement ranks first. Beyond the early stages the chronic inflammation may invade the cortex to produce an osteoperiostitis, and then

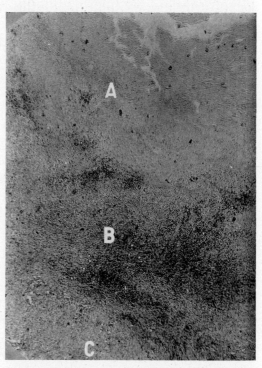

FIGURE 104. Photomicrograph of a gumma (periosteal). *A*. Area of necrosis. *B*. Zone of giant cells and round cells. *C*. Zone of fibrosis.

enter the medullary canal to complete the picture of an osteomyelitis. Actually one rarely sees luetic bone lesions in a pathologic examination that do not to some degree involve all elements of the bone, even though the roentgenogram discloses only a periostitis.

Stokes reported a survey of 239 Mayo clinic cases: there were 57 percent males and 43 percent females; Cranial bone involvement occurred in 42 percent; tibial lesions in 26 percent; sterum and ribs in 10 percent; clavicle in 7.5 percent; femur in 4.5 percent; humerus in 3.5 percent; vertebra in 5 percent. Periostitis was by far the most frequent lesion occuring in 53 percent; osteomyelitis occurred in 20 percent, arthritis in 12 percent. Prior to their admission to the Mayo clinic only 7 percent of the cases were diagnosed as syphilis.

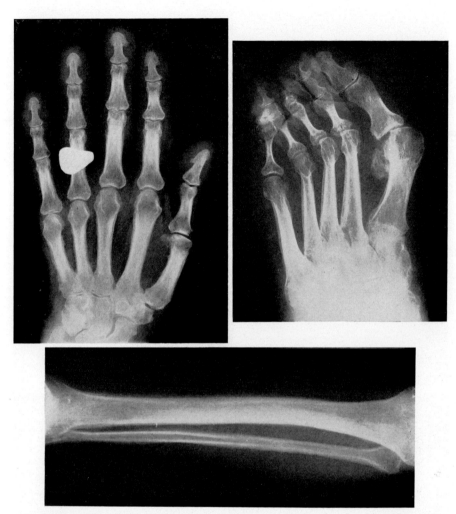

Figure 105. Tertiary acquired syphilis. Male age 52. Had had no treatment. Ossifying periostitis developed in all of the long bones and most of the short bones. A. *(Left)* Hand. B. *(Below)* Tibia. C. *(Right)* Foot.

Types of Bone Syphilis

Periostitis

As has been previously mentioned, periostitis is overwhelmingly the most frequent bone lesion. It occurs in both the skull and long bones, but much more often in the latter. There may be involvement of a circumscribed portion of the shaft, or an entire diaphysis. The perios-

teum becomes edematous and infiltrated by round cells and elevated
to a variable degree by the formation of granulation tissue beneath

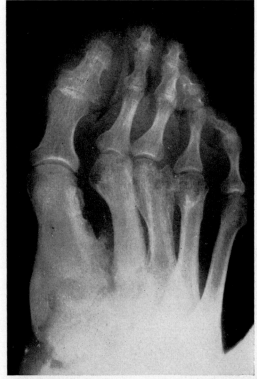

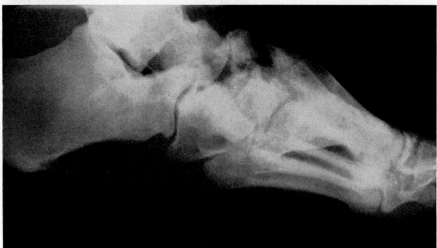

FIGURE 106. Tertiary acquired
syphilis. Roentgenograms showing
luetic osteomyelitis of the foot. A.
(Above) Antero-posterior view. B.
(Below) Lateral view.

and within it. If the granulation tissue does not absorb either spontaneously or as the result of antiluetic therapy, there is the usual transforma-

tion to fibrous tissue. In a later stage, bone forms within this fibrous tissue and generally possesses an irregular lace-like outline. In very late stages, the periosteal bone may become more dense, assimilate with the cortex, and present a smooth outline. In other cases, the chronic inflammatory process of the periostitis may lead to porosis of the underlying cortex, and then spread into the cortex to produce an osteitis.

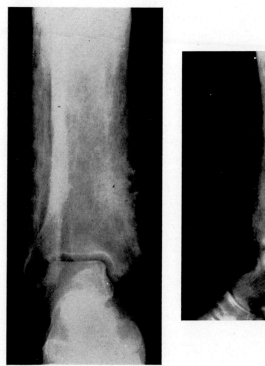
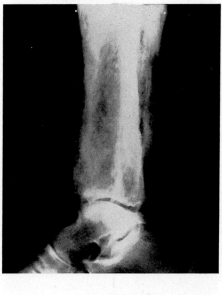

FIGURE 107. Syphilitic gummatous osteomyelitis of the tibia and fibula. A. *(Left)* Antero-posterior view. B. *(Right)* Lateral view.

Osteoperiostitis

This condition is described separately from luetic osteomyelitis, but from the pathologic standpoint this should not be done. Osteoperiostitis as usually described involves all of the bone elements including the medulla. The term luetic osteomyelitis is reserved for that extensive gummatous type of involvement in which there is as much of a destructive phase as proliferative. In both the skull and the long bones a predominance of osteoplastic activity is characteristic, and often is responsible for considerably thickening of bones. The cortex may become sclerotic and so much thickened internally that the medullary cavity becomes narrowed or even obliterated. Freund has shown that in such bones few or no gummata exist. The sclerosis is not often uniform in density but presents spotty irregularities due in part to a wide variation in the extent of osseous necrosis. In the long bones, particularly in the cortex, sequestra are rare; in the outer table of the skull and in the facial bones sequestra occasionally are seen. In

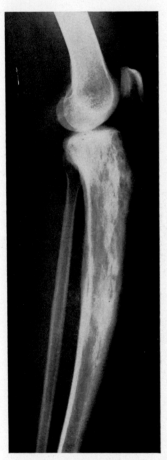

decades past when the therapy was less effective, such sequestra were frequently observed, especially among sailors. Patterns of skull involvement are widely variable, but the major changes generally are limited to the outer cortex and periosteum. Such involvement, if predominately productive, results in the formation of areas of closely placed small nodules. If the process is more destructive than proliferative there are great numbers of shallow, small, rounded pits in the cortex, which usually enlarge as the process becomes a true gummatous osteomyelitis.

Gummatous Osteomyelitis

The most extensive and destructive luetic lesions of both the long bones and the skull represent gummatous osteomyelitis (Figs. 107-111). In the long bones the involvement is more advanced toward the ends of the bone than in the center. When sequestra occur they develop in the cancellous bone of the metaphyseal and epiphyseal regions (Fig. 102A). It is not uncommon for the process to break through into a joint and produce a gummatous

FIGURE 108. Syphilitic osteomyelitis resembling Paget's disease.

arthritis. The many areas of reduced density represent sites of gummata, the gummata causing resorption of the bone directly within and adjacent to them. While the crater-like pits in the skull ordinarily involve the outer table, they have been known to perforate the inner table, allowing the gummata to invade the dura and produce a luetic pachymeningitis. If the multiple small areas of destruction become confluent, the area presents an irregular, serpiginous contour. Areas of bone, even large ones, may become necrotic and subsequently sequestrate. Small sequestra absorb with treatment, but in both skull and long bones, large sequestra may have to be dealt with surgically. In the healing process the skull may become considerably thickened and the diploe replaced by new bone, making differentiation of the skull tables impossible.

Syphilitic Joint Lesions

Joint lesions are not a prominent feature of skeletal system syphilis, but they definitely do occur. In a Mayo clinic survey reported by Stokes there was a ratio of joint-bone involvement of 1:7. While any joint may become involved, the knee is by far the most frequent site. There is confusion concerning the pathology of most luetic joint lesions. Clinical symptoms generally are mild.

Syphilitic Synovitis

This condition is almost always bilateral, involves the larger joints, and occurs more frequently early than late in tertiary syphilis. Occasionally luetic synovitis is observed in the secondary stage. There is an increase in joint fluid but never any pus or the classical signs of inflammation. Motion is not limited unless the lesion is of very long duration. Pathologically there is a lymphocytic and plasma cellular infiltration of the stratum fibrosum and synovialis. After a long period there may be capsular thickening by fibrosis. The articular surfaces are not materially altered.

Luetic Arthritis

The exact pathological changes in this entity are neither clear-cut nor well established. Cases have been reported in which there were punched out areas of destruction

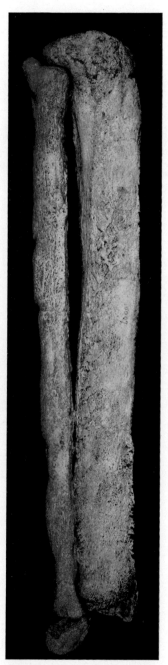

FIGURE 109. Syphilitic periostitis and osteomyelitis of the tibia and fibula. (Courtesy, *U. S. Army Institute of Pathology*. Neg. No. 66252. Acc. No. 10067 P.S.)

in the articular surfaces, but no signs of gummata. Other reported changes resembled those of degenerative arthritis. In fact, the term syphilitic pseudo-arthritis deformans was suggested but not widely accepted. It is believed that many of the reported cases of so-called luetic arthritis have actually represented early Charcot joints or degenerative and proliferative arthritis.

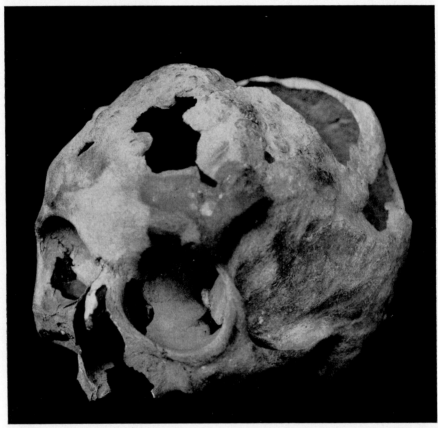

FIGURE 110. Syphilitic osteomyelitis of the skull. Female more than 60 years of age; died of syphilis 1869. (Courtesy, *U. S. Army Institute of Pathology,* Hamilton Collection. Neg. No. 66249. Acc. No. 10032 P. S.)

Gummatous Arthritis

This entity is well established both pathologically and clinically. Gummatous arthritis is said never to be primary, but always the result of direct extension from an adjacent gummatous osteomyelitis or, in rare instances, from adjacent soft tissue gummata. The gummata may extensively destroy the joint capsule, and there are variable degrees of cartilage destruction, but bony ankylosis is not expected, even when destruction is extensive. The knee is the joint most frequently involved, but, in contrast to the bilateral distribution of luetic synovitis, the involvement is unilateral and usually mono-articular. Constitutional reaction is ordinarily mild in spite of considerable swelling and joint damage. Gummata may perforate overlying skin to form an ulcer which frequently ushers in a secondary infection and suppuration. It is rare for gummata to advance across the joint to set up an osteomyelitis in the opposite bone.

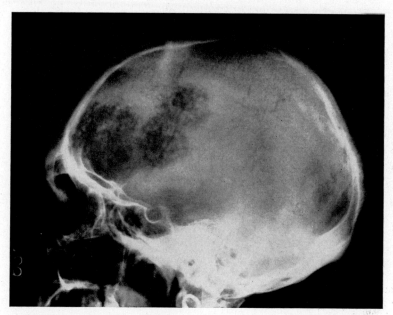

FIGURE 111. Syphilitic osteomyelitis of the skull. Lateral roentgenogram.

Charcot Joint

This condition in times past occasionally was erroneously interpreted as a specific luetic lesion. As is well known, it is not due to a joint invasion by the spirochaeta pallida or its toxins, but represents a neuro-arthropathy caused by lesions of the spinal cord. Tabes dorsalis is the commonest cause of the spinal cord lesions leading to the development of Charcot joints; other conditions, such as syringomyelia, cord trauma, and spina bifida may also lead to arthropathies.

DIFFERENTIAL DIAGNOSIS

Skeletal syphilis must be differentiated from: (1) Tuberculous osteomyelitis and arthritis; (2) Pyogenic osteomyelitis; (3) malignancies; (4) Paget's disease; (5) Actinomycosis; and, (6) Blastomycosis.

Considerable difficulty may be encountered in differentiating skeletal tuberculosis from skeletal syphilis. The only certain differentiation lies in the identification of tubercle bacilli or spirochaeta pallida. Clinically, tuberculosis usually produces more of a systemic reaction than does syphilis. Tuberculosis involves joints much more frequently than bones, whereas the reverse is true in syphilis. Abscesses appear in syphilis only with the advent of a secondary infection; abscesses are the rule in the tuberculosis. In osteomyelitis of the skull, syphilis involves principally the outer table, whereas tuberculosis generally involves the inner table.

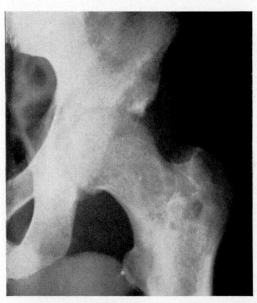

FIGURE 112. Actinomycotic osteomyelitis and arthritis. Male age 26. Occupation: dealer in animal hides. Skin abscesses and lung symptoms 14 months, left hip pain and rigidity seven months. Expired with meningitis. Osteomyelitis trochanteric region, neck and head of femur. Complete destruction of the hip joint. Many actinomyces were found in the bone lesions, but only a few were found in the joint.

By roentgenogram, pyogenic osteomyelitis may at times be confused with syphilitic osteomyelitis, but clinically the differentiation usually is uncomplicated. Pathologically, the diagnosis ordinarily is obvious if adequate material is examined. The ease with which pyogenic organisms may be cultured aids in the differentiation when the lesion at hand is due to one of the pyogenic group.

An important differential diagnosis exists between skeletal spyhilis and bone malignancies. Frequently there is much at stake in such a differentiation. Many amputations have been needlessly performed for skeletal syphilis erroneously diagnosed as sarcoma. Even the histological differentiation of these two conditions may offer difficulty if in a leutic lesion the tissue examined is from an area of active proliferation. As much tissue as possible should be examined, and special stains for the identification of spirochaetes often need to be employed. Of course, the entire picture should be studied, and not merely the histology and roentgenology. Sarcomata usually present only solitary skeletal lesions, whereas luetic lesions are multiple. The bony metastases of carcinomata are often confusing when the primary carcinoma is not evident.

Monostotic Paget's disease may present a problem in differential diagnosis; in fact, there are cases where roentgenological differentiation is impossible (Fig. 108). Generally the coarse trabeculations of luetic osteomyelitis are denser and have less tendency to develop an irregular wave-like contour. Less periosteal new bone formation is expected in

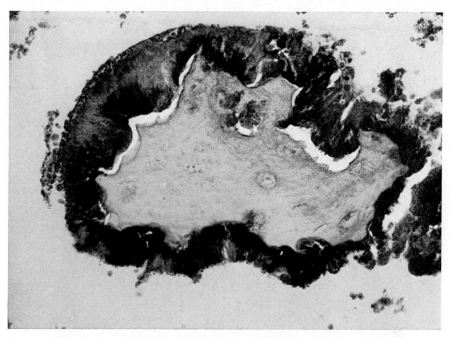

FIGURE 113. Actinomyces (ray fungus). Actinomyces accumulated around a spicule of necrotic bone.

syphilis, and the striking mosaic structure, so prominent in Paget's disease, is not present in luetic bone lesions.

Actinomycosis may be differentiated by the presence of ray fungi and sulphur granules. This condition, together with blastomycosis, rarely presents a differential diagnostic problem, either pathologically or bacteriologically.

ACTINOMYCOSIS

Actinomycosis, a chronic infective granuloma found throughout the United States, occurs most frequently in the upper Mississippi Valley and Northwestern states. It develops in man and in such animals as pigs, cows and horses. In cattle the disease is known as "lumpy jaw." One of the higher fungi known as ray fungus is the cause of the disease. Ray fungus *(actinomycea bovis)* is characterized by the presence of thread-like filaments radiating like actinic rays from a small central colony of club-shaped cells and spores (Fig. 114). These central yellowish masses measuring approximately 1 mm in diameter, are called yellow granules. The presence of ray fungi in an actinomycotic infection may be detected by placing a thin film of the debris, pus or granulation

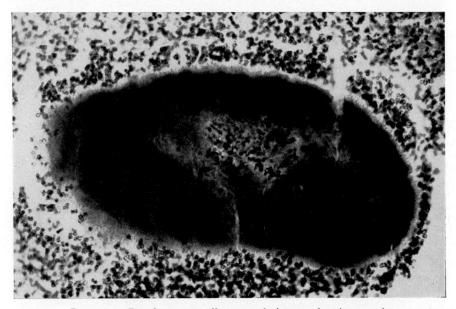

FIGURE 114. Ray fungus or yellow granule in pus of actinomycosis.

tissue, between two small glass slides. When the slides are held up to a light, the sulphur granules become visible.

The method by which the disease is conveyed to man is not known. In spite of the fact that the disease is more common in rural dwellers, there is no proof that man is inoculated directly from animals. Most cases develop during the second and third decades.

SITES OF INVOLVEMENT

More than half of the lesions occur in the head and neck. *(Cervicofacial type)*. Next in frequency is the iliocaecal region, around the appendix. A substantial percentage of cases begin in the lungs or skin. Lymph nodes and blood vessels are conspicuous for their freedom from involvement. This fact is useful in differentiating actinomycosis from other chronic infections. Almost all bone involvement occurs by direct extension from adjacent pathologic involvement of soft tissues. Most primary involvement occurs in subcutaneous and submucous tissues. Very rarely a primary lesion arises in a bone. Cases have been reported of metatases to the skeleton from a primary pulmonary actinomycosis.

PATHOGENESIS

In view of the fact that nearly all skeletal lesions in actinomycosis occur by direct extension, the periosteum is naturally invaded first. The cortex is gradually destroyed and the infection admitted to the medullary canal. While the destructive phase of actinomycosis predominates, there is a definite proliferative phase, and in an occasional case bone proliferation becomes pronounced. The rare primary bone lesions are difficult to diagnose but, notwithstanding, several cases of primary vertebral invasion have been reported. Such cases usually are diagnosed tuberculous spondylitis. Primary joint invasion apparently has not been observed.

The primary lesion develops most frequently in the lower jaw. An indurated brawny mass appears, which breaks down to form abscesses. Within a brief time the involved area becomes perforated with a number of draining sinuses; the multiple draining sinuses are an important characteristic of actinomycosis. Lower jaw muccous membrane infections often extend into the mandible and riddle it. Lung infections may extend into vertebrae and ribs, caecal infections into the pelvis. Actinomycotic infections have a propensity for burrowing, which is accomplished by necrotizing and liquefying nearly every barrier in their path. Soft tissue involvement in the extremities frequently extends to adjacent long bones.

HISTOLOGY

The microscopic picture is that of a granuloma with suppuration superimposed. There is the expected picture of chronic inflammation with numerous round cells, fibroblasts, and foreign body giant cells. Occasionally, there may be a temporary acute phase with increased suppuration, and during such periods the histologic picture is that of acute inflammation. Healing is by fibrosis.

VERTEBRAL LESIONS

Lesions of the vertebral bodies are among the most frequent in the disease. Involvement of multiple areas in several vertebra, and intact intervertebral disks is the rule. Direct extensions of the infection from the lungs usually involve the dorsal vertebra; extensions from the

abdominal viscera involve the lumbar vertebra. Collapse of a vertebral body is rare, even in the presence of extensive destruction. This
characteristic helps differentiate actinomycotic spondylitis from tuberculosis spondylitis. Large paravertebral abscesses may form and ulti-

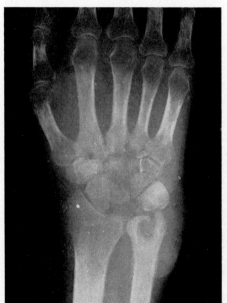
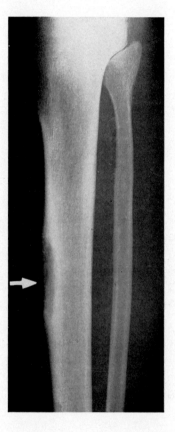

FIGURE 115. Blastomycosis: A. *(Left)* Right
wrist. B. *(Right)* Right tibia. Male age 47. Symptoms 13 weeks at time roentgenograms were
taken. Wrist involvement was hematogenous;
tibial cortex erosion was a direct extension of a
large leg ulcer. No pulmonary involvement. Wrist
abscess was drained surgically. Blostomyces recovered from both lesions. The outcome was a
complete recovery with an ankylosed wrist.

mately attain surface openings. Areas of bone are rendered necrotic,
but sequestration in the true sense does not take place.

PROGNOSIS

Wagensteen emphasizes the fact that the prognosis in the cervicofacial type is good unless too much reliance is placed on the therapeutic
response to iodides and irradiation. He recommends energetic surgical incision and excision whenever it is feasible, pointing out that the
ray fungus is essentially anerobic and should be combatted by open
drainage with excision of dead tissue. The prognosis, when there is
extensive thoracic or abdominal involvement, is poor.

BLASTOMYCOSIS

Blastomycosis was described in the year 1894, with Gilchrist and Busse each reporting a case. The Busse case was a tibial osteomyelitis, the first bone infection from which the double refractile blastomyces were recovered.

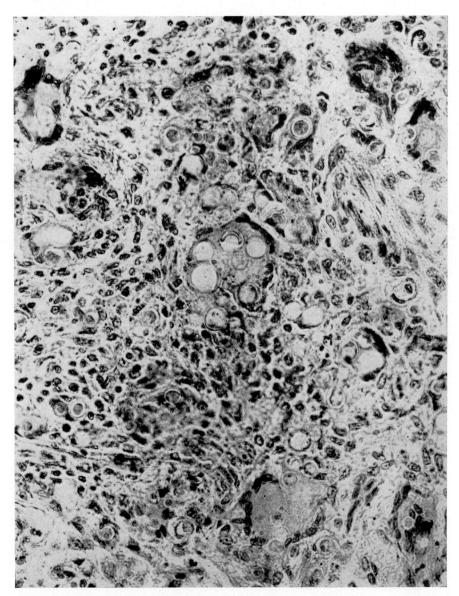

FIGURE 116. Blastomyces. The double refractile character is seen at the periphery of the blastomyces. Several of the organisms have been phagocytosed by giant cells. (Courtesy, A. Purdy Scott, M.D., New York).

The fungus blastomyces causes blastomycosis, and it exists in animals as round, double refractile organisms measuring 15 to 20 micra in diameter (Fig. 116). Blastomyces are found in great numbers both in the pus and involved tissues.

Blastomycosis occurs much less commonly than does either actinomycosis or coccidioides. According to Colonna and Gucker's survey, only 67 cases with bone involvement were reported up to April 1944.

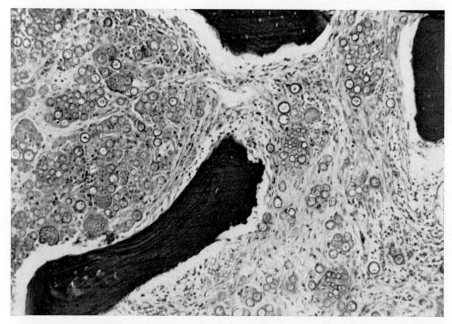

FIGURE 117. Coccidoidal spherules infiltrating marrow spaces. Spherules have double refractile walls and represent the parasitic phase. (Courtesy, *U. S. Army Institute of Pathology.*

Of these cases there were nine males to one female, and the mortality was said to have been 89 percent (only 11 out of the 67 recovered). In order of frequency the involved bones were: vertebrae, skull, ribs, tibia, tarsus, knee, metatarsus and carpus.

TYPES—The disease occurs in two forms:

1. Cutaneous and 2. Systemic.

1. *In the cutaneous type* large suppurating ulcers and sinuses are characteristic, occuring most frequently on the face, backs of hands, and front of legs. Involvement of bones and joints is uncommon, but, when present, develops through direct extension, or from organisms carried to the bones by the blood stream.

2. *In the systemic type* lung involvement is the outstanding manifestation. The bone and joint lesions are similar to those of disseminated coccidioides.

COCCIDIOIDES

Coccidioides is a chronic granulomatous infection caused by the fungus coccidioides imitis. The first case was observed by Posadas and reported by Wernicke in 1892 (Carter). The second and third cases were reported by Rixford and Thorne, respectively, in 1894; Rixford and Gilchrist, in 1896, suggested the name coccidioides imitis. The fungus exists in a saprophytic phase in nature presumably as chlamydospores, and in a parasitic phase in animals, as spherules. As a saphrophyte, the fungus occurs in arid regions; in the United States it is abundant in the San Joaquin Valley of California. As yet, the host of the fungus has not been discovered.

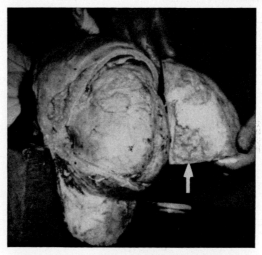

FIGURE 118A. Coccidioidomycosis osteomyelitis of the skull (arrow). Negro age 27.

Spherules of the parasitic phase have a double refractile wall similar to blastomyces (Fig. 117). However, the spherule is larger and multiplies by endosporulation, whereas the blastomyces propagate by budding. The spherule protoplasm is divided radially into endospores, which, upon being released, grow into mature spherules. Spherules reach the many parts of the animal body by traveling in the blood and lymphatic streams.

The fungus gains entrance to the body by way of the respiratory tract, except for an occasional case that is contracted through a break in the skin. Most cases remain localized and eventually heal. According to Smith, only one case in every 500 to 1000 becomes disseminated. Dissemination leads to generalized lesions and usually to a slow death. The lungs, lymph glands, bones and meninges are particularly susceptible. Bone lesions occur in both the localized and disseminated forms but are particularly frequent in the latter. Injection of pus into a guinea pig produces a suppurative orchitis from which a positive diagnosis can be made; culture of the spores reproduces the fungus in either a mycelial form or as spherules.

In animal tissues, nodules form, somewhat resembling tubercles, and they frequently coalesce, caseate, and suppurate to create large abscesses. Chronic inflammatory cells and spherules thickly infiltrate involved tissues.

SKELETAL LESIONS

In contrast to actinomycosis, where the skeleton generally is involved by direct extention, coccidioides invades the skeleton through metastases

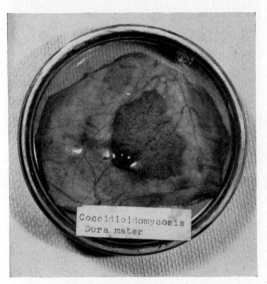

from soft tissue foci. However, bone can become involved by direct extension, particularly from the intractable, deep burrowing skin lesions. Metastatic bone lesions involve cancellous areas except in rare instances. This limits most of the original metastatic lesions to metaphyses and epiphyses. Involvement of diaphyses through extension from metaphyses does occur but is not a prominent feature of the disease. The bone lesions, being predominately destructive and granulomatous, are similar to

FIGURE 118B. Coccidioidomycosis of the dura mater (lesion represented a direct extension from the skull lesion). (Courtesy, Mark P. Beam, M.D.)

those of tuberculous osteomyelitis; however, in coccidioides the bone lesions ordinarily are multiple, a feature relatively uncommon in tuberculosis. Periosteal bone formation is not conspicuous, although it occurs to some degree in most cases (Fig. 119). After surgical drainage, massive periosteal bone may form.

Joint invasion generally develops by direct extension from an adjacent bony focus. In rare instances a joint lesion is primary or may result from an overlying soft tissue focus. Articular cartilage is slowly destroyed by granulation tissue, there being no large numbers of neutrophils to supply a proteolytic enzyme.

Any bone or joint may be invaded. In Carter's cases the ribs were the site of the largest number of lesions. Skull involvement is seen as punched out areas in the outer table, with only minimal inner table damage (Fig. 118). Involvement of the inner table may arise by direct extension from a dural lesion.

The roentgenologist, Ray Carter, surveyed 94 skeletal lesions in 60 cases. All but one lesion arose in cancellous bone, with 30 arising superficially, and 27 arising centrally in the cancellous bone. An epiphyseal line was crossed in 25 cases. Margins of the lesions were circumscribed in 40, and diffuse in 50. Marginal bone production occurred in 28, bone production within the lesions, in 14. Joints adjacent to epiphyseal lesions became involved in 28 cases. Forty percent of the lesions involved bony prominences. The lesions resembled those of blastomycosis more than those of tuberculosis.

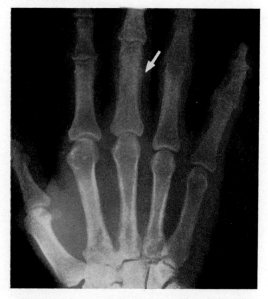

FIGURE 119. Coccidiodal osteomyelitis of the proximal phalanx middle finger. (Courtesy, *U. S. Army Institute of Pathology*, Neg. No. 68685, Acc. No. 62489.)

Goren reported the case of a soldier incurring coccidioides through a laceration of an index finger. The lesion involved the phalanges but remained localized. A cure followed amputation of the finger.

McMaster and Gilfillan, reporting 24 cases, emphasized the high incidence of lesions in such bony prominences as tibial tubercles, malleoli and the olecranon. Thirteen of their 24 cases were fatal, and all of the fatal cases had pulmonary involvement.

SPOROTRICHOSIS

Sporotrichosis is a rare chronic granulomatous infection caused by a sporotrichium, a filamentous spore-bearing fungus. The first case was reported by Shenk at the Johns Hopkins Hospital in 1898, and had involvement of the right upper extremity.

Humans, horses, dogs, and rats are capable of having the disease, and also are able to transmit it.

Both localized and diseminated forms of the disease have been observed. While the infection may last for several years, it rarely is fatal.

Gumma-like nodules with central necrosis are characteristic. At the periphery of the nodules there are epithelioid and giant cells similar to those in syphilitic gummata.

Bone Lesions: Bone lesions are rare but when they occur they may be hematogenous or develop from direct extension of an overlying ulcer or abscess. Multiple hematogenous lesions, predominately destructive, may involve many long bones, the ribs, the skull, and the jaws. Phalan-

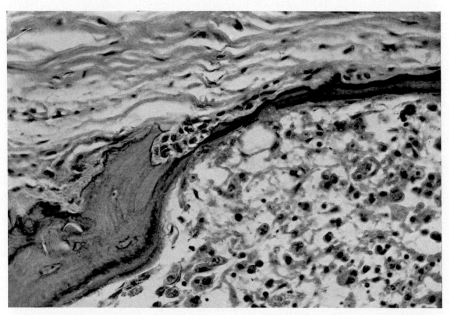

FIGURE 120. Osteolysis in leprosy. Histologic section of a granulomatous bone lesion (X500). (Courtesy, *U. S. Army Institute of Pathology*, Neg. No. 81176, Acc. No. 109630.)

geal lesions produce changes similar to those seen in luetic and tuberculosis dactylitis.

STREPTOTHRICOSIS

Streptothricosis is a rare, chronic, granulomatous infection, in which the lesions in man resemble those of actinomycosis. The disease is due to a mycotic organism called streptothrix, which is characterized by loose clusters of fungus filaments. Concentration of the filaments into granules, as occurs with actinomyces, is not seen with streptothrix.

A few lesions of the head and neck have been observed, but the principal site of involvement is the lungs. All cases complicated by a streptothrix pneumonia have been fatal.

Skeletal lesions cannot be differentiated from those of actinomycosis.

HISTOPLASMOSIS

Histoplasmosis is a fungus infection. Only one case with a skeletal lesion has been reported. Key and Large treated a 47 year old male with a knee lesion resembling tuberculous arthritis. Lung lesions were also found. Ten days following a lower thigh amputation, the patient died of a right lower lobe pneumonia.

TORULOSIS

Torulosis is caused by the fungus, torula. According to Kessler it was first reported by Zenker in 1861; and up to 1935 there had been 45 cases described in the literature. Cutaneous and meningeal involvement are the most frequent. Only one known patient has exhibited a bone or joint lesion, and he was studied and treated by J. C. Wilson and F. M. McKeever. This patient was a 38 year old male who developed symptoms in the left knee similar to those of tuberculous arthritis. In fluid removed from the knee of this patient, Kessler found torula. A cure followed an amputation in the lower one-half of the left thigh.

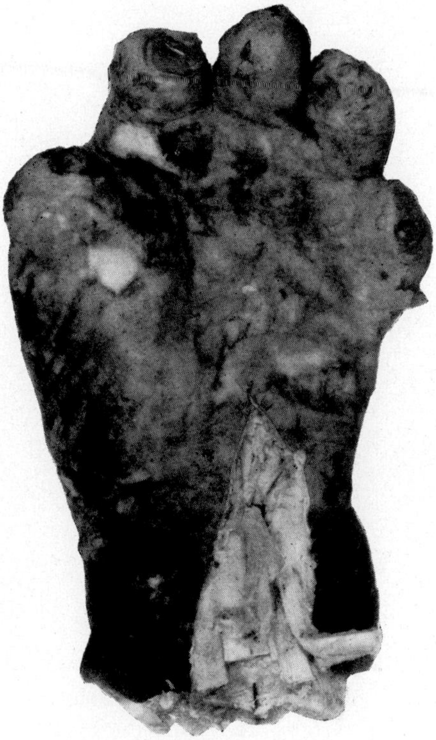

FIGURE 121. Leprosy involving the hand. (Courtesy, *U. S. Army Institute of Pathology*, Neg. No. 38560, Acc. No. 20980.)

LEPROSY

Leprosy is a chronic, infective, contagious granuloma caused by the Bacillus Leprae. Bacillus Leprae was first isolated and described by Hausen in 1873. The disease appears to be transmitted by inhalations, the initial lesions usually developing in the nasal system. Most common in middle aged males, leprosy occurs at all ages, even in children, but develops only after long and intimate contact.

HISTOPATHOLOGY

The microscopic picture of leprosy closely resembles that of tuberculosis and syphilis. The granulomata consist of fibroblastic tissue infiltrated with epithelioid cells, lymphocytes, plasma cells, giant cells, and scattered so-called "lepra cells" which are large cells with clear pale cytoplasm. The baccillus leprae resembles the tubercle bacillus in both its staining reaction and structure. The bacilli may spread throughout the body and become numerous in the blood stream. Honey found nine positive blood streams in 28 lepers.

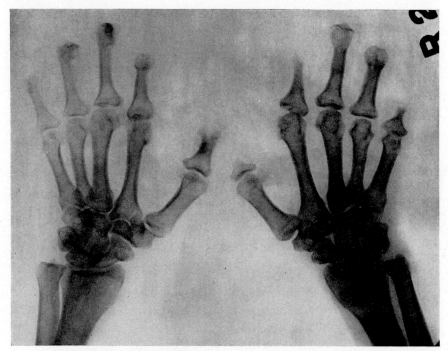

FIGURE 122. Leprosy involving the hands. Antero-posterior roentgenograms. (Courtesy, *U. S. Army Institute of Pathology*, Neg. No. 48550.)

BONE CHANGES

Skeletal system involvement may appear in both forms of leprosy: the nervous or maculo-anesthetic, and the nodular or lepra tuberosa. In 140 cases examined roentgenologically by Murdock and Hatter, 108 disclosed bone lesions. Trophic changes in the bones (Fig. 123) are inevitable when the overlying soft parts become extensively involved. These changes have been described by Chamberlain, Wayson, and Garland as "nicking, slicing, or collar-buttoning." Multiple small cystic-like areas appear, particularly in phalanges, and these areas are filled with fibrous tissue. Leprous periostitis and osteomyelitis also have been described. Through skin ulcerations, the bone lesions may communicate with the surface and become secondarily infected. A minimum of periosteal bone forms over the cortical and cancellous lesions. Bone atrophy, including concentric atrophy, develops in involved regions. As is well known, fingers and toes may be deprived of their blood supply and drop off (Figs. 121 & 123).

YAWS

Yaws, or frambesia, once called *stone age syphilis* and *tropical syphilis*, is an infectious, granulomatous, tropical disease. It is non-venereal,

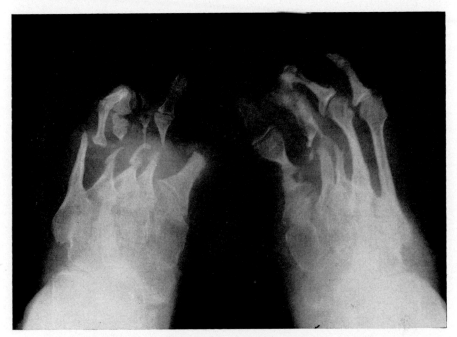

FIGURE 123. Leprosy involving the feet. Antero-posterior roentgenogram. (Courtesy, *U. S. Army Institute of Pathology*, Neg. No. 48467.)

non-hereditary, and is characterized by skin papillomata plus destructive lesions of the skin and bones. Central nervous system lesions do not occur.

The cause of the disease, spirocheta pallidula, also called treponema pertenue, was described in 1905 by Castellani. It closely resembles the spirochete of syphilis.

Craig believes that three stages of the disease can be identified. The initial stage is characterized by a cutaneous granuloma often termed the "mother yaw." A granulomatous skin eruption appears during the secondary stage, and in the "tertiary" stage bone lesions occur in 10 to 20 percent of the cases.

SKELETAL LESIONS

A synovitis may appear during the secondary stage and involve both small and large joints, not unlike early rheumatoid arthritis. Joint destruction does not follow.

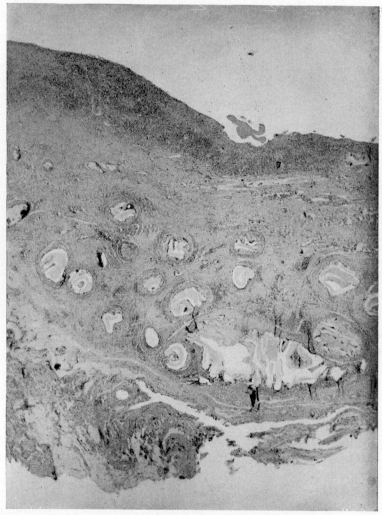

FIGURE 124. Echinococcic cyst. Low power photomicrograph showing the characteristic multilocular structure. (Courtesy, A. Purdy Stout, M.D., New York.)

Bone lesions are a late manifestation. A painful periostitis, characterized by multiple nodes, develops in the long bones, being most likely to appear on the radius, ulna, and tibia. Ossifying periostitis, so advanced over the anterior aspect of the tibia as to produce a "saber shin" has been described. Dactylitis with prominent periosteal bone formation is not unusual. There may be multiple small round or oval areas of absorption, a rarefying osteitis, extensive bone destruction, pathologic

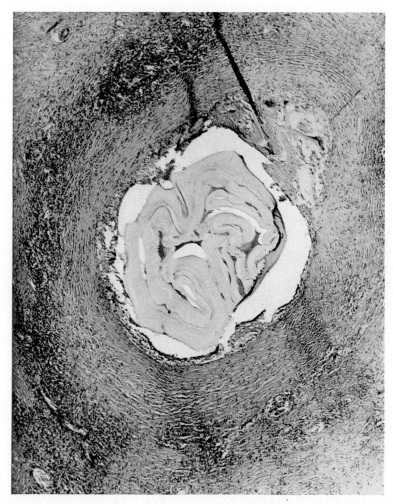

FIGURE 125. Echinococcic cyst. High power photomicrograph showing an individual locule with its acellular laminated membrane. (Courtesy, A. Purdy Stout, M.D., New York.)

fracture and ulceration of overlying skin. A rare but gruesome destruction of the nasopharynx and overlying skin, called Gangosa, is attributed to yaws.

ECHINOCOCCOSIS

Echinococcosis is a parasitic disease caused by larva of the taenia echinococcus (dog tapeworm). Bone lesions occur in approximately 1 percent of cases.

Howorth, in a comprehensive survey of the world's literature on echinococcosis, estimated that up to July 1945 there had been about 1000 cases reported, only ten of which had come from North America.

The disease, endemic throughout the world, is most common in countries such as South America, Australia, New Zealand, and Asia Minor, where sheep raising is widespread.

LIFE CYCLE

Ovum stage: The ova are released from the taenia echinococcus uterus into the faeces of the definitive host, which usually is a dog. Ova carried out in the faeces are deposited on grass or in water. Ultimately the ova are ingested by man or other intermediary hosts such as sheep, goats, cows, hogs and moose. Once in the intestine of the intermediary host, the ova develop into embryos.

Embryo stage: The echinococcus embryos migrate through the intesttinal wall, enter a vein, and are carried in the blood stream to the liver where 50 to 75 percent of the embryos are retained; the remainder are scattered over the body with 1 percent going to the skeletal systm. After three weeks the embryos become larvae.

Larva stage: The larvae exist in the host's body as cysts or hydatids. An echinococcus cyst has a laminated wall and measures one to several inches in diameter. Inside the cyst the scolices with their hooks and suckers grow toward maturity. Cysts form inside of cysts. When a cyst ruptures or is opened scolices are released and may be found in the host's urine, faeces, and sputum. Scolices develop into taenia only if ingested by a definitive host.

Mature cestode stage (taenia echinococcus): If a definitive host, usually a dog, eats viscera infested with scolices, or in any other way acquires the scolices, a taenia echinococcus develops from each scolex inside the definitive host's intestine. The mature worm has three or four segments and measures 2.5 to 6 mm. in length. Within each worm's uterus, 500 to 800 ova develop.

BONE LESIONS

In nine of the ten North American cases, the distribution of the lesions was as follows: one humeral, one vertebral, four cases with pelvic bone lesions, one tibial, one femoral, and one sternal (Howorth). Solitary bone lesions are the rule but adjacent bones may become involved by direct extension. Lesions appear principally in adults in the cancellous bone of epiphyses and metaphyses. The initial bone lesion may remain localized or extend to involve an entire bone. One of Coley's cases involved an entire innominate, and a case of Hiesh's spread through an entire femur. Bones may become involved via the blood stream or by direct extension.

Roentgenologic Features

Roentgenologically the bone lesions appear cystic and multilocular. In some instances these lesions have been mistaken for sarcomas, osteitis fibrous cystica, giant cell tumors, and Paget's disease. Little periosteal bone develops, and very little cortical expansion. Pathological fractures occur, during which the cysts rupture into adjacent soft tissues or externally.

Surgery

Surgical excision, when complete, has been successful in a few instances. If excision is incomplete the lesion recurs. During surgery there is danger of dissemination of the scolices and of anaphalactic reactions to the cyst fluid.

REFERENCES

Pyogenic Osteomyelitis

Brodie, Benjamin: *Pathological and Surgical Observations on Diseases of the Joints.* London, 1807, Longman, 1836.

Compere, E.: Streptococcus viridans osteomyelitis. *J. Bone & Joint Surg., 14*:244 1932.

Ely, L. W.: Inflammation in Bones and Joints. J. B. Lippincott, Philadelphia, 1923.

Knaggs, R. L.: Inflammatory and Toxic Diseases of Bone, page 42. Wm. Woods & Co., 1926.

Kreuscher, P. H. and Hueper, W. C.: The histology of the post-operative healing process in chronic osteomyelitis and its prognostication from biopsy sections. *J. Bone & Joint Surg., 12*:541, 1930.

Larsen, R.: Diaphyseal bone necrosis. *Ann. Surg., 108*:138, 1938.

Milgram, J. E.: Epithelization of cancellous bone in osteomyelitis. *J. Bone & Joint Surg., 12*:319, 1931.

Phemister, D. B.: Chronic fibrous osteomyelitis. *Ann. Surg., 81*:756, 1929.

Phemister, D. B.: Unusual forms of osteomyelitis. *Northwest Med., 27*:460, 1928.

Sever, J. W.: Changes in the epiphysis secondary to infection. *New England J. Med., 209*:62-66, 1933.

Steindler, A.: Osteomyelitis of the spine. *J. Iowa M. Soc., :3*, June 1930.

Wilensky, A. O.: Osteomyelitis of the spine. *Ann. Surg., 89*:561, 731, 1929.

Wilson, J. C. and McKeever, F. M.: Hematogenous acute osteomyelitis in children. *J. Bone & Joint Surg., 18*:323, 1936.

Wilensky, A. O.: *Osteomyelitis.* The Macmillan Co., New York, 1934.

Brucellosis

Harbin, M.: Non-suppurative osteomyelitis. *J. Bone & Joint Surg., 8*:401, 1926.

Koch, S. L.: Osteomyelitis of the bones of the hand. *Surg. Gynec. & Obst.,* Jan. 1937.

McCarroll, H. R. and Key, J. A.: The present status of chronic osteomyelitis. *Surg. Gynec. & Obst.,* June 1939.

Ober, F. R.: Osteomyelitis in children. *Am. J. Surg., 39*:319, 1938.

PHALEN, G. L., PRICKMAN, L. E., and KRUSEN, F. H.: Brucellosis Spondylitis. *J. A. M. A., 118:*859, 1942.
WILENSKY, A. O.: Osteomyelitis of the pelvic girdle. *Arch. Surg.,* Sept. 1938.

TUBERCULOUS OSTEOMYELITIS

ALLISON, N.: Tuberculosis of bone. *Arch. Surg.,* 2:593-626, 1921.
ERDHEIM, J.: Ueber tuberkulose des knochen. *Virchows Arch. f. path. Anat., 283:*354, 1932.
FINDER, J.: The healing process in tuberculous spondylitis. *Surg. Gynec. & Obst., 62:*665, 1936.
FINDER, J.: Subchondral tuberculous sequestra. *Ann. Surg., 104:*1008-1102, 1936.
FRASER, J.: The pathology of tuberculosis of bones. *J. Path. & Bact., 17:*254, 1912.
HSIEH, C. K. and MILTNER, L. J. and CHANG, C. P.: Tuberculosis of the shaft of the large bones of the extremities. *J. Bone & Joint Surg., 16:*545-563, 1934.
PETTER, C. K. and MEDELMAN, J. P.: Tuberculosis of the shafts of long bones. *Am. Rev. Tuberc., 32:*285, 1935.
POTT, PERCIVAL: *Remarks on the Kind of Palsy of the Lower Limbs which is Frequently Found to Accompany a Curvature of the Spine.* London, 1779.
STEINDLER, A.: Diseases and Deformities of the Spine and Thorax, Pathology of Spinal Tuberculosis, pages 352-382. C. V. Mosby Co., St. Louis, 1929.

TUBERCULOUS ARTHRITIS

BRAV and HENCH: Tuberculous rheumatism, a résumé. *J. Bone & Joint Surg., 16:*839-866, 1934.
CLEVELAND, M. and BOSWORTH, D. M.: The pathology of tuberculosis of the spine. *J. Bone & Joint Surg.,* July 1942.
ELY, L.: Inflammation of Bones and Joints. Philadelphia, 1923.
ELY, L.: On the study of joint tuberculosis. *Surg. Gynec. & Obst.,* :561, June 1910.
FELDMAN, W. H.: The histology of experimental tuberculosis in different special. *Arch. Path.* 2:896-913, 1931.
FINDER, J. G.: The healing process in tuberculous spondylitis. *Surg. Gynec. & Obst., 62:*665, 1936.
FINDER, J. G.: Subchondral tuberculous sequestra. *Ann. Surg., 104:*1080, 1936.
GRIEG, D. M.: *Bone Pathology.* Edinburgh, 1931.
HARRIS, I.: The pathology of surgical tuberculosis. *Am. J. Surg., 10:*514-520, 1930.
KNAGGS, R. L.: *Diseases of Bone.* Wm. Woods & Co., New York, 1926.
KOCH, ROBERT: Tuberculous arthritis. *Berlin Klin. Woch.,* No. 15, 1882.
KOENIG, F.: *Die tuberculose der Menschlichen gelenke, Sowie der Brustwand und der Schadel.* Berlin, 1906.
MILGRAM, J. E.: Diagnostic inaccuracy in tuberculosis of bone, joint, and bursa. *J. A. M. A., 97:*232-235, 1931.
NUSSBAUM, A.: Ueber die Gefasse des unteren Femureades und ihre Beziehungen zur Pathologie. *Beitr. z. klin. Chir., 129:*245, 1923.
PHEMISTER, D. B. and HATCHER, C. H.: Correlation of pathological and roentgenological findings in the diagnosis of tuberculous arthritis. *Am. J. Roentgenol., 29:* 736, 1933.
PHEMISTER, D. B.: Changes in the articular surfaces in tuberculous and pyogenic infections of joints. *Am. J. Roentgenol.,* 2:1, 1924.
SMITH, A. DeF.: The early diagnosis of joint tuberculosis. *J. A. M. A., 83:*1569, 1924.

SARCOID

BOECK, C.: Multiple benign sarcoid of the skin. *J. Cut. & G. U. Dis., 17:*543, 1899.
DOUB, H. P. and MENAGH, F. R.: Bone lesions in sarcoid. Roentgen and clinical study. *Am. J. Roentgenol., 21:*149, 1929.
GOECKERMAN, W. H.: Sarcoids and related lesions. Report of 17 cases. *Arch. Dermat. & Syph., 18:*237, 1928.

HUNTER, F. T.: Hutchinson-Boecks disease (generalized sarcoidosis). *New England J. Med.*, *214*:346, 1936.

JUNGLING, O.: Ostitis tuberculosa multiplex cystica. Fortschr a.d. Geb. d. Röntgen-strahlen, *27*:375, 1919-21.

JUNGLING, O.: Uber ostitis tuberculosa multiplex cystoides zugleich ein Beitrag zur Lehre von den Tuberkulidendes Knochens. *Beitr. z. klin, Chir.*, *143*:401, 1928.

KIRKLIN, B. R. and MORTON, S. A.: Roentgenologic changes in sarcoid and related lesions. *Radiology*, *16*:328, 1931.

LONGCOPE, W. T.: Sarcoidosis or Besnie-Boeck-Schaumann disease. *J. A. M. A.*, *117*: 1321, 1941.

SCHAUMANN, J.: Benign lymphogranuloma and its cutaneous manifestations. *Brit J. Dermat.*, *36*:515, 1924; *48*:399, 1936.

SYPHILIS OF BONES AND JOINTS

BECK, C.: Leontiasis ossea with halisteresis. *Surg. Gynec. & Obst.*, *4*:710, 1907.

BROMER, R. S.: Osteochondritis luetica: Comparison with analagous zones in rickets and infantile scurvy. *New England J. Med.*, *200*:524, 1929.

CAMPELL, W. C.: An analysis of bone and joint lesions of known syphilitic origin. *Radiology*, *122*:5, 1925.

CONWAY, F. M.: Syphilis of the clavicle. *Ann. Surg.*, *99*:290, 1934.

FREUND, E.: Uber Knochensyphilis. *Virchow's Arch. f. path. Anat.*, *288*:146, 1933.

HODGES, P. C., PHEMISTER, D. B. and BRUNSCHWIG, A.: *The Roentgen-Ray Diagnosis of Diseases of the Bones and Joints.* Thomas Nelson and Sons, New York, 1938.

HOTZ, A.: *Syphilis der Knochen und Gelenke.* Schinz, Boensch, Friedl Lehrbuch der Roentgen Diagnostik. Chap. 4, 3rd ed. George Thieme, Leipzig 1932.

IVY, R. H. and CURTIS, L.: Congenital syphilitic osteomyelitis of the mandible. *Ann. Surg.*, *100*:535, 1934.

KLING, D. H.: Syphilitic arthritis with effusion. *Am. J. M. Sc.*, *183*:538, 1932.

KNAGGS, R. L.: *Inflammatory and Toxic Diseases of Bone.* John Wright and Sons, Ltd., Bristol, 1926.

PARRUCKER: Knockensyphilis und trauma. *Arch, f. orthop. w. unfall-Chir.*, *28*:46, 1930.

PENDERGRASS, E. P. and BROMER, R. S.: Congenital bone syphilis. *Am. J. Roentgenol.*, *22*:1, 1929.

PICK, L.: Angeborene Knochensyphilis. *Henke-Lubarsch Handbuch der Spec. Anat. und Histologie.*, *9*:240, 1929. J. Spinger, Berlin.

SPEED, J. S. and BOYD, H. B.: Bone syphilis. *South M. J.*, *29*:371, 1936.

STEWART, D. M.: Roentgenological manifestations of bone syphilis. *Am. J. Roent-genol.*, *40*:215, 1938.

STOKES, J. H.: *Clinical Syphilology.* W. B. Saunders Co., 1934.

SUTHERLAND, G. F. and MITCHEL, J. H.: Effects of treatment on bone lesions in con-genital syphilis. *J. A. M. A.*, *81*:1752, 1923.

TODD, A. H.: Syphilitic arthritis. *Brit. J. Surg.*, *14*:260, 1926-27.

UNGERMAN, A. H., VICARY, W. H. and ELDRIDGE, W. W.: Luetic osteitis simulating malignant disease. *Am. J. Roentgenol.*, *40*:224, 1938.

WEGNER, G.: Ueber hereditäre Knockensyphilis bei jungen kindern. *Virchow's Arch. f. path. Anat.*, *50*:305, 1870.

WILLIAMS, H. U.: The origin and antiquity of syphilis: The evidence from diseased bones. *Arch. Path.*, *13*:779, 1932.

ACTINOMYCOSIS

ALLENBACH, E., SARTORI, A. and ZIMMER, M.: Actinomycose ossense primitive. *Rev. d'orthop.*, *18*:572, 1931.

KROGIUS, A.: Zur Kenntnis der hamatogenen aktinomycose des lavgen Rohrenknock-en. *Acta chir. Scandinav.*, *63*:121, 1928.

PARKER, C. A.: Actinomycosis and blastomycosis of spine. *J. Bone & Joint Surg.*, *5*: 759, 1923.

SIMPSON, W. M. and McINTOSH, C. A.: Actinomycosis of vertebrae (actinomycotic Potts disease). Report of 4 cases. *Arch. Surg.*, *14*:116, 1927.

ZISKIN, D. E., SHOHAM, J., and HANFORD, J. M.: Actinomycosis. Case report. *Am. J. Orthodontics, 29*:193, 1943.
LOVETT, R. W. and WOLBACH, A. B.: Diagnosis and pathology of some obscure cases of bone lesions. *Surg., Gynec. & Obst., 31*:111, 1920.
WATSON, W. W.: Human Actinomycosis. *Surg. Gynec. & Obst., 34*:482, 1922.
LUBERT, M.: Actinomycosis of the vertebra. *Am. J. Roentgenol., 51*:669, 1944.

BLASTOMYCOSIS

COLONNA, PAUL A. and GUCKER, T.: Blastomycosis of the skeletal system. *J. Bone & Joint Surg., 26*:322, 1944.
COOPER, C. N.: *J. Iowa State M. Soc., 21*:119, 1931.
LEWISON, M. and JACKSON, H. A.: *Arch. Int. Med., 13*:575, 1914.
STOBER, A. M.: *Arch. Int. Med., 13*:509, 1914.
CHURCHILL, T. and STOBER, A. M.: *Arch. Int. Med., 13*:568, 1914.
MARTIN, D. S. and JONES, R. R.: *Surgery, 10*:931, 1941.
MARTIN, D. S. and SMITH, D. T.: Blastomycosis (review of literature). *Am. Rev. Tuberc., 39*:275, 488, 1938.

COCCIDIOIDES

BENNIKGHOVEN, C. D. and MILLER, E. R.: Coccidioidal infection of bone. *Radiology, 38*:663, 1942.
BOWMAN, W. B.: *Am. J. Roentgenology, 6*:547, 1919.
CARTER, R. A.: Infectious granulomas of bones and joints with special reference to coccidioidal granuloma. *Radiology, 23*:1, 1934.
CARTER, R. A.: Coccidioidal granuloma. Roentgenological diagnosis (Review of Literature). *Am. J. Roentgenol., 25*:715, 1931.
DICKSON, E. C.: Coccidioidonycosis. The preliminary infection with fungus coccidioides. *J. A. M. A., 111*:1362, 1938.
GOREN, M. L.: Localized coccidioidomycosis of bone. *J. Bone & Joint Surg., 28*:157, 1946.
McMASTER, P. E. and GILFILLAN, C. F.: Coccidioidal osteomyelitis. *J. A. M. A.,* April 1, 1939.
POSADAS, A.: Psorospermiose infectante generalisee. *Rev. de Chir., 20*:277, 1900.
RIXFORD, E. and GILCHRIST, T. C.: Two cases of protogoan (coccidioidal) infection of the skin and other organs. *Bull. Johns Hopkins Hosp., 1*:209-267, 1896.
SMITH, C. E.: Parallelism of coccidioidal and tuberculous infections. *Radiology, 38*:643, 1942.
SMITH, C. E.: Coccidioidomycosis. *M. Clin. N. Am., 27*:790, 1943.
TAYLOR, R. G.: *Am. J. Roentgenology, 10*:551, 1923.
THORNE, W. S.: A case of protzoic skin disease. *Occidental M. Time, 8*:703, 1894.

SPOROTRICHOSIS

SCHENK: *Bull. Johns Hopkins Hosp., 2*:286, 1898.
FOERSTER, H. R.: Sporotrichosis. *Am. J. M. Sc., 167*:54, 1924.

STREPTOTHRICOSIS

MUSGRAVE, W. E., CLEGG, M. T. and POLK, M.: Streptothricosis with special reference to the etiology and classification of mycetomas. *Philippine J. Sc., 3*:447, 1908.

HISTOPLASMOSIS

KEY, J. A. and LARGE, A. M.: Histoplasmosis of the knee. *J. Bone & Joint Surg., 24*:28, 1942.

TORULA

KESSEL, J. F. and HOLTZWART, F.: Experimental studies with torula from a knee infection in man. *Am. J. Trop. Med., 15*:467, 1935.
MITCHEL, L. A.: Torulosis. *J. A. M. A., 106*:450, 1936.

Leprosy

Honey, J. A.: Bone changes in leprosy. *Am. J. Roentgenol., 4*:494, 1917.

Chamberlain, W. E., Wayson, N. E. and Garland, L. H.: Bone and joint changes of leprosy. A roentgenological study. *Radiology, 17*:930, 1931.

Murdock, J. R. and Hutter, H. J.: Leprosy: A roentgenological survey. *Am. J. Rontgenol., 28*:598, 1932.

Yaws

Craig, C. F.: Yaws (Frambesia) in Tice, *Practice of Med,* Vol. IV, page 703. W. F. Prior Co., 1932.

Maul, H. W.: Bone and joint lesions of yaws. *Am. J. Roentgenol., 6*:421, 1919.

Wilson, P. W. and Mathis, M. S.: Epidemiology and pathology of yaws. Based on study of 1423 consecutive cases in Haiti. *J. A. M. A., 94*:1289, 1930.

Echinococcus

Coley, B. L.: Echinococcus disease of bone. Report of 2 cases involving pelvic girdle. *J. Bone & Joint Surg., 14*:477, 1932.

Hsieh, C. K.: Echinococcus involvement of bones. Report of case with x-ray examination. *Radiology 14*:562, 1930.

Howorth, M. B.: Echinococcus of bone (includes review of the literature). *J. Bone and Joint Surg., 27*:401, 1945.

Osler, Wm.: On echinococcus disease in America. *Am. J. M. Sc., 84*:475, 1882.

Magath, T. B.: Hydatid (echinococcus) disease in the United States and Canada. *Am. J. Hygiene, 25*:107, 1937.

Harris, H.: Hydatid Disease of bone. *Am. J. Roentgenol., 6*:277, 1919.

Hood, M., Lamberg, C. N. and Thomas, H. B.: Hydatid cyst of the bone. A case Report. *J. Bone & Joint Surg., 22*:986, 1940.

Sinberg, S. E.: Echinococcus cyst of the sternum. *Radiology, 27*:736, 1936.

Stone, R. S.: Echinococcus involvement of bone with a case report. *Radiology, 14*:557, 1930.

CHAPTER IV

Aseptic (Avascular) Osseous Necrosis

Contents

The several entities that have osseous aseptic necrosis as their basic pathologic alteration constitute an important part of bone pathology and orthopedic surgery. Perhaps the first to recognize what we now term aseptic necrosis was Alexander Munro in 1738. In 1870 Sir James Paget described aseptic necrosis as "quiet necrosis," and referred to a loose body that separated from a femoral condyle as having "exfoliated without acute inflammation." But the first comprehensive dissertation on the subject was by König in 1888.

A vast and confused literature has grown up around this interesting subject. But all is not confusion, the pathogenesis is now well understood, even though the etiology of most of the epiphyseal osteochondritides remains a mystery. A great impetus to the study and recognition of osseous aseptic necrosis came with the discovery of the roentgen-ray. In determining the diagnosis and in following the pathogenesis, the roentgenogram is indispensable.

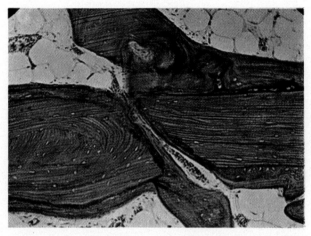

FIGURE 126. Microscopic appearance of osseous aseptic necrosis. Osteocytes are missing; lacuane are "empty tombs."

Classification

I. Unknown etiology
   1. Osteochondritis of growing epiphyses
   2. Osteochondritis of small short bones
   3. Osteochondritis dissecans
II. Known etiology
   1. Aseptic necrosis of the femoral head resulting from—
      a. Fracture of the hip
      b. Dislocations of the hip
      c. Slipping of the capital epiphysis
   2. Aseptic necrosis of the proximal fragment of the carpal navicular after fracture
   3. Aseptic necrosis of all fracture surfaces, and certain fracture fragments e.g., head of humerus and astragalus
   4. Aseptic necrosis in autogenous bone grafts
   5. Caisson disease
   6. Roentgen-ray and radium radiation necrosis

OSTEOCHONDRITIS OF GROWING EPIPHYSES

Nearly every secondary epiphysis and many of the primary epiphyses in the body have been observed as the site of an osteochondritis. Unfortunately each original observer has had his name appended to the epiphysis he described. As a result there has been confusion—confusion leading to the belief that in each epiphysis the disease represented a different entity. Harbin and many others have recommended that for unity in our concept of this subject we should abandon the practice of referring to osteochondritis of the various epiphyses by the names of individuals. Hodges, Phemister and Brunschwig point out that there is much to be said in favor of this stand, but that, "Some of the older terms however, have won a permanent place in medicine, and is should be remembered that they were introduced long before the histology was known, the etiology guessed, or the group relationship suspected." We now consider the pathology and pathogenesis of all of the epiphyseal osteochondritides to be essentially the same. More than likely when the etiology is discovered it too will be fundamentally the same for the entire group.

ETIOLOGY

Numerous theories have been offered to explain the etiology, but there is little convincing evidence to support any one of them as an explanation of all cases. Trauma appears rather definitely to have been a factor in many instances; in as many other instances there has been no evidence whatever of unusual trauma. A low grade pyogenic (streptococcus) infection is believed by some to be the principal etiologic factor. Phemister, Brunschwig, and Day found streptococci when they cultured biopsy specimens in six cases involving the tarsal scaphoid, the carpal lunate and the capital femoral epiphysis.

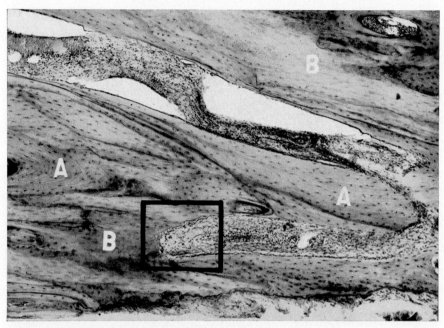

FIGURE 127. Photomicrograph of a section of necrotic compact bone in the process of being regenerated by creeping substitution. Young fibrous tissue fills the enlarged haversian canals. A. Viable bone. B. Necrotic bone.

An endocrine unbalance appears to be a factor in certain cases. However, some of the supposed osteochondritides in pituitary and thyroid disturbances are not aseptic necrosis. What appears by roentgenogram to be an osteochondritis frequently has been only an irregular ossification of the epiphysis by multiple small centers. Cavanaugh, Shelton and Sutherland observed a high incidence of associated metabolic disturbances, and secured an early restoration of normal epiphyseal structure after thyroid (thyroxin) therapy.

An obliteration of the epiphyseal blood supply often stands out as a prominent feature, but the cause of the obliteration defies analysis in most cases (Legg). When epiphyseal aseptic necrosis follows a fracture or dislocation, the mechanism of the interference with the blood supply usually is obvious. Much experimental work on animals has been done to determine the type of vascular interference necessary to reproduce epiphyseal osteochondritis. Miltner and Hu in dog experiments produced changes in the capital femoral epiphysis similar to those seen in Legg-Perthe's disease. This was accomplished by ligation of the ligamentum teres and stripping of the femoral neck periosteum. Flattening of the femoral head and retarded growth took place when Leriche tied the ligamentum teres of rabbits.

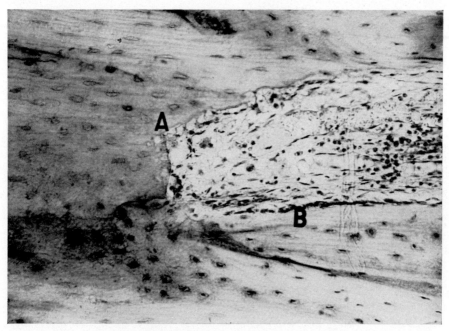

FIGURE 128. Photomicrograph showing osteoclastic and osteoblastic phases in the regeneration of compact bone. (High power of square marked on Figure 127.) A. Osteoclastic (bone resorption). B. Osteoblastic (new bone apposition).

An heritary constitutional factor has been long suspected. Frequently several etiologic factors are evident in the same case. It is not unlikely that more than one factor is necessary to precipitate an osteochondritis.

SITES OF INVOLVEMENT

The following list presents most of the epiphyses in which idiopathic aseptic necrosis is observed, together with the name of the original investigator, and the date of the original report.

1. Tibial tubercle *(Osgood-Schlatter's disease)*
   Osgood—1903

2. Patella—primary epiphysis.
   Kohler—1908
3. Tarsal navicular.
   Kohler—1908
4. Capital epiphysis femur *(Osteochondritis deformans juvenilis; Legg-Perthe's disease)*
   Legg—1909
5. Apophysis tuber os calcis
   Sever—1912
6. Second metatarsal head
   Freiberg—1914
7. Patella—secondary epiphysis
   Sinding-Larsen—1921
8. Vertebral bodies—secondary epiphyses
   Scheuermann—1921
9. Vertebral bodies—primary epiphysis
   Calve—1925
10. Head of humerus
    Lewin—1930

No attempt has been made to make this list complete. The epiphyses added since about 1930 generally are not referred to by the name of an individual. These epiphyses include the iliac crest, symphysis pubis, tuberosity of the ischium, capitellum humeri, carpal navicular (not associated with a fracture), metatarsal heads other than the second, the base of the 1st metatarsal, the upper tibial epiphyses, and several sesamoids of the foot. There appears to be no reason to believe than any epiphysis is immune from an osteochondritis.

Rapid growth is believed to make an epiphysis more vulnerable to osteochondritis. Primary epiphyses ordinarily become involved during infancy and childhood, a time when they are ossifying and rapidly enlarging. Secondary epiphyses generally become involved during puberty, the period of their most rapid growth.

PATHOGENESIS

The pathogenesis of the osteochondritides has been followed in detail from the onset of the necrosis to complete healing. For descriptive purposes the sequence of events may be divided into three stages: (1) early stage, (2) regenerating stage, and, (3) healed stage. These stages are not sharply defined, but are useful in visualizing the sequence of the various changes.

Early Stage

This stage represents the onset of necrosis. By some manner the etiologic factor presumably obliterates the blood supply of the epiphysis. The reactions that follow derive from nature's attempt to replace the necrotic elements with viable ones. In the beginning it would be readily possible to identify the necrotic state of the epiphysis by patho-

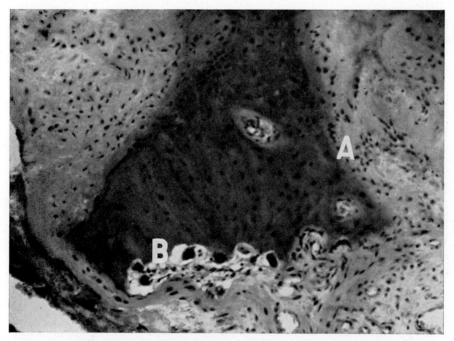

FIGURE 129. Microscopic appearance of regenerating cancellous bone. Osteoblasts are active on one surface of the trabeculum (A), and osteoclasia is active on another surface (B).

logic study, but not by roentgenogram. Microscopically, the osteocytes show either advanced necrobiotic changes or complete destruction. Although the osteocytic lacunae become "empty tombs" (Fig. 126), the bony architecture at the outset is in no way altered. This accounts for the normal appearing roentgenogram during early stages. The marrow elements do not retain their form and identity but transform quickly into an oily, formless debris.

Soon after the onset of necrosis the neighboring bone elements develop an active hyperemia which becomes manifest by osteoporosis. The hyperemia supplies many of the necessary elements with which to construct a bed of capillaries, and, brings in an army of phagocytes with which to invade and absorb the necrotic bone and marrow.

At this stage the necrotic bone begins to be demarcated roentgenographically from neighboring viable bone; this occurs because the necrotic area
does not take part in the osteoporosis (Fig. 130A). This is entirely reasonable since a blood supply is absolutely essential to producing an
osteoporosis. By contrast the necrotic bone appears increased in
density, but ordinarily there is little or no increase in the density of
the dead bone.

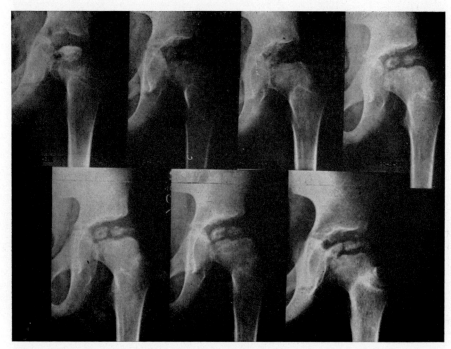

FIGURE 130A. Osteochondritis deformans juvenilis *(Legg-Perthes disease)*. Sequence
of changes at intervals of two to four months.

The overlying articular cartilage may or may not become necrotic.
In most instances it remains viable on the basis of its ability to derive
adequate nutrition from the synovial fluid; however, necrosis of parts
of the cartilage may occur in late stages, particularly with the advent of
degenerative arthritic changes.

Regenerative Stage

The manner by which nature is able to substitute viable bone
elements for necrotic ones, and simultaneously maintain most of the
original architecture, is truly impressive. Capillaries project themselves
into the peripheral marrow spaces of the necrotic epiphysis, accompan-

ied by a young fibrous stroma. Phagocytes, both mononuclear and multinuclear, absorb the necrotic debris of the dead marrow elements.

Osteoclasts and osteoblasts soon enter the picture (Figs. 128 & 129). Bone formation and resorption occur simultaneously to the extent that microscopically one may observe osteoclasia on one side of a necrotic trabeculum, and on the opposite surface find osteoblasts overlying an osteoid "seam." By this process both form and architecture are preserved during the period of "creeping substitution." The process as it occurs in compact bone deserves additional description. When the invading granulation tissue enters the haversian canals with the purpose of reconstructing a new haversian system, it does its work in two phases (Fig. 128). The first phase is marked by osteoabsorption. Osteoclasis of the canal wall gradually enlarges the canal to several times its original size. It seems that when a certain degree of enlargement has been attained, the osteoclastic phase gives way to the osteoblastic. The osteoblastic phase continues until the canal is again restored, layer upon layer, to normal proportions. Little

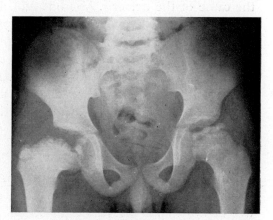

FIGURE 130B. Bilateral osteochondritis deformans juvenilis.

by little the entire haversian system is rebuilt. If viewed microscopically there may appear to be no order or orientation to the regenerative process. This complex and confusing picture results from the micro-section's cutting across the haversian canals at many different angles. Small bits of necrotic bone may appear totally isolated, but they are not as isolated as they seem. Eventually these seemingly neglected fragments are replaced with new bone. Complete regeneration may require many months or even many years, especially in compact bone. If new capillaries have access to the necrotic area along a wide margin, regeneration proceeds much more rapidly than when only a narrow part of the necrotic tissue is accessible. For example, when the entire capital femoral epiphysis dies, regeneration is slow and consumes many months since only a narrow zone of the periphery is readily accessible (polar regeneration as seen in the roentgenogram).

There is considerable variation in the pattern of the regenerative process. The so-called fragmentation, commonly observed roentgeno-graphically, represents the result of numerous small tongue-like in-roads of granulation and fibrous tissue projecting into the necrotic area. This phenomenon is best observed in the capital femoral epiphysis where the necrotic elements are attacked simultaneously by vessels entering via the ligamentum teres, capsule, periosteum of femoral neck, and even through the epiphyseal plate, which may become perforated to permit vessels to enter from the metaphysis.

Subchondral fractures frequently are observed in the necrotic bone after the necrosis has lowered the mechanical resistance (Fig. 142). Some observers have believed these fractures to be the primary lesion and the cause of the necrosis. Micro-motion between the fracture surfaces gives them smooth surfaces. Marrow spaces adjacent to the fracture site become filled with a calcified amorphous material and with many tiny bone spicules through friction between the fractured surfaces. Fracture lines may or may not pass through the articular cartilage. The cartilage islands that are occasionally found in the epiphysis probably represent fractured off fragments of articular cartilage or epiphyseal plate.

Healed Stage

During the regenerative stage the newly formed bone is soft. If the epiphysis is subjected to pressure stresses such as those incurred during weight bearing, considerable distortion is likely to occur. Flattening of the medial and superior aspects of the femoral head in Legg-Perthes' disease is a familiar example (Fig. 130). Distortion of contours, which unfortunately is the rule rather than the exception, has much to do with the sequence of events during the healed stage.

Irregularities in the contour of articular surfaces cause definite and consistent adaptive changes that are manifest as degenerative arthritis. These changes may be mild and may never give rise to clinical symp-toms, or they may be severe and lead to serious disability. Degenerative arthritic changes rarely become manifest clinically for many years after the osteochondritis has healed.

OSTEOCHONDRITIS OF THE CAPITAL FEMORAL EPIPHYSIS

Osteochondritis of the capital femoral epiphysis was first described by Arthur Legg in 1909; it was described independently somewhat later by Perthes and by Calvé. The classical report by Perthes in 1913 is one of the best descriptions of the condition yet recorded; it was in this report that he suggested the name Osteochondritis Deformans Juvenilis.

There is a much higher incidence in boys than girls. While it may occur in younger children, it is most common between the ages of eight and twelve. Bilateral involvement is rare. Residual deformation of the femoral head may occur regardless of the age of the patient at the onset; however, as Moller has emphasized, the younger the patient the better the prognosis for a good anatomical restoration of the head.

Aseptic necrosis ordinarily takes place in the entire capital epiphysis, but is some instances it involves only the central or subchondral area.

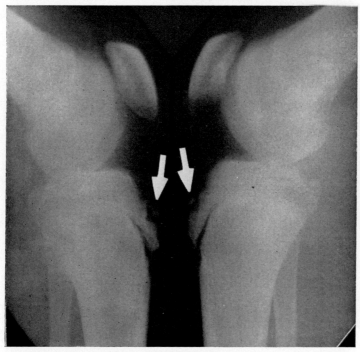

FIGURE 131. Osteochondritis of the epiphysis of the tibial tubercle. *(Osgood-Schlatter's disease.)*

Similar aseptic necrosis in a circumscribed area of the acetabulum or femoral neck is not uncommonly associated with the epiphyseal lesion.

Roentgenographic Correlation

When regeneration is established, the necrotic bone becomes demarcated and then gradually diminishes in size as necrotic bone at the margin is substituted for viable bone. The basis for the appearance of fragmentation has been described. In the anterposterior roentgenogram there often is evidence of flattening of the femoral head. Part of this flattening is real and part is represented by an increased cartilage width.

In the lateral roentgenogram, showing the sagital plane, the head contour is much nearer normal (Slocum), and this is true even when the flattening shown in the frontal plane (A.P.) is pronounced.

Retarded ossification of the growing epiphysis is manifest by the involved capital epiphysis becoming relatively smaller than the normal epiphysis on the opposite side. This disparity in size often proves to be one of the earliest diagnostic signs.

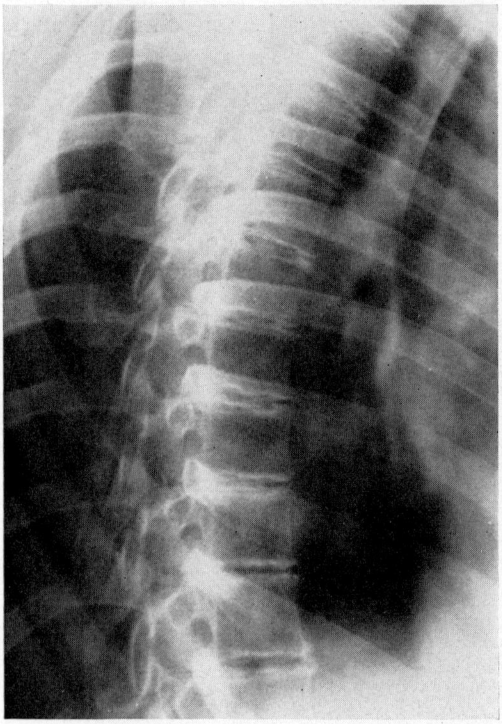

Degenerative arthritis changes are inevitable when the femoral head becomes deformed. Narrowed cartilage space, marginal osteophytes, and subchondral eburnation may encompass the joint when the patient is twenty to thirty years of age.

OSTEOCHONDRITIS OF THE TIBIAL TUBERCLE

Osteochondritis of the epiphysis of the tibial tubercle was first described by Robert Osgood in 1903, and independently by Schlatter in the same year.

FIGURE 132. Kyphosis vertebralis juvenilis *(Scheuermann's disease).*

Prior to its ossification, the tubercle epiphysis exists as a beak-like cartilaginous process pointing distalward from the anterior aspect of the proximal tibial epiphysis. A center of ossification appears in the tubercle during puberty; a separate center for the distal tip of the tubercle may also appear (Fels). Complete ossification of the tubercle and fusion to its tibial bed takes place near the age of twenty.

During an osteochondritis the tubercle enlarges, principally through thickening of overlying soft tissues. In the roentgenogram a relative increase in density and fragmentation appear during regeneration just as in osteochondritis elsewhere.

During the process of regeneration, a small fragment of the epiphysis may separate and form a body in the patellar tendon (Fig. 131). These

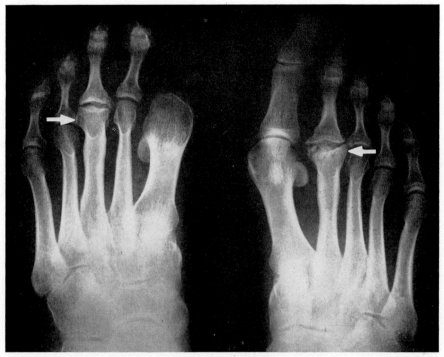

FIGURE 133. Osteochondritis of the 2nd metatarsal head *(Freiberg's disease)*, on the left, and of the 3rd metatarsal head on the right.

bone formations are round or oval, usually single, and are separated from the tibia by a zone of dense fibrous tissue or fibro-cartilage. Ex-

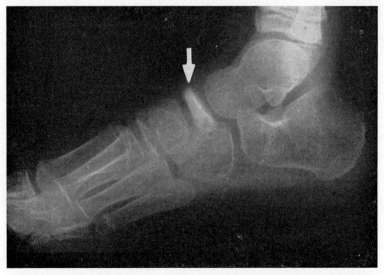

FIGURE 134. Osteochondritis of the tarsal navicular *(Kohler's disease)*.

cision of such a bony body is indicated when it causes disabling pain that cannot be relieved by conservative measures. Histologic study of several of these specimens revealed scattered microscopic islands of necrotic bone. A tibial tubercle in an early state of aseptic necrosis has not been available for study.

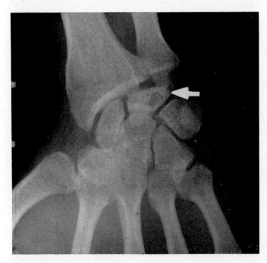

FIGURE 135. Osteochondritis of the carpal lunate *(Kienböck's disease)*.

OSTEOCHONDRITIS OF SECONDARY EPIPHYSES OF VERTEBRAL BODIES

Scheuermann described the changes in juvenile dorsal kyphosis as an osteochondritis of the secondary epiphyses of vertebral bodies. What appears as fragmentation of the epiphyses may be due in many instances to growth disturbances, and, as Schmorl has pointed out, to protrusions of intervertebral discs, and extrusions of the nucleus pulposes. The kyphosis reflects the anterior vertebral body compression and anterior narrowing of the intervertebral discs (Fig. 132).

OSTEOCHONDRITIS OF THE SECOND METATARSAL HEAD

In 1914 Freiberg reported six cases in which there was an osteochondritis of the second metatarsal head. Since then many cases have been observed and many second metatarsal heads have been

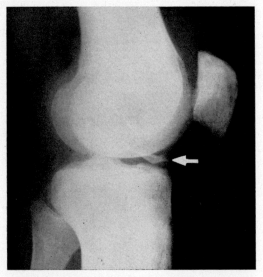

FIGURE 136A. Osteochondritis dissecans. Lateral roentgenogram.

excised. Flattening of the head occurs consistently during the process of regeneration (Fig. 133). Extensive damage to the metatarso-phalangeal joint is associated with adhesions and pannus formations. Cartilage changes are more advanced and the contour much more altered on the metatarsal head than on the base of the proximal phalanx. Small, free, cartilaginous joint bodies often are observed.

Since the second metatarsal is the longest of the metatarsals, it is subject to considerable trauma. This anatomical fact probably plays a part in the etiology.

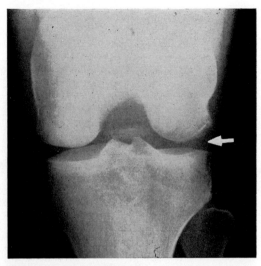

FIGURE 136B. Osteochrondritis dissecans. Flexed knee postero-anterior roentgenogram.

When regeneration of the necrotic metatarsal head leaves the joint severely damaged and with disabling persistent pain, excision of the head is indicated.

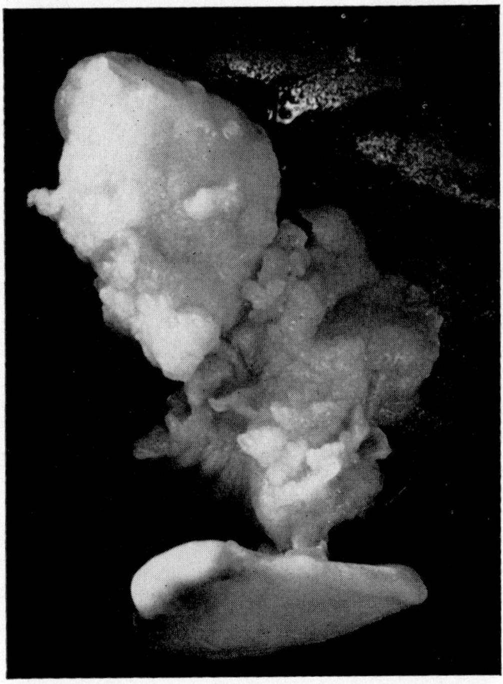

OSTEOCHONDRITIS OF THE TARSAL NAVICULAR

FIGURE 136C. Osteochondritis dissecans. Loose body with its synovial pedicle and a portion of the infrapatellar fat pad.

In 1908 Kohler described changes in the tarsal navicular, characteristic of an osteochondritis. Since Kohler's disease is a primary epiphysitis, it develops in young children usually before the age of six. The nucleus of ossification in the navicular ceases to grow and soon shows the roentgenographic osseous condensation seen in the other osteochondritides (Fig. 134). In spite of the pronounced shearing and pressure stresses on the navicular, a normal anatomical restoration is the rule.

Apophysitis of the Tuber Os Calis

Sever in 1912 described aseptic necrosis of the secondary epiphysis

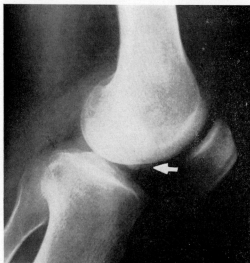

FIGURE 137. Osteochondritis disse-
cans of the medial femoral condyle.
A. *(Above)* Lateral roentgenogram.
B. *(Below)* Section of loose body,
A, lying in its bed, *B*.

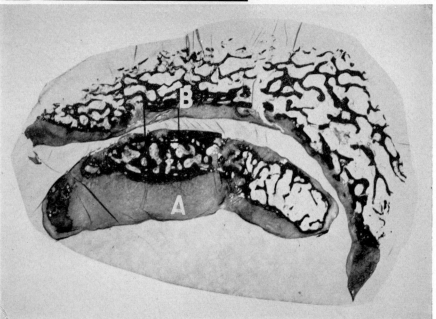

of the tuber os calcis. This entity is seen between the time ossification
appears at about the age of eight years and the time the epiphysis fuses

with the os calcis at age 14. Regeneration proceeds to completion without significant anatomical alteration.

OSTEOCHONDRITIS OF THE CARPAL LUNATE

In 1911 Kienbock described aseptic necrosis of the lunate. In his cases the bone became compressed during regeneration, as is characteristic of the disease when it occurs in the lunate. Trauma has so consistently preceded the necrosis that many (including Kienbock) have be-

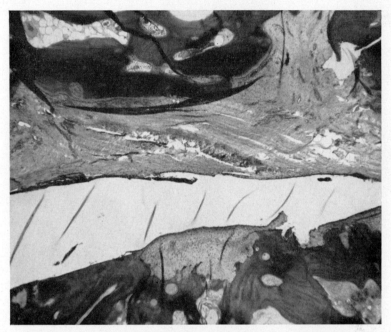

FIGURE 137. *(Continued)* C. Magnification of area in square marked on B.

lieved the changes were the result of an invisible fracture or a severe sprain. Residual deformity (Fig. 135) from collapse of the bone invite degenerative arthritis and disabling pain. Excision of the lunate frequently is indicated.

OSTEOCHONDRITIS DISSECANS

In contrast to the extensive area of necrosis in epiphyseal osteochondritis, osteochondritis dissecans involves only a small, well circumscribed, superficial area. In susceptible areas on certain joint surfaces, a fragment of articular cartilage, usually together with adjacent subchondral bone, becomes partially or totally separated from its bed. This lesion is most frequently observed on the medial femoral condyle near the intercondylar notch (Figs. 136 & 137). It is also observed at the superior aspect of the femoral head (Fig. 139), in the elbow joint where it generally involves the capitellum (Fig. 138), on the superior aspect of the astragalus, and on the head of the humerus.

Osteochondritis dissecans is observed most commonly in young adult males but occurs in both sexes, and may develop at any age beyond childhood. An hereditary factor seldom has been evident, notwithstanding Waggoner and Cohn's three cases from the same family. König described the first case (in an elbow joint) in 1888 and gave the condition its present name of osteochondritis dissecans.

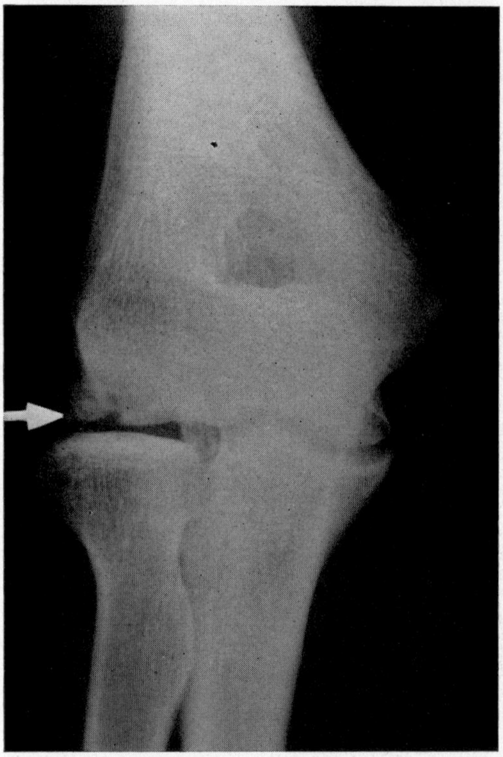

FIGURE 138. Osteochondritis dissecans of capitellum.

ETIOLOGY

The etiology is still uncertain. Many investigators believe the condition can be attributed entirely to trauma. Although there is considerable evidence in favor of this explanation, the lesion could not be reproduced on cadavers. Fairbank believes it is a fracture pure and simple, resulting from violent internal rotation of the tibia on the femur, driving the tibial spine against the medial femoral condyle. Axhausen's embolic theory met with considerable favor for a time but unfortunately there has been no definite pathological and anatomical confirmation.

PATHOLOGIC ANATOMY

As in epiphyseal osteochondritis the pathogenesis is understood. No evidence of an infection has been observed, the process appearing entirely aseptic. One of four fates may befall the joint body:

1. It may remain permanently in its bed and if undisturbed subse-

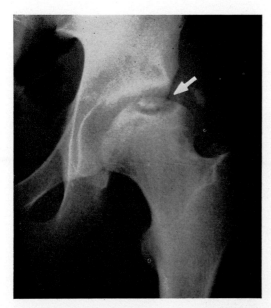

FIGURE 139. Osteochondritis dissecans of femoral head.

quently regenerate. The articular cartilage over the body may remain intact or may be broken and heal by fibrous tissue and fibrocartilage.

2. The body may drop into the joint but retain a pedicle from its bed and from it derive a blood supply.

3. The body may drop free into the joint and remain a free body.

4. The body may drop free into the joint but subsequently acquire a synovial pedicle, receive a blood supply and regenerate.

Although the bone elements die for want of a blood supply, the articular cartilage survives. As previously mentioned, the cartilage secures nourishment from the synovial fluid by diffusion. The microscopic picture of necrotic bone and marrow need not be repeated. After entering the joint the bony surface of the body soon becomes smooth. This is accomplished by a fibrocartilaginous pannus extending over the bony surface as a continuation of the perichondrium-like structure enveloping the articular cartilage element of

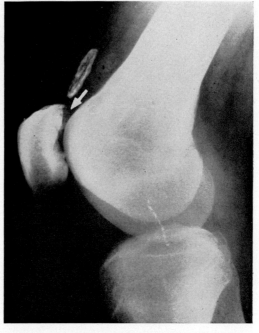

FIGURE 140. Osteochondritis dissecans of the patella. Part of the loose body remains in its bed (arrow).

the body. The cartilage portion of the joint body may proliferate and contribute materially to the size of the body. The bone element remains necrotic and indefinitely unaltered unless the fragment acquires a blood supply through a synovial attachment. With the advent of a new blood supply the bone is regenerated by "creeping substitution."

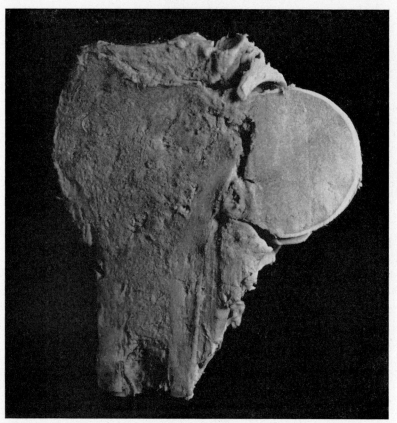

FIGURE 141. Aseptic necrosis of the femoral head following pathologic fracture from osteolytic carcinoma metastases. Head is white and retains its original density.

ASEPTIC NECROSIS OF FRACTURE FRAGMENTS

Some degree of osseous aseptic necrosis occurs in all fractures; the minimum is represented by a millimeter or so of necrotic bone on the fracture surfaces. Entire fragments may become necrotic as in certain types of fractures of the astragalus, carpal-scaphoid, neck of the femur, the lower humerus and tibia, and the head of the humerus. In all instances the necrosis results from traumatic obliteration of blood vessels. Regeneration occurs by creeping substitution. Delayed union is the rule, and complete failure of healing is common.

Aseptic Necrosis of Femoral Head Following Trauma

Aseptic necrosis of the femoral head is a frequent complication of traumatic dislocations and of subcapital fractures of the femoral neck. In these instances the necrosis follows a partial or total obliteration of the blood supply to the femoral head. In subcapital fractures the vessels in the ligamentum teres may remain intact, but they are inadequate to maintain viability in most of the head. However, these vessels may hypertrophy and play a part in regeneration, especially in younger individuals. Aseptic necrosis of the head occurs more frequently fol-

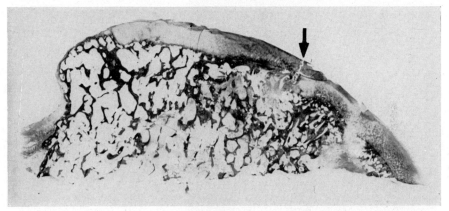

FIGURE 142. Section from a femoral head that lost its blood supply as a result of a fracture of the neck of the femur. Articular cartilage is degenerated, and is fractured at arrow.

lowing subcapital fractures than after dislocations (Fig. 141). In both instances extensive capsular tears do most of the damage.

Pathologic Features

The pathologic changes are essentially the same as those described for epiphyseal osteochondritis, particularly Legg-Perthes' disease. There may be more degenerative articular cartilage changes consequent to a fracture than after Legg-Perthes' disease; the older age period in which fractures occur is responsible. After a femoral neck fracture in an adult there may be resorption of articular cartilage from below, and softening on the surface. Occasionally a fibrous tissue pannus forms and absorbs the articular cartilage beneath it.

The following conclusions by Phemister present an excellent summary of the problem:

1. The head may retain an adequate blood supply through the

ligamentum teres and intact parts of periosteum, and survive, especially in children.

2. The head though alive may fail to unite. Both fragments are then porotic.

3. Lacking adequate blood supply, the head may die and retain its density in contrast to the osteoporosis that develops in the neck, shaft and pelvis. This reduces, but does not preclude the possibility of union, and, when union does occur in this circumstance, there is gradual disintegration and removal of dead bone by "creeping substitution." If weight is borne during this stage, the head may suffer severe collapse. Motion without weight bearing hastens replacement.

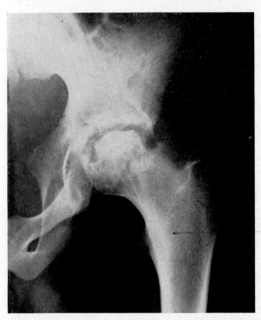

FIGURE 143. Aseptic necrosis in an adult femoral head. Etiology unknown.

4. The head may die and fail to unite with the neck, remaining for years as a dense foreign body. Eventually the head may be resorbed and in part replaced by living bone. Cavitation of the head is apt to result in the end.

ASEPTIC NECROSIS OF THE PROXIMAL FRAGMENT
AFTER FRACTURE OF THE CARPAL-NAVICULAR

All of the nutrient arteries of the carpal navicular frequently enter the bone in its distal one half. A transverse fracture through the waist or proximal pole of such a navicular inevitably inflicts an avascular necrosis on the proximal fragment. Bony union in the presence of the necrosis is not impossible, but delayed or non-union are the rule. Regeneration is a long, slow process and is associated with degenerative changes in the articular cartilage. Adhesions often form and limit mobility of the wrist. Excision of the necrotic fragment or the insertion of some type of bone graft is a popular form of treatment, but the end results are discouraging.

Aseptic Necrosis in Autogenous Bone Grafts

Bone grafts will be discussed in detail in the next chapter on Fractures. Some degree of aseptic necrosis may be seen in all cortical bone grafts; the thicker the graft, the more extensive the necrosis. Surface

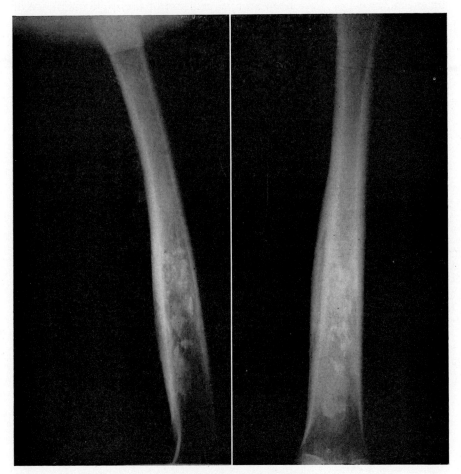

FIGURE 144A. Caisson Disease Femur.

layers usually have access to sufficient nutrition to remain viable. Deeper in the graft, osteocytes degenerate and die since there is no blood circulation, and nutrition through imbition proves inadequate. Thin cortical grafts and many cancellous grafts survive. When there are areas of aseptic necrosis in autogenous grafts, such areas are slowly regenerated by a process of "creeping substitution." Viable elements in the graft assist in the regeneration of necrotic elements. In obeyance of Wolff's Law certain areas of a graft may be absorbed in place of being substituted; other areas may be heavily reinforced.

CAISSON DISEASE

Caisson disease has been recognized since Aristotle's time, but only in recent years has there been an appreciation of the high incidence of skeletal involvement.

Virtually all body systems may become involved and produce symptoms. Skeletal symptoms have proved to be among the most frequent; they arise from either microscopic or massive areas of aseptic necrosis.

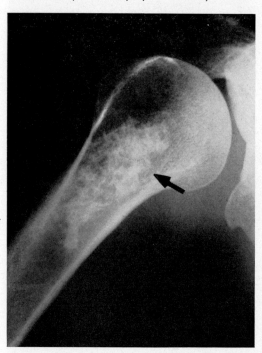

FIGURE 144B. Caisson Disease Humerus.

ETIOLOGY

Under increased atmospheric pressure the blood absorbs an excess of nitrogen from the lungs; the blood and body tissues become supersaturated with nitrogen. When the increased air pressure is too rapidly returned to normal, the lungs are unable to excrete the excess nitrogen fast enough; as an outcome, the overload of nitrogen appears in the blood stream in gaseous form as many small bubbles. These nitrogen bubble emboli are capable of blocking smaller arteries and creating infarcts. Tissues with the highest lipoid content have the greatest capacity for nitrogen absorption, and therefore become the sites of major involvement. These tissues include the fatty bone marrow, the brain and spinal cord, and intestinal mesenteric fat.

BONE LESIONS

Bone lesions occur predominately in the long bones; a high incidence of infarcts appears in both the diaphyses and the epiphyses. Lesions may involve only one localized area of a bone or extend throughout the bone (Fig. 144). Involvement of bones of the lower extremities is considerably more frequent than upper extremity involvement.

Bilateral Lesions are the Rule

Small areas of aseptic necrosis may be readily regenerated through the usual process of creeping substitution. In the larger infarcts a considerable area of bone may be killed and regeneration may be obstructed. A margin of fibrous tissue and fibrous bone frequently forms around large bone infarcts; this is followed by some degree of calcification of the necrotic marrow within the infarct.

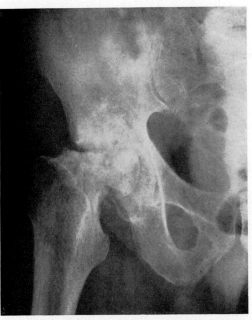

JOINT LESIONS

Joint symptoms have their origin in the altered contours of articular surfaces, and are not due to capsular infarcts. Epiphyseal involvement which ordinarily is at the knees, hips, and shoulders may be so extensive that partial collapse of the articular surface occurs during regeneration (Bassoe).

FIGURE 145. Aseptic necrosis and collapse of a femoral head following roentgen therapy for a carcinoma of the uterus. (Courtesy, Leo Levi, M.D., Los Angeles.)

Osteoarthritis develops in response to the trauma incident to articulating in the presence of irregular joint contours.

RADIATION NECROSIS OF BONE

Soon after Roentgen discovered the x-ray, efforts were made to determine the damage the rays could exert upon living tissues. Perthes in 1903 found that the rays would retard bone growth in the wings of young chickens. Recaimier's experiments in 1905 also demonstrated the inhibitory influence of roentgen radiation on bone growth. Cluzet radiated fractures in 1909 and noted a delay in callous formation. Wilkins and Regan in 1934 reported a pronounced reduction of phosphatase activity in bones and at fracture sites of growing dogs after moderate doses of roentgen-ray radiation.

Aseptic osseous necrosis from roentgen-ray radiation is relatively common, and in a few instances has led to fractures. Phillip reported five cases of fracture of the neck of the femur in women, following roentgen-ray treatments for carcinoma of the uterus.

PATHOGENESIS

Numerous reports of radium necrosis of bone have appeared in medical literautre. In 1926 Ewing pointed out that radium killed the osteocytes and altered the lamellar structure of bone. In the same year Phemister demonstrated that an area of bone killed by radium undergoes sequestration, and is slowly absorbed provided the dead bone is not needed by the host bone for mechanical support. If the area of necrotic bone is needed for support, it is not sequestrated, but is slowly replaced by viable bone through the process of creeping substitution. In 1939 Watson and Scarborough reported that of 1819 cases of jaw malignancies treated by radium at the New York Memorial Hospital, 235, or 13 percent, developed radio-osteonecrosis.

Both roentgen-rays and radium radiations in sufficient dosage create an aseptic necrosis in the area of bone radiated. The reaction of neighboring tissues to the presence of the necrotic bone depends upon the size and location of the area of necrosis, the condition of adjacent soft tissues and the status of the neighboring blood vessels. In the majority of instances the overlying soft tissues and blood vessels are damaged thus delaying regeneration. Where the mandible and maxilla are involved, a break in the oral mucous membrane frequently adds a secondary infection, transforming the avascular bone lesion into a pyogenic osteomyelitis.

Bone absorbs more radiation than other tissues; and secondary radiations develop inside bone, increasing the damage. There is evidence that the secondary rays represent a transformation of the primary rays by the calcium phosphate in bone.

The periosteum may be killed, but more frequently it shows hyaline degeneration, edema and diminished cellular activity. Periosteal blood vessels may be extensively damaged and obliterated.

Ewing divided the reaction of bone to irradiation into five stages or degrees, based upon the dosage of the radiation. With light irradiation growth was briefly retarded, and the osteocytes showed a short period of diminished vitality. With somewhat more irradiation a second stage reaction followed and was manifested by a productive osteitis in which there was thickening of the bone and a "fuzzy" periosteum. In the third stage there was osteosclerosis, and the increased fragility was reflected by a higher incidence of fractures. With the next increase in irradiation, the fourth stage, there were aseptic necrosis and sequestration. A fifth stage was added for cases such as jaw malignancies, in which secondary infection and osteomyelitis frequently become superimposed upon the radiation necrosis.

REFERENCES

AXHAUSEN, G.: Köhler's disease and Perthes' disease. *Ztschr. f. Chir., 50*:553, 1923.

AXHAUSEN, G.: Konig's osteochondritis dissecans. *Klin Wchschr., 3*:1057, 1924. (Abstr. *J. A. M. A., 83*:228, 1924.)

BERNSTEIN, M. A.: Osteochondritis dissecans. *J. Bone & Joint Surg., 7*:319, 1925.

BURMAN, M., WINKLE, I. V. and LANGSAM, M. J.: Adolescent osteochondritis of the symphysis pubis. *J. Bone & Joint Surg., 16*:649, 1934.

CALVE, J.: Localized affection of spine suggesting osteochondritis of vertebral body with clinical aspects of Potts' disease. *J. Bone & Joint Surg., 7*:41, 1925.

CAVANAUGH, L. A., SHELTON, E. K. and SUTHERLAND, R.: Metabolic studies in osteochondritis of the capital femoral epiphysis. *J. Bone & Joint Surg., 18*:957, 1936.

CHRISTIE, A. C.: Review of osteochondritis or epiphysitis. *J. A. M. A., 87*:528, 1926.

FAIRBANKS, H. A. T.: Osteochondritis dissecans. *Brit. J. Surg., 21*:67, 1933.

FREIBERG, A. H.: Infraction of the second metatarsal bone. *Surg. Gynec & Obst., 19*:191, 1914.

FREUND, E.: Bilateral aseptic necrosis of the femoral head. *Ann. Surg., 104*:100, 1936.

GELLMAN, M.: Osteochondritis of the patella. *J. Bone & Joint Surg., 16*:95, 1934.

HARBIN, M.: Focal and multiple osteochondritis. *Am. J. Roentgenol. 29*:763, 1933.

HARBIN, M. and ZOLLINGER, R.: Osteochondritis of growth centers. *Surg. Gynec. & Obst., 51*:145, 1930.

HENDERSON, M. S.: Chronic osteitis of the semilunar bone (Kienböck's disease). *J. Bone & Joint Surg., 8*:504, 1926.

KIENBOCK, R.: Uber traumatische Maladie des Mondbeins. *Fortsch, a.d. Geb. d. Röntgenstrahien, 16*:77, 1910.

KING, E. S. J.: *Localized Rarefying Conditions of Bone.* Wm. Wood & Co., Baltimore, 1935.

KOHLER, A.: Uber die haufigen Krankheiten des Kinderknochen. *München med. Wchschr., 55*:1923, 1908.

KOHLER, A.: Eine typische Erknorrung. *München med. Wchschr., 67*:1289, 1920.

KONIG, F.: Uber freie Korper inden Gelenken. *Deutsche Ztschr. f. Chir., 27*:90, 1888.

LEGG, A.: An obscure affection of the hip joint. *Boston M. & Surg. J., 162*:202, 1910.

LERICHE, M. R.: Exper. research on the mechanism of the formation of osteochondritis of the hip. *Lyon Chir., 31*:5, 1934.

LIPPMANN, R. K.: Pathogenesis of Perthes' disease based upon pathological findings in a case. *Am J. Surg., 6*:785, 1929; *4*:169, 1928.

MILTNER, L. J. and HU: Osteochondritis of head of femur; experimental study. *Arch. Surg., 27*:645, 1933.

MOUAT, T. B., WILKIE, J. and HARDING, H. E.: Isolated fracture of the carpal semilunar and Kienböck's disease. *Brit. J. Surg., 19*:577, 1932.

MOORE, R. D.: Aseptic necrosis of the capital femoral epiphysis. *Surg., Gynec. & Obst., 801*:199, 1945.

OSGOOD, R. B.: Lesions of tibial tubercle occuring during adolescence. *Boston M. & Surg. Jr., 148*:114, 1903.

OVERTON, L. M.: Osteochondritis of growth centers. *Ann. Surg., 101*:1062, 1935.

PERTHES, GEORG: Uber osteochondritis deformans juvenilis. *Arch. f. klin. Chir., 101*:779, 1913.

PHEMISTER, D. B.: Recognition of dead bone based on pathological and x-ray studies. *Ann. Surg., 72*:466, 1920.

PHEMISTER, D. B.: Repair of bone in the presence of aseptic necrosis resulting from fractures, transplantations, and vascular obstruction. *J. Bone & Joint Surg., 12*:769-787, 1930.

SCHEUERMANN, H.: Kyphosis dorsalis juvenilis. *Ztschr. f. Orthop.*, *41*:305, 1921.

SCHLATTER, C.: Verletzungen des Schienbeinformigen Fortsatzes d. oberen Tibia Epiphyse. *Beitr. z. klin. Chir.*, *38*:874, 1903.

SEVER, J. W.: Apophysitis of os calcis. *N. Y. State J. Med.*, *95*:1025, 1912.

SINDING-LARSEN, C. F.: Hitherto unknown affections of the Patella. *Acta. Radiol.*, *1*:171, 1921.

SLOCUM, D. B.: Coxa plana. *Northwest Med.*, *40*:233, 1941.

ZERMANSKY, A. P.: The pathology and pathogenesis of Legg-Calve-Perthes' disease. *Am. J. Surg.*, *4*:169, 1928.

CAISSON DISEASE

BASSOE, P.: Late manifestations of compressed air disease. *Am. J. M. Sc.*, *145*:522, 1913.

BERNSTEIN, A. and PLATE, E.: Uber chronische Gelekveraenderungen eustavden durch Presslufterkrakung. *Fortsch. a. d. Geb. d. Röntgenstrahlen*, *17*:197, 1911.

COLEY, B. L. and MOORE, M.: Caisson disease in bones and joints. *Ann. Surg.*, *111*:1065, 1940.

KAHLSTROM, S. C., PHEMISTER, D. B., and BURTON, C. C.: Bone and joint changes in Caisson disease, including infraction and deforming arthritis. *Surg. Gynec. & Obst.*, *68*:129, 1939.

RENDICH, R. A. and HARRINGTON, LEO: Roentgen findings in Caisson disease, with case reports. *Radiology*, *35*:439, 1940.

WALKER, W. A.: Aseptic necrosis of bone occurring in Caisson's disease. *J. Bone & Joint Surg.*, *22*:1080, 1940.

RADIATION NECROSIS

BAKER, L. D.: Spontaneous fracture of the femoral neck following irradiation. *J. Bone & Joint Surg.*, *23*:354, 1941.

BROOKS, B. and HILLSTROM, H. I.: Effects of roentgenrays on growth and bone regeneration. Experimental. *Am. J. Surg.*, *20*:599, 1933.

CLUZET: Action of x-rays on the development of callus. *Lyon Med.*, *114*:22, 1910.

DALBY, R. G., JACOX, H. W., and MILLER, N. F.: Fractures of the femoral neck following irradiation. *Am. J. Obst. & Gynec.*, *32*:50, 1936.

PHILLIP, E. T.: Five cases of femoral neck injury in women after x-ray treatment for carcinoma of the uterus. *Strahlentherapie*, *44*:363, 1932.

PHEMISTER, D. B.: Radium necrosis of bone. *Am. J. Roentgenol.*, *16*:340, 1926.

RECAMIER: Action des rayons X sur le tissue osseux en voie de developpment. *Arch. d'electric Med. Bordeaux*, *13*:853, 1905.

WATSON, W. L. and SCARBOROUGH, J. E.: Osteoradionecrosis in intraoral cancer. *Am. J. Roentgenol.*, *40*:524, 1939.

WILKINS, W. E. and REGEN, E. M.: Effect of roentgen irradiation of the entire animal on phosphatase activity and electrolytic content of its water extract. *Radiology*, *23*:443, 1934.

CHAPTER V

Fractures

Contents

"The surgeon who attempts to treat fractures without a full knowledge of the pathology of bones and joints is faced with insuperable difficulties." (Sir Reginald Watson-Jones.)

Decidedly improved fracture treatment has grown out of a better understanding of the pathogenesis of fracture repair. Few fields have been more earnestly investigated. While many of the experiments in this field have been only of academic interest, others have had significant and far reaching clinical application.

Fracture repair will be discussed under the following headings:

1. Normal union
2. Delayed union
3. Non-union
  a. Fibrous union
  b. Neoarthrosis

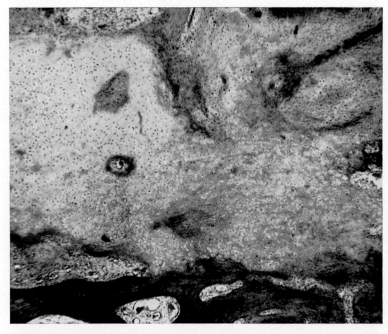

FIGURE 146. Hyaline cartilage and fibrocartilage in the early external callus.

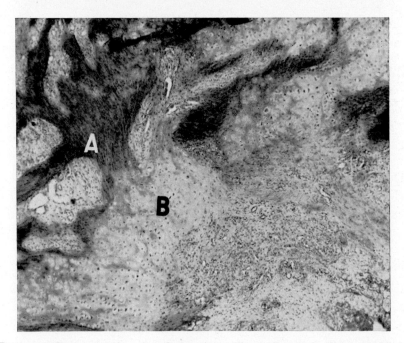

FIGURE 147. Bony trabeculae, *A*, replacing the cartilage callus, *B*, by direct metaplasia.

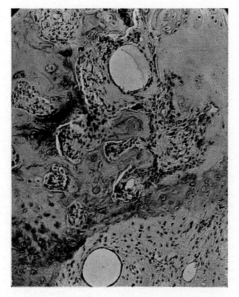

FIGURE 148. Section through callus to show zone of calcified cartilage at the junction of the bone and cartilage

This chapter will also include a discussion of the interesting history and histology of bone grafts and the reaction of bone to metal plates, screws and pins.

NORMAL UNION

A fracture severs blood vessels in the medullary canal, the bone proper, the periosteum, and also frequently in the overlying muscles. Preservation of the hematoma that follows is important. A firm, abundant hematoma whose fibrin enables it to bridge the fragment ends gives the healing process a good start.

Organization of the hematoma is under way within 24 hours; myriad capillaries grow into the periphery of the clot from the periosteum, endosteum, haversian canals, marrow, and even from adjacent muscles. With the neighboring hyperemia and the leukocytic infiltration the picture is that of traumatic inflammation. Fibroblastic granulation tissue, replacing the hematoma, joins the fragment ends. In long bones, granulation tissue fills the marrow canal for a short distance at each fragment end; granulations also fill in the space between the elevated periosteum and the cortex. As with all healthy granulation tissue, fibrous condensation takes place, and it is then that chondrification and ossification become possible.

Areas of fibrocartilage and hyaline cartilage are prone to form in the young fibrous tissue by metaplasia. Most of the metaplastic cartilage appears at the periphery—in the external callus (Fig. 146). There is a wide variation in the proportions of the cartilage callus; it may be exuberant, or there may be none. "Cartilage callus" forms more abundantly in the young than in the old, more in animals than in humans, and more when there is motion at the fracture site than when there is immobilization.

Since the hyperemia of the fracture area involves the bones as well as soft tissues, there is a progressive osteoporosis of all viable fragments. Superficial cortical absorption of fracture fragments takes place as part of the process of deossification. Calcium salts are released as the bone atrophies, and are retained locally to aid in calcifying the bony callus as it forms. Leriche and Policard refer to this local accumulation of calcium salts as the "calcific surcharge."

Bony trabeculae forming in the primary callus are the membranous type and appear first in the proliferating cambium layer of the periosteum (Fig. 149). Trabeculae develop proximal and distal to the fracture site at the outset, then gradually extend to, and into the fracture cleft, replacing the fibrous tissue and cartilage encountered in their path. Urist and McLean have demonstrated that under optimum con-

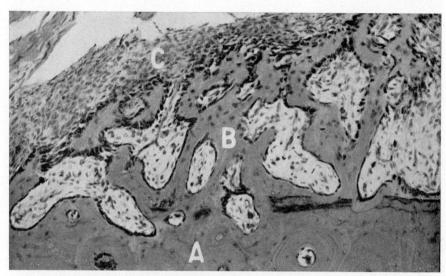

FIGURE 149. Primary bony callus. Section is through the periosteal callus. *A*. Cortex. *B*. Periosteal bone. *C*. Cambium.

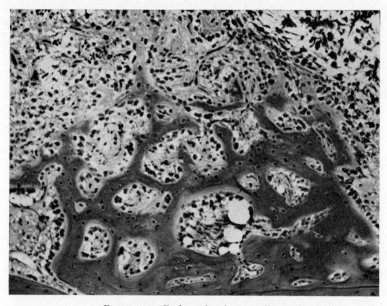

FIGURE 150. Endosteal primary callus.

ditions the newly forming trabeculae calcify as they are laid down. An osteoid stage exists only in the malacic diseases, and on other occasions when local conditions develop in which the supply of calcium does not keep pace with the needs of the new trabeculae. Urist and McLean have also pointed out that random calcification of the "cartilage callus" does not occur. The cartilage calcifies only along the junction between the cartilage and the newly forming bony trabeculae

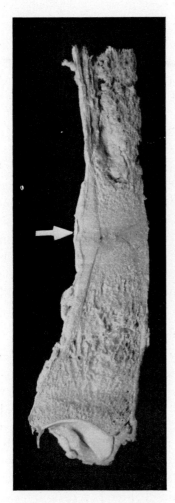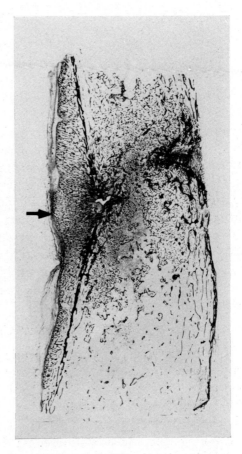

FIGURE 151. Primary bony callus in a buckling type of fracture of a tibia softened by osteomalacia. A. (Left) Specimen. B. (Right) Histologic section.

(Fig. 148). Replacement of the cartilage occurs principally by direct metaplasia of the cartilage to bone; however, a primitive disorderly type of enchondral ossification may also be seen. Fibrous tissue within the callus undergoes metaplasia to bone, but simple calcification of fibrous tissue is not seen.

The bony trabeculae of the primary callus form rapidly, and under normal conditions form abundantly. Except in intraarticular fractures, where there is no appreciable periosteal callus, the primary callus becomes most extensive in the periosteum. When a new trabeculum forms, osteoblasts cover its surface, and layer upon layer of new bone is applied. Lines of stress through the fracture site do not dictate the alignment of trabeculae in the primary callus.

Early Reduction of Fractures Versus Delayed Reduction

Murray, Watson-Jones and others crusade for the prompt reduction of fractures and undisturbed immobilization. In the face of this crusade Moore waits for several days before reducing fractures and has good results to support his contention. On the basis of the histopathology observed during the healing of fractures, there appears to be a solid foundation for the Clay Ray Murray, Sir Reginald Watson-Jones teaching. The hematoma must become organized to establish healing, this important step is obviously disturbed and even disrupted by delayed or repeated manipulation of the fracture fragments. Granulation tissue replacing the hematoma is not ossifiable. It must undergo fibrous condensation and thereby reduce its hyperemia before it becomes an "ossifiable medium." With repeated manipulations or with persistent motion at the fracture site, new granulation tissue continues to form, perpetuating the hyperemia, the osteoporosis, and the acid reaction of the local tissue fluids—all of which are incompatible with calcification and ossification.

Secondary Callus

The primary callus is not mechanically constructed to bear heavy stresses and must be replaced by the mature lamellar bone of the secondary callus. Most of the external primary callus is not replaced, but simply absorbed. And in tubular bones the same is true of endosteal callus. Primary callus uniting cortical walls is replaced by a process resembling creeping substitution. As the primary fibrous bone is absorbed, lamellar bone is laid down in line with the predominating lines of stress, which in long bones run parallel to the longitudinal axis. Haversian systems are reconstructed around blood vessels by the formation of lamellar plates, applied one upon the other. When cortical walls are restored to near-normal dimensions and the medullary canal is re-established, fibrous tissue in the marrow spaces is replaced by fatty or hematogenous marrow elements.

If the fracture heals with an angulation or displacement deformity, the internal architecture of the bone slowly adapts and realigns itself to the new lines of stress, according to Wolff's law.

DELAYED UNION

Although much has been written about systemic causes of delayed healing of fractures, local causes are far more significant and infinitely

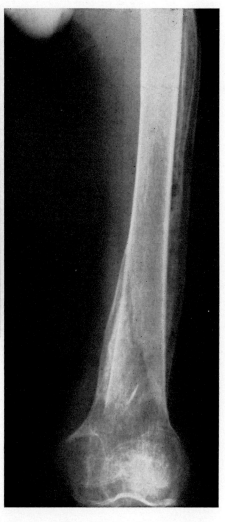

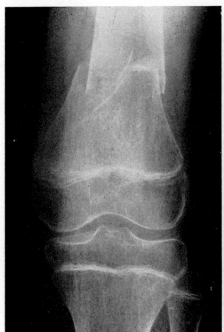

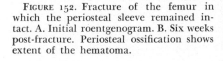

FIGURE 152. Fracture of the femur in which the periosteal sleeve remained intact. A. Initial roentgenogram. B. Six weeks post-fracture. Periosteal ossification shows extent of the hematoma.

more frequent; among the local causes, those having a mechanical or physical basis are the most important.

I. MECHANICAL CAUSES OF DELAYED UNION

1. *Inadequate immobilization:* When casts or splints are loose or are too short, motion develops at the fracture site and is capable of protracting the healing process tremendously. The trend toward wider

use of non-padded casts has grown out of the numerous instances of delayed union associated with inadequate splinting. Repeated change of casts, tractions, or splints when accompanied by rough handling of the fracture site, also delays union.

2. *Distraction of the fragments:* With the advent of skeletal traction and transfixion pin splints there were innumerable instances of long delays in bony union, due specifically to distraction of the fragment ends. Delayed union on this basis was so widely experienced that efforts are now made to avoid at all costs, distraction of the fragments.

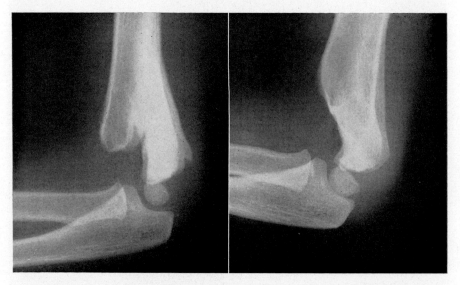

FIGURE 153. Wolff's law functioning in a supracondylar fracture of the humerus. A. *(Left)* Four months post-fracture. B. *(Right)* One year post-fracture.

From a histologic standpoint it is difficult to explain the pronounced delays in healing that can follow even slight distraction of the fragments. The answer to this question awaits further experimental observations.

3. *Displacement and angulation of the fragments* can cause delayed union, particularly at such sites as the neck of the femur, the carpal scaphoid and the tibial malleolus.

4. *Repeated manipulations or changes of traction:* One of the most frequent sources of delayed union lies in the tendency of many surgeons to manipulate and meddle with the fragments. New hemorrhage and new granulation tissue follow each disturbance, causing the healing process to begin anew in much or all of the fracture area. Since the local reaction tends to be acid during the granulation tissue stage and

alkaline during the ossifying fibrous connective tissue stage, it can be readily realized why calcification and ossification are temporarily halted each time hemorrhage and granulation tissue pervade the fracture site.

5. Cowan emphasized the point that union is delayed *when the periosteum is severed sharply and not elevated by traumatic stripping.* In this circumstance periosteal bone does not develop to any appreciable

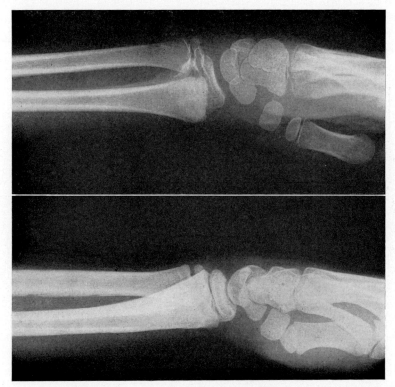

FIGURE 154. Epiphyseal separation of the distal radial epiphysis. A. *(Above)* Twenty days post-fracture. B. *(Below)* Nine months post-fracture.

extent; thus, the healing is limited to osteal and endosteal bridging. This situation exists in most transcervical fractures of the femur. Since the periosteum strips with much more difficulty in the elderly, it follows that less periosteal elevation is to be expected in older individuals.

II. Infection

A pyogenic infection at a fracture site can seriously disrupt and delay fracture healing. The local calcium concentration, if it forms at all, may be lost through suppuration. An infection does not necessarily spell doom to fracture repair. The reason healing often fails instead of simply being delayed resides in the inadequate immobilization so frequently associated with a splinting arrangement that allows for dressing the draining wound. It is not difficult to recall the instances in the past when one could look through the window of a cast at an infected wound exposing a long bone fracture site and see the fragments move each time the patient contracted his muscles. During World War II a great deal was accomplished in improving the treatment of infected fractures. With proper excision of sequestrated bone and debris, prompt plastic repair of the soft tissue defect, and dependable immobilization, the

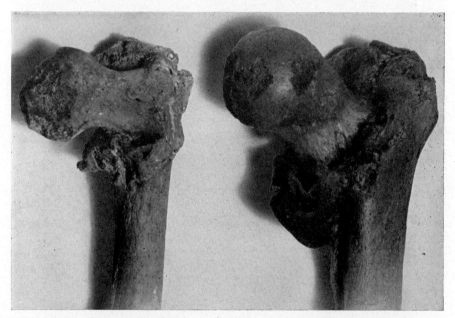

FIGURE 155. Intertrochanteric fractures. Dried specimens showing the abundant external callus that forms in fractures at this level.

results were amazingly good. This was one of the gratifying experiences of military orthopedic surgeons during World War II.

Callus is able to form in the presence of a low grade infection, particularly when pus and necrotic debris do not accumulate.

III. CIRCULATORY IMPAIRMENT

Avascular necrosis of a fracture fragment delays union in that the necrotic fragment can neither contribute capillaries to organize the hematoma nor its share of calcium to the "calcific surcharge." Healing of the fracture is accompanied by regeneration of the necrotic bone, a process that appears to divert materials and energy from the fracture repair.

IV. Defective Hematoma

Crushing injuries damage the local circulation by actually destroying part of the blood vessels and causing thrombosis of others. A poorly

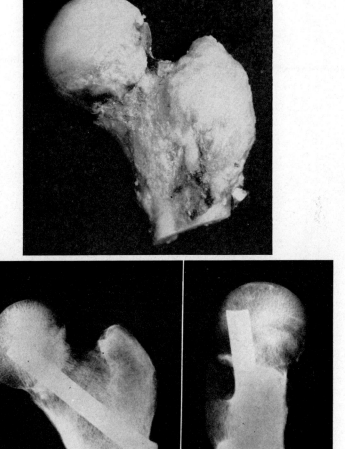

FIGURE 156. Subcapital fracture of the neck of the femur, six weeks post-fracture. Fracture was promptly pinned. Patient expired after six weeks from a vascular accident. A. *(Above)* Post-mortem specimen. B. *(Below)* Roentgenograms.

formed hematoma often is associated with crushing of the bone and overlying soft tissues.

In compound fractures much of the hemorrhage that would ordinarily collect to form the hematoma may be lost through the communication of the surface wound with the fracture site.

Occasionally a pocket of fluid collects between the fragments, be-

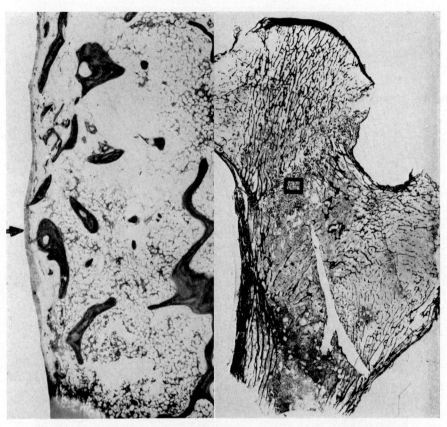

FIGURE 156. *(Continued)* C. *(Left)* Thin Layer of reactive fibrous tissue along path of Smith-Peterson pin (arrow). (Kulowski, J. and Luck, J. V.: *J. Bone and Joint Surg., 23:17,* 1941.) D. *(Right)* Histologic section of the entire specimen.

comes walled off, and delays union by displacing the hematoma and by acting as a barrier to the ingrowth of fibroblasts.

V. SYSTEMIC CAUSES OF DELAYED UNION

Of the numerous systemic causes to which delayed union has been attributed, only two will be mentioned: senility and starvation. Most fractures heal slowly during senility, but the delay is more physiologic than pathologic. Anabolism is relatively more retarded than catabolism, and this is decidedly evident in osteoblastic and gonadal activity. During starvation all body processes are slowed, including the repair of fractures. Protein deficiencies often profoundly impair bone metabolism.

NON-UNION

All of the significant causes of failure to form a bony bridge across a fracture are mechanical. There are no systemic causes of non-union. Non-union of a fracture invariably can be traced to: (1) loss of apposition between the fragments, and/or (2) motion between the fracture fragments during the period of healing.

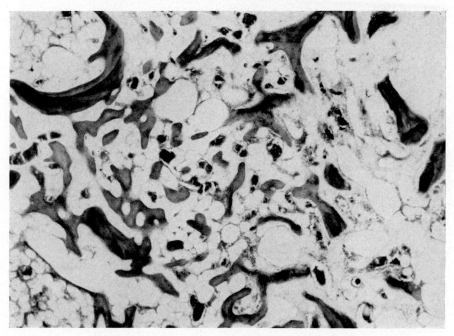

FIGURE 156. *(Continued)* E. Primary bony callus in square marked on C.

Loss of Apposition of the Fragments

Malposition of the fragments with loss of continuity of the hematoma between the fragment ends. Granulation and fibrous tissues form and may even ossify, but build only a cap over each fragment, achieving no bridging of the fracture.

Avulsion of a fragment: This may occur in compound diaphyseal fractures of long bones, with a loss of one to several inches of the bone, creating a gap that leads to non-union.

Interposition of fibrous connective tissues: This occurs in displaced fractures of the patella, olecranon, epicondyles of the humerus, and the tibial internal malleolus. Interposition of a small amount of muscle is compatible with fracture healing, and this is particularly true when there is a minimum of fascia and fibrous septa included with the muscle.

Distraction of the fragments: This is a leading cause of non-union. When soft tissues are interposed and when the fragments are widely displaced, something usually is done about it, but a slight distraction of the fragments appears of no concern to the uninitiated and is allowed to remain.

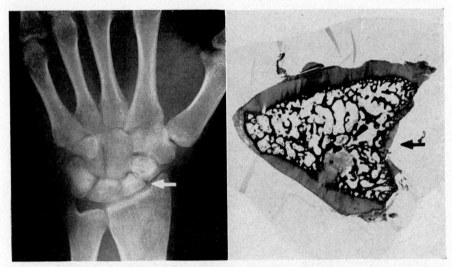

FIGURE 157. Ununited fracture of the carpal navicular. A. *(Left)* Roentgenogram before surgery. B. *(Right)* Excised proximal pole. Friction and pressure had created a layer of fibrocartilage on the fracture surface (arrow).

MOTION OF THE FRAGMENTS DURING THE PERIOD OF HEALING

Motion at the fracture site may occur as the result of either inadequate splinting or no splinting. With defective immobilization or with too short a period of fracture protection, a widely variable degree of motion develops between the bone ends in response to the various stresses acting upon the fragments. All forms of motion can disrupt reparative processes, but in general the most damaging are shear and torsion movements. Pressure, up to a certain point, can stimulate healing. Bending at the fracture site produces compression on the concave side of the bend, and tension stresses on the convex side. Very slight movements may not produce a non-union, but the idea that motion at the fracture site stimulates good healing and is to be encouraged is a gross error and one that has inflicted a great deal of suffering upon a great many people.

Torsion stresses are particularly damaging to ossification within the fracture cleft. This type of stress causes many cases of non-union on account of its existence without detection inside the cast or splint. A cast applied to the leg and thigh with the knee extended does not pro-

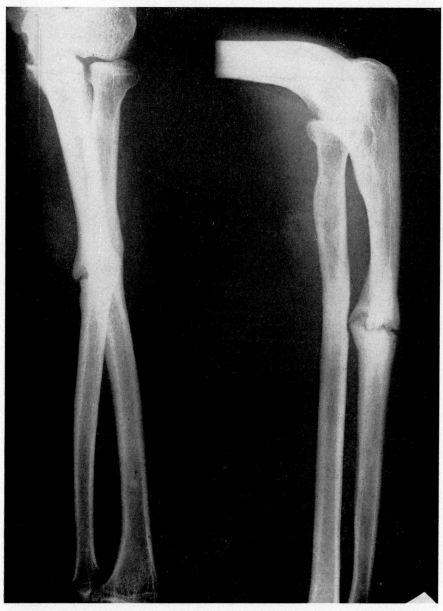

FIGURE 158A. Non-union of a fractured ulna. Pro and supination of the wrist were permitted inside of the original splint; the resulting torsion stresses explain the failure of healing.

tect a fractured tibia against torsion stresses; the knee must be flexed
to prevent torsion. A few degrees of pronation and supination of the
wrist during the healing of a fractured ulnar shaft consistently causes

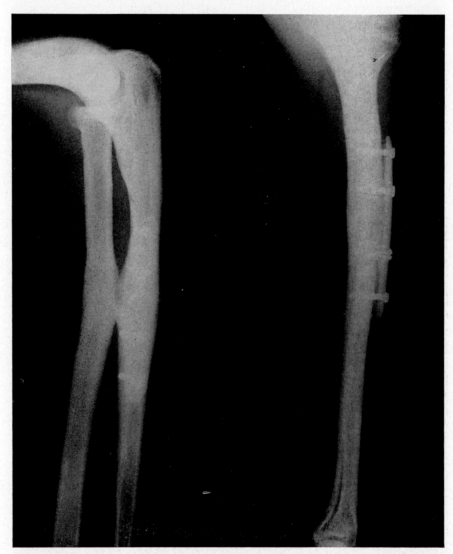

FIGURE 158B. Eight weeks after application of an onlay tibial bone graft.

the young fibrous tissue between the fragments to go on to maturity
without ossifying.

Shearing stresses are readily detected in that displacement of the
fragments occurs when the fracture is not protected from shear. Shearing stresses are manifest in all oblique fractures of long bones. While

most transverse fractures have only a small shear component in their stress pattern, transverse fractures of the neck of the femur may have 100 per cent shearing stresses directed upon them. Until the advent of the Smith-Petersen pin we had no dependable method of eliminating the displacing action of the shear factor. In reconstructing the upper femur after a non-united fracture of the neck, it is imperative to transform as much of the shearing stress as possible into a pressure stress. This may be accomplished by any one of several operative procedures.

PATHOGENESIS

A non-united fracture always presents a fibrous tissue bridge between the fracture fragments. Substantial motion at the site of the non-union produces changes in the fibrous tissue that ultimately may create a "new joint," called a nearthrosis.

FIBROUS UNION

If the fragments are in apposition and a non-union ensues, it is generally always because the fracture was inadequately immobilized (Figs. 157-161). As a result of combinations of bending, twisting, tension, pressure, and shear in the fracture cleft, the young fibrous tissue fails to become an "ossifiable medium." Bony trabeculae do not form in the primary callus, the fibrous tissue remaining barren of calcification and ossification. As time passes, the interposed fibrous tissue matures into an adult form of dense fibrous tissue with more and more

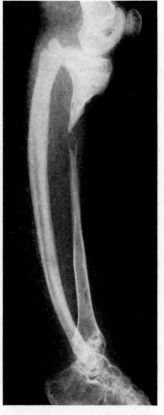

FIGURE 159. A pathologic fracture followed removal of a large osteomyelitic sequestrum. Weight bearing through the fibula has caused it to hypertrophy. Later the fibula was transplanted into each end of the tibia in a two stage operation.

collagen and a diminishing number of cells. Ossification may take place in the periosteum but it does not bridge the fracture. Ossification also occurs in the medullary canal and ultimately blocks the canal with a bony plug in each fragment end. Sclerosis of the bone ends represents the response of the bone to pressure stresses associated with function continued in spite of the non-union.

In a non-union developing from loss of contact by the fragment ends, the ossification process evolves independently over each fragment end, as already mentioned. Bridging of the fracture cleft by bone fails simply from loss of continuity of ossifiable tissues between the fragments. Among civilized peoples there rarely is any reason why fracture fragments cannot be brought into apposition by one method or another. With adequate immobilization and the fragments in good contact,

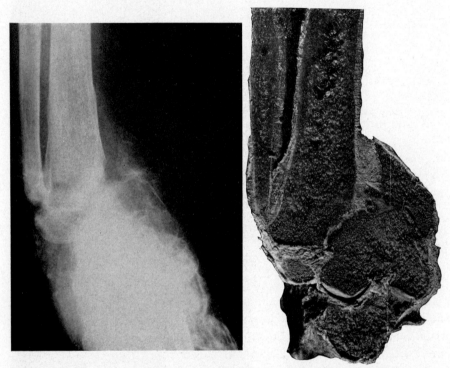

FIGURE 160. Fracture-dislocation of the right ankle. A. *(Left)* pre-amputation roentgenogram. B. *(Right)* Frontal section of the specimen. The ankle joint articular surfaces were replaced by fibrous tissue and joined together in a fibrous ankylosis. (See Figure 185 for histologic section.)

virtually all fractures heal. Watson-Jones and Coltart reported a remarkable series of 804 fractures of the shafts of the tibia and femur in which there was not a single non-union.

NEARTHROSIS

This is the type of non-union that ultimately develops when considerable motion occurs at the fracture site over a period of months or years. Through pressure and friction the fibrous issue covering the bone ends differentiates into fibro-cartilage and eventually into hyaline cartilage. At the outset, large fissures and splits appear in the interposed fibrous tissue. With continued motion between the fragments a cavity develops and encloses the fragment ends. Synovial-like cells line the cavity and secrete a lubricating, cartilage-nourishing fluid to complete the nearthrosis. Wide variation exists in nearthroses. In general, the greater the mobility, and the longer its duration, the more nearly the nearthrosis resembles a joint. Nearthrosis of the femoral neck may attain more mobility than remains between the femoral head and acetabulum (Fig. 161). A non-union of any long bone or of certain of the short bones may develop into a nearthrosis. Some of the more common sites are the middle one-third of the clavicle, the waist of the carpal scaphoid, the humeral diaphysis, the ulnar diaphysis, and the middle one-third of the tibia. The neck of the femur headed the list, prior to the widespread use of internal fixation.

March Fractures

March fractures (Figs. 166 and 167) are spontaneous fractures, and they have their highest incidence in the metatarsals. The term *March fracture* evolved

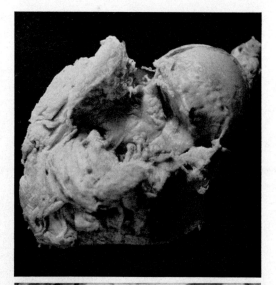

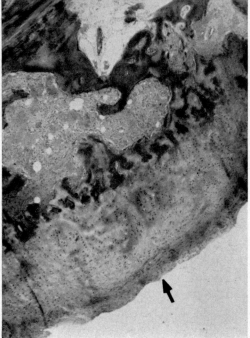

FIGURE 161. Nearthrosis of the neck of the femur. A. *(Above)* The neck has been absorbed and in its place, as a result of proximal migration of the shaft with each step, is a large nearthrotic cavity lined with synovia and filled with fluid. Photograph shows femoral head, nearthrosis, and greater trochanter. B. *(Below)* Section from the fracture surface of the femoral head showing the transformation of fibrous tissue to an articular cartilage (arrow).

from the relatively frequent occurrence of the fracture in soldiers subjected to long marches. Although most frequently observed in the foot
bones, March fractures are also seen in the tibia, fibula, and femur.
There have been numerous descriptions of this entity in medical literature; the first was by Breithaupt in 1855. The many synonyms that appear in these descriptions include stress fracture, spontaneous fracture,
soldier's fracture, fatigue fracture, exhaustion fracture and insidious
fracture.

Numerous explanations of the etiology have been suggested, the most
acceptable theory attributes the fracture to an abnormal concentration

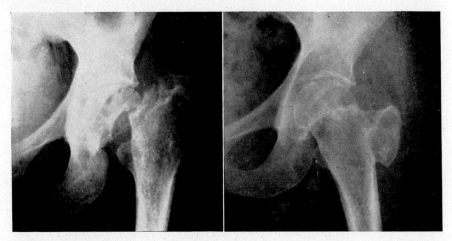

FIGURE 162. Reconstructed upper left femur for an ununited fracture of the neck. The
"table top" principle of the Thompson-Stephens operation was applied to the Brackett
reconstruction. A. *(Left)* Pre-operative roentgenogram. B. *(Right)* Six months post-operative. (Author's article: *J. Iowa M. Soc.,* Dec. 1938.)

of stresses plus loss of the protective action of the muscles from fatigue.
Overloading together with the repeated trauma finally cause the bone
to yield. No displacement occurs. Continued activity is the rule in spite
of pain.

Healing may be delayed but non-union is not seen. A fusiform-shaped
callus appears in most instances. If the patient continues to walk on
the foot during the healing stage, the callus becomes exuberant.

PATHOLOGIC ANATOMY

A small number of cases have been studied histologically. Straus
studied a metatarsal that was excised because of an erroneous diagnosis
of osteogenic sarcoma. He stated that there was nothing specific or
unusual, the picture was that of a typical healing response to a typical
non-displaced fracture. There was no evidence whatever of an infection.

Dodd also reported a March fracture that had been erroneously diagnosed as sarcoma. In this case the leg had been needlessly amputated. Nothing unusual was found in a study of the fracture site.

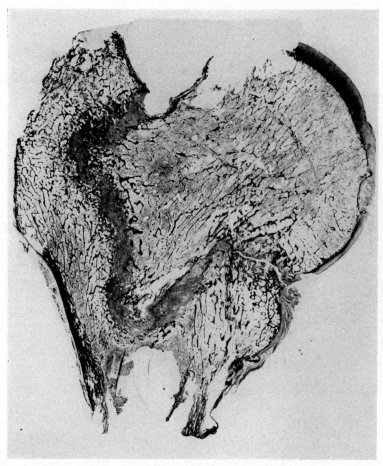

FIGURE 163. Fibrous union of a fracture at the base of the femoral neck. The femoral neck is telescoped into the greater trochanter. Impingement of the femoral head against the lesser trochanter has led to localized reactive osteosclerosis.

PSEUDOFRACTURES

McCullough classified the spontaneous non-displaced fractures and fissures in pathologic bones, particularly those in the malacic diseases, as pseudofractures. He emphasized the point that they are to be distinguished from March fractures by the fact that the latter occur in normal bones. March fractures generally exhibit more periosteal bone during healing than do pseudofractures.

Macey reported the case of a 36 year old white male who had pseudofractures in both femora and scapulae, the right tibia and fibula, left ulna, several ribs, and in several bones of the feet. A brother of the patient also had pseudofractures. Phosphatase was absent by test until after a bone graft had been implanted in the femur.

Weaver and Francisco described pseudofractures of the upper tibia in two males, ages 12 and 23, and of the external malleolus of a 21 year old male. In all three cases biopsies are said to have shown histologic evidence of chronic low grade inflammation. No organisms could be cultured. The authors concluded that pseudofractures in their cases were a manifestation of non-suppurative osteomyelitis.

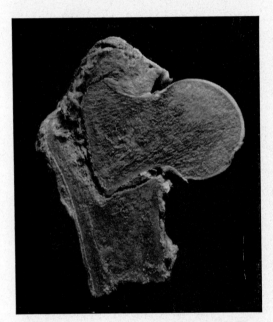

FIGURE 164. A rare instance in which a telescoped intertrochanteric fracture has developed into a nearthrosis.

PATHOLOGIC FRACTURES

Many of the details and most of the illustrations of pathologic fractures are included in the chapters presenting the subjects of chronic osteomyelitis, aseptic osseous necrosis, arthropathies, malacic diseases, congenital defects in skeletal ossification, bone cysts, and bone tumors.

A fracture frequently offers the first opportunity to identify the existence of a local or generalized pathologic process. It therefore is important for physicians treating fractures to have a knowledge of the various disease entities that at times are responsible for pathologic fractures. Keen judgment is required in selecting the proper therapy, and the very foundation of good judgment is a knowledge of pathologic anatomy.

The defects in bone structure that lead to pathologic fractures may be divided into: (1) Localized defects; (2) Regional defects; and, (3) Generalized defects.

LOCALIZED DEFECTS

This is a large group since it includes solitary bone cysts, and all of the bone tumors and dysplasias that create a defect in the bone. Virtually all bone tumors produce a defect in the host bone except the osteomas and exostoses. Localized defects leading to a pathologic fracture may also be created by adjacent soft tissue tumors or by an aneurysm.

It was long held that a fracture through an uncomplicated bone cyst led to healing of the cyst and reossification of the defect. It is now recognized that complete healing of a cyst following a fracture is rare. Frequently, however, a fracture does cause a cyst to diminish in size. If of sufficient size to warrant surgery, the cyst may be obliterated by curretage and insertion of bone chips.

Aseptic necrosis may lead to compression fractures of the head of the femur during regeneration, as already described. Fractures of the femoral neck have occurred at the site of aseptic necrosis from radiation therapy. Fibrous union has been the rule.

REGIONAL DEFECTS

Paget's disease creates defective osseous structure by regions; it is never generalized throughout the skeletal system. Pathologic fractures occur during two periods of the disease: (1) During the period in which osteoclasis predominates, the bone becomes soft and may collapse. (2) After a period in which new bone apposition

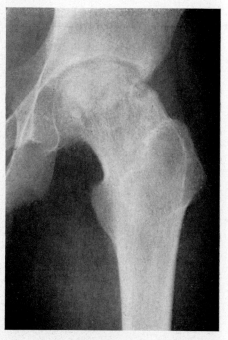

FIGURE 165. The end-result of a slipped upper femoral epiphysis. Following the displacement a pannus formed over much of the femoral head causing a fibrous ankylosis. An arthroplasty was done later.

predominates, the bone becomes sclerotic and may fracture from brittleness. Such fractures are generally transverse. Healing occurs on schedule if immobilization is adequate.

Regional defects may be caused by fibrous dysplasia, there being a regional distribution of osteoporosis and bone defects. Pathologic fractures through large bone defects often require bone transplants in order to restore continuity.

While senile osteoporosis may be generalized, it is more frequently regional, involving the spine in the majority of cases. Pathologic compression fractures of vertebral bodies are common, and are caused by the fragility of the porotic bone.

Disuse-atrophy of bone is ordinarily regional in its distribution. Pathologic fractures in such bone heal well.

GENERALIZED DEFECTS

This group may be divided into a congenital type which includes osteogenesis imperfecta and osteopetrosis, and an acquired form which includes rickets, osteomalacia, and hyperparathyroidism. Pathologic fractures are common in all forms of generalized defective bone structure. In spite of the pronounced alteration of the bones, pathologic fractures heal well in both osteogenesis imperfecta and osteopetrosis (marble bones). Healing of fractures takes place in rickets and osteomalacia, but the callus does not harden properly since the trabeculae remain in the osteoid stage. Pathologic fractures in hyperparathyroidism heal much better after the excessive parathyroid secretion is controlled through excision of the adenomatous of hyperplastic gland. In instances where cysts and brown tumors have destroyed a segment of a diaphysis, reossification may be impossible without excision of the cysts and the insertion of autogenous bone grafts.

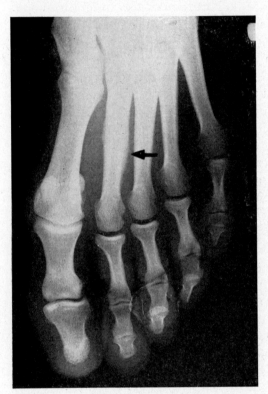

FIGURE 166. March fracture of the second metatarsal (arrow).

BONE GRAFTING

The use of bone grafts has attained such an important place in the treatment of fractures that a discussion of the interesting history of the subject as well as the histologic changes in bone grafts is in order. With increasingly reliable operating room facilities and an improved armamentarium, the uses of autogenous bone grafts have steadily broadened. The results have been gratifying.

HISTORY

Ollier in 1858, being the first to report the use of autogenous bone grafts, is referred to as the father of bone graft surgery. He recommended taking both the periosteum and the endosteum with the graft. On the basis of a great many experiments he came to the dual conclusion that the periosteum was osteogenic and contributed a great deal to the nutrition of the graft.

In 1893 Barth pointed out, in the bone graft experiments he had conducted, that all of the osteocytes in the bone transplants became necrotic. It was his view that the graft served only as an osteoconductive scaffold. Therefore he concluded that heterogenous grafts were as satisfactory as autogenous grafts. Naturally he claimed that there was no virtue in retaining the periosteum and endosteum.

Axhausen, Barth's contemporary, was impressed by what he considered osteogenic properties of the periosteum and endosteum. If allowed to remain intact on a bone graft the periosteum and endosteum survived and contributed substantially to the regeneration of the graft. He agreed with Barth that compact bone

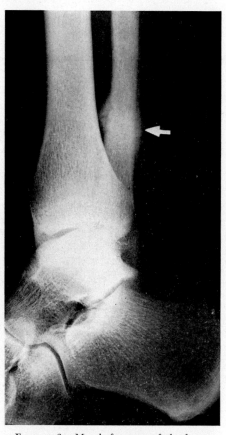

FIGURE 167. March fracture of the lower fibula (arrow).

grafts underwent aseptic necrosis and creeping regeneration.

Macewen heaped fuel upon the periosteum polemic in 1911 by contending that the periosteum was only a limiting membrane. When used to bridge fractures his bone grafts, denuded of both periosteum and endosteum, were rapidly followed by solid bony union.

In 1914 Phemister reported the results of numerous bone grafting experiments on the dog ulna. He demonstrated that osteogenesis takes place in bone grafts regardless of the integrity of the periosteum and endosteum, but when left intact, regeneration of the graft occurs more rapidly. He also observed that fractures through bone grafts heal by abundant callus. Aseptic necrosis developed throughout his cortical grafts with the exception of surface cells close to a source of nutrition. Another report in 1914 by Haas also emphasized the important part played by the periosteum and endosteum in the regeneration of bone.

In 1926 Leriche and Policard contended that the new bone forming in and around bone transplants was dependent upon resorption of the transplant for minerals.

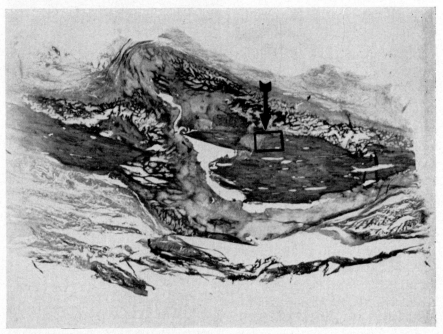

FIGURE 168. A. A fracture through an Albee bone graft of the spine for tuberculous spondylitis. The fracture site is filled with fibrous tissue and cartilage. Excessive bending stresses caused absorption in the center of the graft, and then a fracture.

Ghormley and Stuck in 1934 studied bone grafts that had been utilized in fusing the spines of dogs. Their conclusions include the following: " (1) Periosteal grafts in old animals do not produce new bone. (2) Cortical transplants do not completely die but unite slowly with the bone of their host, and decreased calcification is seen roentgenographically at the end of three months. (3) Cancellous bone unites more quickly and more firmly than cortical bone, whether taken from the cancellous bone of the ilium or from the endosteum of the tibia. It gives evidence of increased calcification roentgenographically at the end of three months."

In 1939 Franceschelli reported clinical and pathologic observations on four autogenous bone grafts examined 32 days to one year after the original surgery. He noted an intimate fusion to the host bone even after 32 days. All grafts oozed when cut but microscopically had large areas of necrosis. Reconstruction of the grafts began promptly after they were transplanted, with osteoclasis predominating at the outset and osteogenesis predominating during the later stages.

PERIOSTEUM OF THE GRAFT

Disagreement regarding the value of retaining the periosteum on bone transplants centers principally around the fibrous layer of the

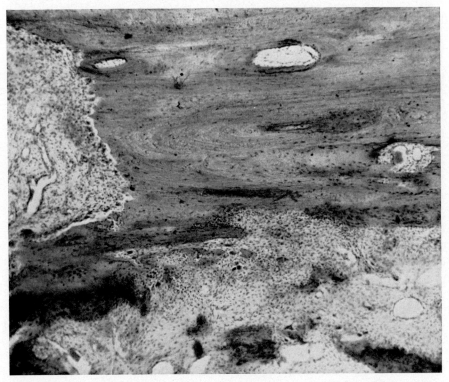

FIGURE 168. *(Continued)* B. Photomicrograph of the area in the square marked on A. The fracture surface of the graft is lined with osteoclasts.

periosteum. On the point that the cambium layer is useful to the graft there is agreement. Hey Groves refers to the cambium layer as the epiosteum and considers it to be a part of the bone. This leaves only the fibrous layer as the true periosteum, which all agree is neither osteogenic nor essential to health and nutrition of the graft. Since it is difficult to remove all of the fibrous periosteum without disturbing areas of the cambium layer (or epiosteum), it is recommended that a thin portion of the fibrous layer be left attached to the graft.

In children there is a line of cleavage between the fibrous and cambium layers, and blunt stripping of the periosteum leaves most of the cambium cells with the cortex. In a healthy environment both layers of the periosteum readily regenerate after excision.

Periosteal bone forms on the surface of a bone graft in the same manner as at a fracture site; it is primary fibrous bone at the outset and later is replaced by secondary lamellar bone. Periosteal and endosteal bone play an essential part in fusing the graft to its bed.

Types of Autogenous Bone Grafts

There is no concurrence as to the best type of autogenous graft to employ. The osteogenic potentialities of the various types of grafts have been intensively investigated. Cortical grafts have been compared to cancellous grafts; multiple small grafts, compared to the single solid graft; and grafts from the tibia, compared with grafts from the ilium.

McWilliams believes that the multiple small grafts have a better opportunity to survive. Phemister and Keith stress the importance of function in stimulating new bone, and this they believe demands that the graft be both solid and mechanically fixed. Solitary large cortical grafts give immediate fixation and stability, not possible with cancellous or fragmented grafts. Ghormley and Stuck demonstrated that cancellous grafts fused better to the host bone and were much more rapidly regenerated.

When stability at the site of the graft must be secured through internal fixation, it is necessary to use a solid graft of compact bone, a metal plate, or both. Cancellous chip grafts may be packed around the fracture site when a plate is used. In the past the solitary cortical graft has been the most popular, but the pendulum is now swinging toward a wider use of cancellous bone. This change to multiple cancellous bone grafts has a sound basis both in experimental results, and clinical practice. The rapid regeneration of cancellous bone plus the large osteogenic element that is able to remain viable, makes it more effective in bridging bone defects. War surgery has played a part in raising the stature of cancellous grafts.

Aseptic Necrosis in Bone Grafts

Since the turn of the century there has gradually evolved a widespread agreement on the point that in cortical bone transplants much of the bone (although not all) undergoes aseptic necrosis. This is due of course to removal of the bone from its blood circulation. Imbibition serves to maintain life only in those cells that lie close to the surfaces of the graft. As already described, the necrotic areas are replaced by "creeping substitution" made possible through the ingrowth of adjacent cellular and vascular elements. Thin cortical grafts have necrosis in a smaller proportion of their area than have thick cortical grafts. Cancellous bone generally undergoes less necrosis than compact bone. An area of necrosis in a cancellous graft is much more rapidly regenerated than a similar-sized area in a cortical graft.

HETEROGENOUS BONE GRAFTS, IVORY, AND COW'S HORN

Beef bone grafts and such materials as ivory and cow's horn have been employed with variable success. Henderson observed no unfavorable reactions to beef bone. The beef bone is said to be slowly replaced by living bone. Ivory pegs have been used, and, in Groves' experiments on cats, were well tolerated. No absorption and replacement occurs with ivory. In the use of cow's horn transplants, Siegling and Fahey were unable to demonstrate any significant absorption after seven and one-half months, and there was no stimulation of osteogenesis. Autogenous grafts and refrigerated grafts

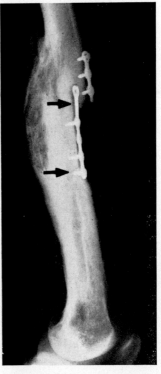

FIGURE 169. Osteitis around a metal plate (arrows). The plate is too narrow, the screws too short, and the metal is electrolytic.

are far superior in the way they are tolerated and their capacity to stimulate osteogenesis. Beef bone and ivory pegs and screws have been largely replaced by nonelectrolytic metal screws and pins.

REACTION OF BONE TO METALS

Metals long were used as a means of securing internal fixation of fractures in spite of an unexplained high incidence of osteitis around the metal. In 1927, Dahl-Iverson reported that a reactive osteitis had occurred in 28 per cent of 174 cases in which Lane plates had been employed. Lambotte, in 1911, stated that it had been necessary to remove 46 per cent of the metal plates in the series of cases that he reviewed.

In 1937, Venable, Stuck and Beach demonstrated that the corrosion of the metal plates, pins, and screws that had been used in bone surgery was due principally to electrolysis. The metals had promoted electrolysis in the body fluids, thereby creating an electric battery in the bone. Adjacent tissue fluids became the electrolyte, and in time galvanic action produced metallic salts that were irritating to the tissues. An osteitis followed, together with an impairment of osteogenesis. Venable and Stuck, in several reports, described experiments with different metals in their search for a metal that would be electrically neutral in the body fluids. They found that a combination of cobalt, chromium, and tungsten, called vitallium, was the most nearly 100 per cent inert and was entirely immune from corrosion. It has been discovered that, when a metal is electrically inert in a given fluid, the metal surface protects itself from damage through the creation of a "molecular veil" that covers the metal.

Stainless steels of the type having 18 percent chromium and 8 percent nickel have been widely used. Key found S.M.O. 18-8 stainless steel to be better tempered, less brittle and less expensive than vitallium. He concluded that its mechanical advantages outweighed its slight tendency to corrosion. In a later paper Key pointed out that it is unwise to mix stainless steels in the same operative site. A reactive osteitis developed in several of his cases when one type of stainless steel was used in the plate and another type in the screws.

Certain metals such as chromium, copper and manganese, when set free through electrolysis or through chemical reaction can form poisonous metallic salts. Bothe, Beaton and Davenport did multiple metallic implants and observed numerous toxic reactions to the implants.

Pure metals are electrically inert in the tissues. The local and systemic reactions that occur between pure metals and the tissue fluids are chemical reactions, in which a part of the metal is dissolved by acids in the tissue fluids.

REFERENCES

FRACTURES

ANNERSTEN, S.: Fracture healing. Alkalinization in callus. *Arch. f. klin. Chir., 203*:122, 1942.

BANCROFT, J. W.: Process of union after fracture. *Ann. Surg., 90*:546, 1929.

BERG, R. and KUGELMASS, I. N.: Calcification in callus formation and fracture repair. *Ann. Surg., 93*:1009, 1931.

BLAISDELL, F. E. and COWAN, J. F.: Healing of simple fractures. An experimental study. *Arch. Surg., 12*:619, 1926.

BOTTERELL, E. H. and KING, E. S. J.: Phosphatase in fractures. *Lancet, 1*:1267, 1935.

BRUSH, H. V.: The effects of thyroxin and stilbestrol on healing of fractures in the rat. *Am. J. Anat., 76*:339, 1945.

COMPERE, E. L., HAMILTON, B. and DEWAR, M.: The influence of Vit. D upon bone repair. The healing of fractures of rachitic bones. *Surg. Gynec. & Obst. 68*:878, 1939.

Downs, W. B., Jr. and McKeown, R. M.: Histology of healing fractures in rats on normal diets. *Arch. Surg., 25*:94, 1932.

Goisman, J. and Compere, E. L.: The healing of fractures of atrophic bones. *J. Bone & Joint Surg., 20*:587, 1938.

Granger, R. C.: The effect of viosterol on periosteum in experimental fractures. *Arch. Surg., 25*:1035, 1932.

Groves, E. W. H.: *Modern Methods of Treating Fractures.* 2nd Ed. Wm. Woods & Co., New York, 1922.

Groves, E. W. H.: Repair of bone injuries. *Brit. M. J., 10*:440, 1922.

Haldeman, K. O.: The role of periosteum in the healing of fractures. An experimental study. *Arch. Surg., 24*:440, 1932.

Haldeman, K. O. and Moore, J. M.: Influence of local excess of calcium and phosphorus on the healing of fractures. *Arch. Surg., 29*:385, 1934.

Ham, A. W.: Early phases of bone repair (after experimental fracture). *J. Bone & Joint Surg., 12*:827, 1930.

Ham, A. W., Tisdall, F. F., and Drake, T. G. H.: Experimental non-calcification of callus simulating non-union. *J. Bone & Joint Surg., 20*:345, 1938.

Keith, Sir A.: Bone growth and bone repair. *Brit. J. Surg., 5*:685, 1917; *6*:19, 1918; *6*:160, 1918.

Key, A.: The effect of a local calcium deposit on osteogenesis and healing of fractures. *J. Bone & Joint Surg., 16*:176, 1934.

Kulowski, J. and Luck, J. V.: Microscopic changes after internal fixation of transcervical fracture of the femur. *J. Bone & Joint Surg., 23*:17, 1941.

Kushner, A.: Evaluation of Wolff's law of bone formation. *J. Bone & Surg., 22*:589, 1940.

Leriche, R. and Policard, A.: *The Normal and Pathological Physiology of Bone.* Translation by Moore, S. and Key, J. A. C. V. Mosby, St. Louis, 1928.

Levander, G.: A study of bone regeneration. *Surg. Gynec. & Obst., 67*:705, 1938.

Levander, G.: An experimental study of the role of the bone marrow in bone regeneration. *Acta chir. Scandinav., 83*:545, 1940.

Lindsay, M. K.: Observations on fracture healing in rats. *J. Bone & Joint Surg., 16*:62, 1934.

Lindsay, M. K. and Howes, E. L.: Breaking strength of healing fractures. *J. Bone & Joint Surg., 13*:491, 1931.

Luck, J. V.: A reconstruction operation for pseudarthrosis and resorption of the neck of the femur. *J. Iowa M. Soc., 28*:620, 1938.

McGaw, W. H. and Harbin, M.: The role of bone marrow and endosteum in bone regeneration. *J. Bone & Joint Surg., 16*:816, 1934.

McLean, F. C. and Bloom, W.: Calcification and ossification. Calcification in normal growing bone. *Anat. Rec., 78*:333, 1940.

Moritz, A. R.: The Pathology of Trauma. Lea and Febiger, Philadelphia, 1942.

Morrison, G. M.: Promotion of fracture repair. *J. Bone & Joint Surg., 19*:425, 1937.

Morton, D. J. and Engle, E. T.: Passive hyperemia as a means of hastening or obtaining union. *J. Bone & Joint Surg., 13*:381, 1931.

Murray, C. R.: Healing of fractures; its influence on the choice of methods of treatment. *Arch. Surg., 29*:446, 1934.

Murray, C. R.: The pathological process following fracture and treatment methods. *Indust. Med., 10*:171, 1941.

Murray, C. R.: The time of fracture healing. *J. Bone & Joint Surg., 23*:598, 1941.

Phemister, D. B.: Bone growth and repair. *Ann. Surg., 102*:261, 1935.

Phemister, D. B.: The repair of bone in the presence of aseptic necrosis resulting from fractures, transplantations, and vascular obstruction. *J. Bone & Joint Surg., 12*:769, 1930.

Potts, W. J.: The role of the hematoma in fracture healing. *Surg. Gynec. & Obst., 57*:318, 1933.

Ravdin, I. S. and Jonas, L.: Calcium and phosphorus metabolism in the fracture of bones. *Ann. Surg., 84*:37, 1926.

SPEED, K. and RIDER, D. L.: Experimental healing of bone after parathyroidectomy. *Arch. Surg., 21*:679, 1930.

STIRLING, R. I.: The report of an investigation into the process of the healing of fractured bones, with some clinical applications. *Edinburgh M. J., 39*:203, 1932.

SWART, H. A.: Effect of irradiated ergosterol on healing of experimentally produced fractures in animals. *J. Bone & Joint Surg., 21*:360, 1930.

TODD, T. W.: The role of cancellous tissue in healing bone. *Ann. Surg., 72*:452, 1920.

TODD, T. W. and ILER, D. H.: The phenomenon of the early stages of bone repair. *Ann. Surg., 86*:715, 1927.

URIST, M. R.: The role of local transfer of bone salt in the calcification of the fracture callus. *South. M. J., 24*:48, 1942.

URIST, M. R. and McLEAN, F. C.: I. Calcification and ossification. *J. Bone & Joint Surg., 23*:1, 1941.

URIST, M. R. and McLEAN, F. C.: Calcification and ossification. II. Control of calcification in the fracture callus in rachitic rats. *J. Bone & Joint Surg., 23*:283, 1941.

URIST, M. R.: Calcification and ossification. III. The role of local transfer of bone salt in the calcification of fracture callus. *J. Bone & Joint Surg., 24*:47, 1942.

URIST, M. R. and JOHNSON, R. W.: Calcification and ossification. IV. The healing of fractures in man under clinical conditions. *J. Bone & Joint Surg., 25*:375, 1943.

WATSON-JONES, R.: Fractures and Joint Injuries, 3rd Ed. Williams and Wilkins Co., Baltimore, 1944.

DELAYED AND NON-UNION

ANDERSON, R. and BURGESS, E.: Delayed union and non-union. *J. Bone & Joint Surg., 25*:427, 1943.

COWAN, J. F.: Non-union of fractures: An experimental and clinical study. *Ann. Surg., 88*:749, 1928.

FREUND, E.: Histologie der nearthrose nach Shenkelhalbrüchen. *Beitr. z. path. Anat. u. z. allg. Path., 85*:101, 1930.

McMURRAY, T. P.: Delay in the union of fractures. *Brit. M. J., 1*:8, 1942.

MOORE, J. R.: Delayed reduction of fractures. *J. Bone & Joint Surg., 26*:151, 1944.

MURRAY, C. R.: Delayed and non-union in fractures in the adult. *Ann. Surg., 93*:961, 1931.

MURRAY, C. R.: The basic problems in bone grafting for un-united compound fractures. *J. Bone & Joint Surg., 26*:437, 1944.

ROADS, J. E. and KASINSKAS, W.: The influence of hypoproteinemia on the formation of callus in experimental fractures. *Surgery, 11*:38, 1942.

SPEED, K.: Non-union after fracture. *Ann. Surg., 90*:574, 1929.

WATSON-JONES, R. and COLTART, W. D.: Slow union of fractures of shafts of tibia and femur. *Brit. J. Surg., 30*:260, 1943.

MARCH FRACTURES

BREITHAUPT, H. S.: Zur pathologie des menschlichen Fusses. *Med. Ztg. Berlin, 24*:169, 1855.

CHILDRESS, H. M.: March fractures of the lower extremity. *War Medicine, 4*:152, 1943.

DODD, H.: Pied forcé or march foot. *Brit. J. Surg., 21*:131, 1933.

HARTLEY, J. B.: Fatigue fractures of the tibia. *Brit. J. Surg., 30*:9, 1942.

MYERDING, H. W. and POLLOCK, G. A.: March fracture. *Surg. Gynec. & Obst., 67*:234, 1938.

PETERSON, L. R.: March fracture of the femur. *J. Bone & Joint Surg., 24*:185, 1942.

SPEED, J. S. and BLAKE, T. H.: March foot. *J. Bone & Joint Surg., 33*:373, 1933.

STRAUS, F. H.: Marching fractures of metatarsal bones with report of pathology. *Surg. Gynec. & Obst., 54*:581, 1932.

PSEUDOFRACTURES

MACEY, H. G.: Pseudofractures. A case report. *Proc. Staff Meet., Mayo Clin., 15*:789, 1940.

McCULLOUGH, J. A. L.: Pseudofractures in diseases affecting the skeletal system. *Proc. Staff Meet., Mayo Clinic, 15*:785, 1940.
WEAVER, J. B. and FRANCISCO, C. B.: Pseudofractures: A manifestation of non-suppurative osteomyelitis. *J. Bone & Joint Surg., 22*:610, 1940.

BONE GRAFTING

ALBEE, F. H.: Fundamentals in bone transplantation. *J. A. M. A., 81*:1429, 1923.
ALBEE, F. H.: Evolution of bone graft surgery. *Am. J. Surg., 63*:421, 1944.
AXHAUSEN, G.: Histologische untersuchunger uber knochentransplantation am menschen. *Deutsche Ztschr. f. Chir., 91*:388, 1908.
BANCROFT, F. W.: The use of small bone transplants in bridging a bone defect. *Ann. Surg., 67*:457, 1918.
BARTH, A.: Ueber osteoplastik. *Arch. f. klin. Chir., 48*:466, 1894; *86*:859, 1908.
GALLIE, W. E.: Transplantation of bone. *Brit. M. J., 2*:840, 1931.
GALLIE, W. E. and ROBERTSON, D. E.: The transplantation of bone. *J. A. M. A., 70*:1134, 1918.
GHORMLEY, R. K.: Choice of graft methods in bone and joint surgery. *Ann. Surg., 115*:427, 1942.
GHORMLEY, R. K. and STUCK, W. B.: Experimental bone transplantation. *Arch. Surg., 28*:742, 1934.
GROVES, E. W. H.: Methods and results of transplantation of bone. *Brit. J. Surg., 5*:185, 1917.
HAAS, S. L.: The importance of the periosteum and endosteum in the repair of transplanted bone. *Arch. Surg., 8*:535, 1924.
HALDEMAN, K. O.: The influence of periosteum on the survival of bone grafts. *J. Bone & Joint Surg., 15*:302, 1933.
HELLSTADINS, A.: The ability of bone tissue to survive in pedicled grafts. *Acta chir. Scandinav., 86*:85, 1942.
HUGHES, C. W.: Rate of absorption and callus stimulating properties of cowhorn, ivory, beef bone, and autogenous bone. *Surg., Gynec. & Obst., 76*:665, 1943.
INCLAN, A.: Use of preserved bone graft in orthopedic surgery. *J. Bone & Joint Surg., 24*:81, 1942.
McWILLIAMS, C. A.: The periosteum in bone transplantations. *J. A. M. A., 62*:346, 1914.
McWILLIAMS, C. A.: The values of the various methods of bone graftings judged by 1390 reported cases. *Ann. Surg., 74*:286, 1921.
MACEWEN, W.: The osteogenic factors in the development and repair of bone. *Ann. Surg., 6*:289, 1887.
MACEWEN, W.: Intrahuman bone grafting and reimplantation. *Ann. Surg., 50*:959, 1909.
MAY, H.: The regeneration of bone transplants. *Ann. Surg., 106*:441, 1937.
OLLIER, LEOPOLD: *Traité des la régénération des os. Traité des réséctions.* Paris 1891.
PHEMISTER, D. B.: The fate of transplanted bone and regenerative power of its various constituents. *Surg., Gynec. & Obst., 19*:303, 1914.
POLLOCK, G. and HENDERSON, M. S.: Value of periosteum in grafting operations. *Proc. Staff Meet., Mayo Clinic, 15*:443, 1940.
POLLOCK, W. E., McKENNEY, P. W. and BLAISDELL, F. E.: The viability of transplanted bone; an experimental study. *Arch. Surg., 18*:607, 1929.
STEWART, W. J.: Experimental bone regeneration using lime salts and autogenous grafts as a source of available calcium. *Surg., Gynec. & Obst., 59*:867, 1934.

REACTION OF BONE TO METALS

BOTHE, R. T., BEATON, L. E. and DAVENPORT, H. A.: Reaction of bone to multiple metalic implants. *Surg., Gynec. & Obst., 71*:598, 1940; *74*:231, 1942.
BURKE, G. L.: Tantalum. *Canad. M. A. J., 43*:125, 1940.
DAHL-IVERSON, E.: Later examination of 66 cases of surgically treated fractures. *Hospitalstid, 70*:449, 1927.

KEY, J. A.: Stainless steel and vitallium in internal fixation of bone: A comparison. *Arch. Surg.*, 1941.

VENABLE, C. S., STUCK, W. G. and BEACH, ASA: The effects on bone of the presence of metals; based upon electrolysis. *Ann. Surg., 105*:917, 1937.

VENABLE, C. S. and STUCK, W. G.: Three years' experience with vitallium. *Ann. Surg., 114*:309, 1941.

VENABLE, C. S. and STUCK, W. G.: *The Internal Fixation of Fractures.* Charles C Thomas, Springfield, 1947.

VON BAEYER, H.: Foreign bodies in the tissues. *Beitr. z. klin. Chir., 58*:1, 1908.

CHAPTER VI

Chronic Arthritis

Contents

This chapter will be devoted principally to a description of two immensely important types of chronic arthritis—osteoarthritis and rheumatoid arthritis. These chronic arthritides, their differentiation so frequently misunderstood, present vast differences in their pathogenesis and pathologic anatomy. An understanding of the pathology of these diseases is mandatory to the proper interpretation of clinical manifestations and an intelligent administration of therapeutic measures.

OSTEO-ARTHRITIS

Osteo-arthritis has been recognized in man and numerous other vertebrates for centuries, and unquestionably had its origin in prehistoric times. Although formerly associated exclusively with senility, we now know that it frequently occurs in the middle aged and occasionally in the young. The terminology of this form of arthritis continues to be confusing and for a good reason. Since the etiology is unknown the many investigators who have written about this disease have used a variety of criteria for their terms. The clinician has used the symptomatology as a basis, the pathologist the gross and microscopic pictures, and

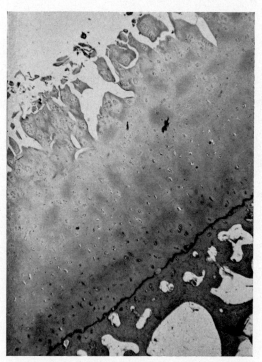

FIGURE 170. Early degenerative changes in the articular cartilage manifest by fibrillation and Weichselbaum's lacunae in superficial layers and mottled calcification of the deep layers (Erdheim's law of protectio-calcification).

the roentgenologist his roentgenograms. Since Virchow, the Germans have called the disease arthritis deformans; the English, following the Garrods, have called it osteoarthritis; and the French, after Charcot, called it partial chronic articular rheumatism.

In the United States the several new terms that have been added to designate this joint syndrome include Nichols and Richardson's term, degenerative arthritis; Goldthwait's term, hypertrophic arthritis; Ely's term, Type II arthritis; the term used by Hodges, Phemister and Brunschwig, chronic osteoarthrosis; and the term suggested (1936) by Bauer and Bennett, degenerative joint disease. To the laity the disease is simply rheumatism. When most laymen think of arthritis they think of the rheumatoid type. Were the author to yield to temptation to add another to the already long list of confusing synonyms, he would call the disease chondromalacic arthrosis. Out of respect for the monumental contributions of Nichols and Richardson in 1909, and because their terminology is based upon pathologic studies, their term, degenerative arthritis, has been widely used by pathologists. After giving the matter thorough consideration the American Rheumatism Association has recommended the Garrod terms: osteo-arthritis and rheumatoid arthritis. These terms will be the ones used in this treatise.

ETIOLOGY

The etiology of osteo-arthritis is unknown, but many of the contributing factors are well understood and may be outlined as follows:

1. Senescence *(Senescent osteo-arthritis)*
2. Trauma *(Traumatic osteo-arthritis)*
3. Static deviations *(Static osteo-arthritis)*
4. Constitutional predisposition *(Constitutional osteo-arthritis)*

1. **Senescent osteo-arthritis:** Every joint develops some degree of osteo-arthritis during senility; in fact, the disease has been termed senile arthritis. With the advent of senescence, degeneration and malacia take place in the articular surfaces, more so in the weight bearing joints than in the non-weight bearing joints. There is profound variation in the degree of osteo-arthritis encountered in a given age group. One individual may have advanced generalized changes at 50 and another, minimal changes at 70. But in general the older the individual, the more generalized and advanced are the degenative joint changes. This is not to imply that all aging individuals have symptoms from their senescent joint changes. Actually only a small percent have disability beyond moderate stiffness and some "creaking."

2. **Traumatic osteo-arthritis:** Trauma, in a broad sense, is a factor in the development of all osteo-arthritis, but in this category will be included only those cases in which a specific known trauma has played a part in the joint changes. Trauma to joints may be sizeable and solitary or microscopic and multiple. For example, a fracture may enter a joint and represent a single great trauma; whereas, changes wrought in the joint surfaces by the fracture may inflict micro-traumata upon the joint during each joint movement for the duration of the patient's life. Trauma to a joint may come in a thousand forms: from the vibration of pneumatic trip-hammers, the heavy loads of longshoremen, loose bodies or torn menisci in the joint, contusions, torn ligaments, dislocations, etc. Charcot joints in advanced stages are caricatures of osteo-arthritis, and the traumatic factor plays a tremendous part in the genesis of the pathologic anatomy.

3. **Static osteo-arthritis:** When a joint is malaligned from a deformity or malposture, it can be expected to develop degenerative changes earlier than similar joints having normal mechanics. For example, when a knee is in a valgus position (knock-knee) the weight bearing stresses are concentrated in the lateral condyles of the tibia and femur.

This increased load eventually leads to degenerative changes in the lateral half of the joint from excessive wear and tear. Pronated or cavus feet, valgum or varum of the ankle, knee or hip, and an acute lumbo-sacral angle are all examples of static deviations that subject the involved joints to excessive wear and tear through an improper distribution of stresses over the articular surfaces. Congenital bone and joint defects, obesity and nutritional deficiencies often lead to static degenerative arthritis.

4. **Constitutional osteo-arthritis:** There is reason to believe that all articular cartilage is not of uniform quality. In some individuals the articular surfaces wear thin by middle age; whereas in others little wear and tear is evident even in old age. This observation refers to the generalized type of osteo-arthritis, not the localized form accruing from a joint injury or mechanical abnormality. The wide variation in the age period when degenerative joint changes appear has led many observers to assume that a constitutional factor exists that determines the intrinsic wearing capacity of the articular cartilage.

Other theories: That the foregoing etiologic factors overlap and do not include certain other much discussed factors is readily admitted. Senescence of the cartilage and a traumatic factor exist in all forms of osteo-arthritis, but, from a didactic viewpoint, it is helpful to classify cases of osteo-arthritis according to the factor that appears dominant in the known aspect of the etiology.

Innumerable theories have been offered through the years to explain the etiology, many of which have been completely discarded or else found tenable for the explanation of only rare and exceptional cases. The *infection theory* has been discarded, since no evidence exists in the pathologic studies to suggest the presence of inflammation. Focal infection has appeared to aggravate clinical symptoms in certain cases of degenerative arthritis, but this too is being challenged. Etiologic theories based upon intestinal stasis, amoebic infections, arterio-sclerosis and other vascular diseases, and endocrine unbalance have been widely abandoned. Aseptic necrosis in a small or large area of subchondral bone may lead to alterations in joint contour, and set the stage for the ultimate development of osteo-arthritis. But to explain osteo-arthritic changes on the basis of aseptic necrosis in the cartilage or underlying bone has no foundation in fact.

A joint infection from a pyogenic organism or involvement by proliferative arthritis may subside short of complete joint destruction, and be followed by restoration of function. Osteo-arthritis develops in such joints from the damage wrought by the burned-out inflammation, but it must not be concluded that the inflammation actually caused the osteo-arthritis. The residual damage from the inflammation predisposed the joint to early chondromalacia through a process of premature cartilage degeneration.

As will be described later, gout and hemophilia may also damage joints and establish the sequence of events that terminate in chondromalacic arthrosis.

It is tempting to attribute osteo-arthritis to ovarian and other endocrine deficiencies. Many cases of generalized osteo-arthritis in women

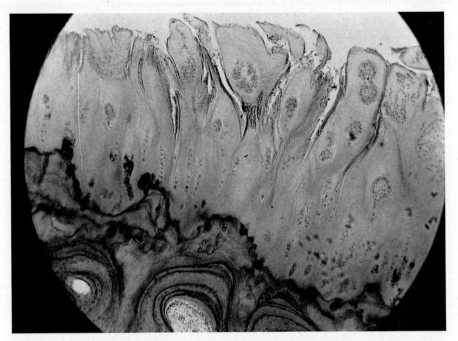

FIGURE 171. Advanced fibrillation of the articular cartilage and increased density of the articular cortex (Femoral head, Figure 174, at arrow).

become symptomatic during the menopause. However, neither an endocrine nor a metabolic etiologic factor has as yet been definitely established.

PATHOLOGIC ANATOMY AND PATHOGENESIS

A vast literature has grown out of the great number of studies and experiments that have been carried out to elucidate the pathology of arthritis. The following investigators are among the many to whom we are indebted for our present knowledge of this important subject: Nichols and Richardson, Pommer, Heine, Heberden, Weichselbaum, Charcot, the Garrods, Wm. Hunter, Virchow, Echner, Volkmann,

Schmorl, Erdheim, Knaggs, Fisher, Adams, Goldthwait, Ely, Keefer, Freund, Bauer and Bennett, Allison and Ghormley, and Key.

Early Stage

The initial lesion is manifest, not in the capsule or bone, but in the articular cartilage, and is believed to represent an impairment of elasticity. This assumption is logical but has not been proved. The first visible change is manifest as degeneration of the non-calcified hyaline articular cartilage, and the sequence of events which follows softening of the cartilage is thought to result from impairment of the shock-absorbing action possessed by normal articular cartilage. In the early stage gross examination discloses some interesting surface changes. Whereas normal articular cartilage is wet, smooth, glistening and hyaline in appearance, degenerating cartilage appears dry, dull, granular, opaque and yellowish. Microscopically, the earliest evidence of the degeneration appears in the form of Weichselbaum's lacunae (Fig. 170). The cartilage cells proliferate within their lacunae and simultaneously encroach upon the wall of matricial substance enclosing them, thereby greatly enlarging the lacunar space. Ten to twenty cartilage cells are often seen in a single large Weichselbaum's lacuna. The cells themselves may later undergo degeneration and become stellate shaped. The next alteration of the cartilage is seen as a flaking off of the superficial or gliding layer of the articular surface, and is brought about by the friction of joint motion. Some of the Weichselbaum's lacunae then open at the joint surface, giving the surface an irregular pitted outline.

Degenerative changes in the hyaline matrix disrupts the binding material of the collagenous fiber bundles, rendering many collagenous bundles visible microscopically (Fig. 171). These fibers, it will be recalled, run in a direction radial to the articular surface. As the degenerative process advances, many of the collagenous bundles separate, giving rise to the familiar picture of fissures and fibrillation. Fibrillation is best observed in non-weight bearing portions of the articular cartilage, such as the femoral trochlea. Placed under water, the fibrils may float erect and waver resembling plush. In weight-bearing areas the delicate collagen fibrils are quickly worn off. Small cyst-like areas of mucoid degeneration are sometimes seen in the deeper layers of the cartilage. With the formation of clefts or fissures, the synovial fluid has a ready access to deeper layers. This is believed by some investigators to furnish additional nourishment, which accounts for the frequently observed cartilage proliferation in the fissure walls. A local piling up of cartilage may result, giving rise to an irregular, infolding surface.

Rather commonly a body of cartilage is gradually crowded out to become a joint mouse. Shaddock has called these cartilage formations epiarticular ecchondroses.

Calcification occurs in the degenerating articular cartilage in an irregular inconsistent manner, and is most evident in the deeper layers. Erdheim referred to this as protective calcification and considered it an attempt to reinforce the deteriorating articular cartilage.

SUBCHONDRAL RESPONSES: As the cartilage alterations develop, some important changes make their appearance in the subchondral bone

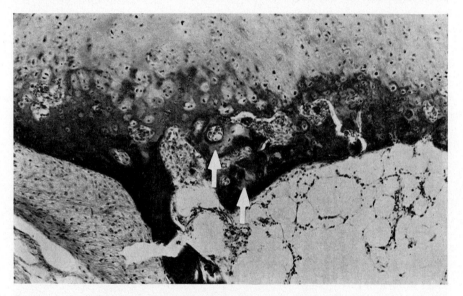

FIGURE 172A. Articular cartilage with reactivated enchondral ossification. (Arrows point to intratrabecular islands of calcified cartilage.)

and marrow. The bone tends to increase in density beneath weight-bearing areas, and to decrease in density outside of these areas. Varying degrees of marrow fibrosis evolve. **In adults a reactivation of enchondral ossification takes place as pointed out by Pommer.** Osteoclastic cells in the subchondral marrow spaces begin resorbing notch-like inroads in the subchondral lamellar plate. The notches ultimately become perforations that expose the zone of provisory calcification, which is then invaded. Osteoblasts lay down osteoid along the borders of the microscopic channels just as occurs in normal enchondral ossification. The deeper cartilage cells frequently assume a column arrangement. Cartilage matrix between the cartilage cell columns calcifies to reform the zone of provisory calcification (Fig. 172).

CAPSULE: The capsule undergoes little or no visible change during the early stage of osteo-arthritis.

Moderately Advanced Stage

As function in the joint continues, the adaptive changes developing in response to the chondromalacia, assert themselves in several different ways. The cartilage, soft and fibrillated, becomes progressively thinner in those areas subjected to the friction of articulating. In time, even the

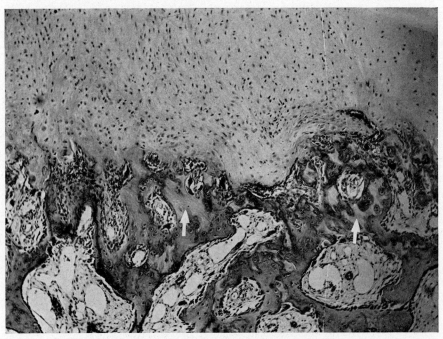

FIGURE 172B. Enchondral ossification in a marginal osteophyte.

zone of provisory calcification may be worn off, leaving areas where the articular cortex is entirely denuded.

While the above alterations in the articular cartilage are evolving, marginal osteophytes make their appearance. These marginal osteophytes or exostoses, vary widely in size and shape. Their origin has been variously explained. Many have believed them to be from perichondrium and periosteum; Nichols and Richardson supported this belief. Pommer has shown us that these osteophytes arise from reactivation of enchondral ossification. In his functional theory of degenerative arthritis Pommer attributes the changes to function. Without function, true osteo-arthritic changes do not appear. There is much clinical and pathologic evidence to support this theory. Immobility in the presence of degenerated articular cartilage does not promote true degenerative arthritic changes. The size and form of marginal osteophytes seems intimately linked with the activity and mechanical stresses to which the joint is subjected.

PATHOGENESIS OF MARGINAL EXOSTOSES: With reactivation of enchondral ossification, length growth is attempted, but does not succeed to a significant degree. The only place where new growth does not meet prohibitive resistance is at the periphery. The mother tissue that creates the cartilage for the process of reactivated enchondral ossification develops in the deep layers of the articular cartilage, or just peripheral to the articular cartilage. At the periphery the mother tissue develops from a reflection of synovial membrane, or from periosteum transformed to perichondrium. A marginal lip of cartilage forms and is replaced by cancellous bone; the enchondral process continues in this manner until the marginal osteophyte ceases growing. The density of a marginal exostosis varies from a state of osteosclerosis to one of pronounced porosis, depending upon the stresses to which it is subjected. At times an osteophyte appears "blown up," consisting of a thin lamellar cortex filled with fatty marrow and thin trabeculae. A thin layer of fibrocartilage may cover the surface. If the osteophyte takes an active part in the articulation it may become covered by a fairly thick layer of hyaline cartilage.

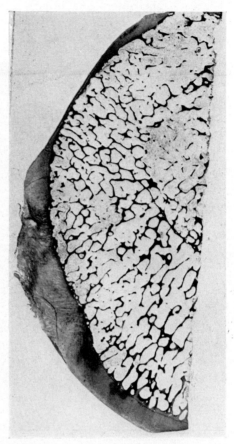

FIGURE 173. Osteoarthritic changes in the femoral head. The articular cartilage has worn thin in the superior half of the head without associated sclerosis of the articular cortex.

The extent to which new bone has formed by the reactivated enchondral ossification may frequently be determined by finding a permanent landmark left by the old articular cortex or by the old zone of provisory calcification. Portions of the transverse lamellar bony plate that formerly constituted the articular cortex may remain behind and may include with it variable amounts of calcified cartilage. These landmarks are more evident peripherally than centrally.

CAPSULAR CHANGES: Not uncommonly after the early stage the capsule undergoes conspicuous changes that are the result of hyperplasia. The proliferation causes the synovial membrane to form fringes and folds.

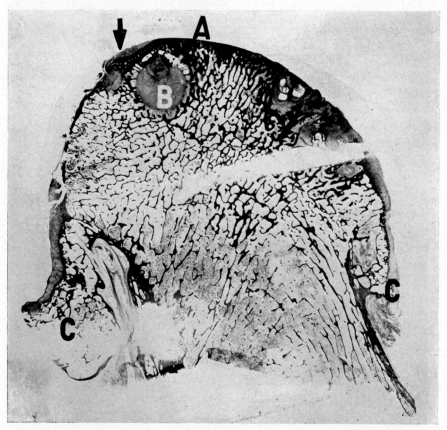

FIGURE 174. Histologic section of a femoral head involved in far advanced osteoarthritic changes. *A*. Eburnation of the articular cortex. All articular cartilage has worn off, except at site of arrow (see Figure 171). *B*. Subchondral "cyst" filled with dense fibrous tissue. *C*. Large marginal osteophytes.

The villi opposite the joint may undergo hyperplasia to the extent that primary villi with their numerous secondary villi hang from the synovialis like microscopic clusters of grapes. A rather pronounced hyperemia may be present, especially during function. But it needs to be said that it is not unusual to see a virtually normal capsule in the presence of even advanced cartilage changes.

CAPSULAR OSTEOCHONDROMATA: Nests of cartilage cells may make their appearance in the synovial membrane and develop into few or many cartilage bodies. Their origin is a matter of speculation. The most tenable theory explains their origin on the basis of mesenchymal cell rests. As described in Chapter I, the capsule shares a common embryologic origin with the perichondrium and periosteum. Another theory states that capsular chondromata form by direct metaplasia of capsular tissue to cartilage.

As the capsular chondromata enlarge they often calcify centrally. Following the deposition of calcium, blood vessels penetrate the cartilage body and make their way to the zone of calcification.

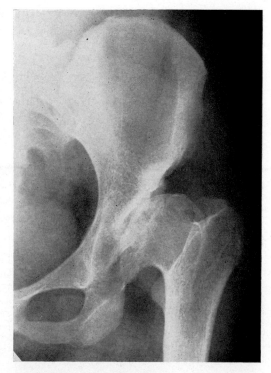

FIGURE 175. Osteoarthritis developing in a young adult due to a congenitally shallow acetabulum and a defective femoral head.

Chondroclasts then resorb the calcified cartilage, and new bone is laid down along the paths of cartilage resorption. This process of primitive enchondral ossification continues and gives the cartilage body a core of cancellous bone. Ossification eventually may replace the major portion of the cartilage (Fig. 180).

Advanced Stage

As the articular cartilage degenerates and wears away, the subchondral bone prepares to meet the situation.

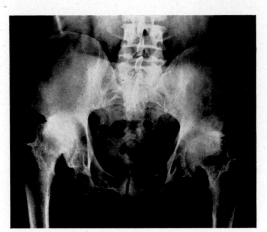

FIGURE 176. Far advanced osteoarthritis of the hips (malum coxae senilis). Eburnation, loss of cartilage space, subluxation, and large marginal osteophytes are the prominent features.

The articular bony cortex and adjacent trabeculae become the site of active new bone apposition, making the marrow spaces progressively smaller. Haversian systems take form when dense compact bone replaces the cancellous trabeculae. This process is most active in weight-bearing joints.

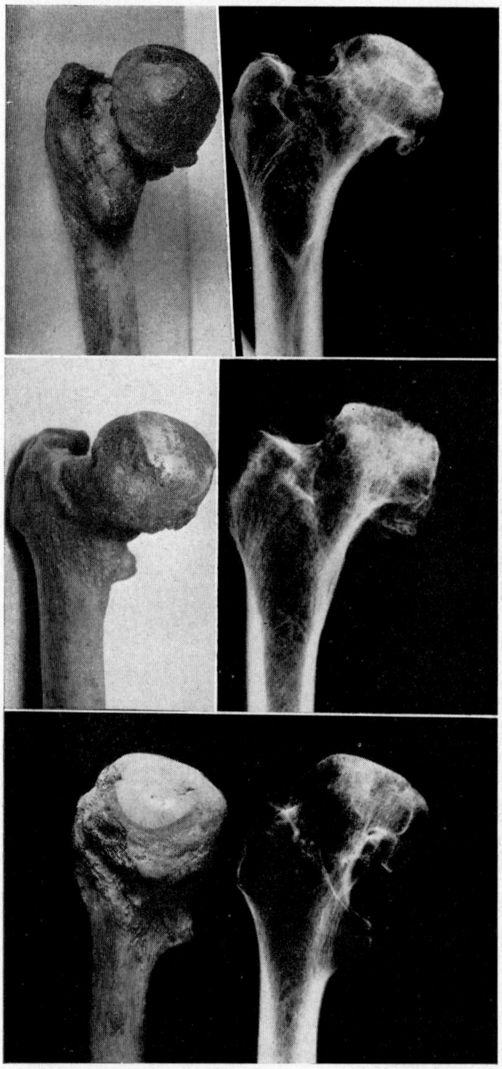

Marginal exostoses continue to enlarge during the advanced stage. When they project from their host for a considerable distance, as they sometimes do in such locations as the head of the femur, buttresses or struts of bone develop between the exostosis and the adjacent cortex. These buttresses make their appearance when the exostosis takes part in the articulation and shares the pressure and tension stresses of function.

FIGURE 177. Far advanced osteoarthritic changes in three femoral heads. Photos of the dried specimen and their roentgenograms. All show flattening of the head, eburnation and large marginal osteophytes.

EBURNATION: As the adaptive process advances, much of the articular cortex may become completely denuded of its cartilage cap (Fig. 174). By the time this stage is reached the articular cortex usually is extremely dense. With the friction of continued joint function, the exposed portions of articular cortex become smooth, polished, and occasionally grooved (Fig. 177). The term eburnation fits the picture exceedingly well.

SUBCHONDRAL FRACTURES: Subchondral fractures are frequently observed. They are usually minute, and they readily heal. The subchondral islands of cartilage occasionally observed are believed by many to represent proliferating remains of cartilage callus which remained behind after the healing of a minute subchondral fracture. Other theories have been proposed to explain these bits of subchondral cartilage, but they are untenable.

SUBCHONDRAL CYSTS: Subchondral so-called cysts rather consistently in advanced cases and have aroused considerable theorizing. These cysts, usually found in areas of osteosclerosis, often contain a mucoid material. Occasionally they are filled with fibrous tissue or necrotic debris (Fig. 174). The most logical explanation of such cysts credits them to osteoclasia prompted by excessive mechanical stresses. Subchondral cysts are almost always aligned with points of great stress. Up to a certain definite limit mechanical stresses stimulate osteoblastic bone apposition, but beyond this limit it is osteoclastic activity that receives an impetus. If the resorptive activity became localized, subchondral cysts would then form. Pommer conceived of the cysts as being due to localized hemorrhages which become encapsulated during an abortive attempt at resorption. Subchondral cysts are looked upon as one of the pathognomic signs of osteo-arthritis.

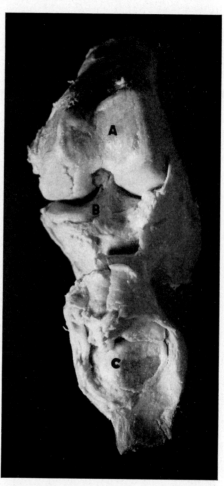

FIGURE 178. Osteoarthritis, far advanced, in the patellar articulation. *A.* Denuded and eburnated femoral trochlea. *B.* Tibial plateau. *C.* Patellar articular surface with a denuded, eburnated area of cartilage.

Axhausen believed that in many cases of degenerative arthritis the primary lesion appeared in the subchondral bone rather than in the articular cartilage. Much experimental work was produced to confirm this conviction. It is now the concensus that such cases likely do exist but are exceptional.

MORBUS COXAE SENILIS: In former years the term morbus coxae senilis of Smith was applied to osteoarthritis of the hip joint observed in elderly individuals. It was long classified as a separate entity, but we now know that it should not be so considered; it also occurs in middle age and even occasionally in young adults. Profound alterations involve the head of the femur and the acetabulum (Fig. 176). With reactivated enchondral ossification and the formation of soft new bone, the shearing stresses on the head of the femur may cause the head to migrate proximally. The superior rim of the acetabulum and capsule also migrate proximally, the end-result being proximal subluxation and extreme malformation of the joint. A large buttressed exostosis frequently projects from the inferior margin of the femoral head. In other instances the femoral head may move deeper into the acetabulum and become bullet shaped. In such cases the overhang-marginal osteophytes of the acetabulum sometimes lock the femoral head in its socket.

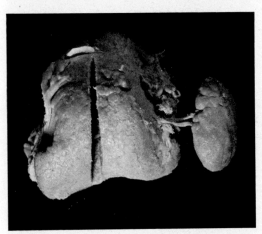

FIGURE 179. Large free body in an osteoarthritic knee joint. Joint body has a pedicle attached to the lateral femoral condyle.

ARTHRITIC JOINT BODIES: The chondromata and osteochondromata which form in the capsule remain buried in the synovial membrane or else pedunculate to hang into the synovial sac. These pedunculated bodies not infrequently become severed from their attachment and drop free into the joint. Their life in the joint is interesting. If there is a nucleus of bone it dies when divorced from the blood supply it received by way of the pedicle. The cartilage element not only subsists but is able to proliferate through the nourishment extracted from the synovial fluid. The bony core remains inert while the overlying cartilage, through the action of an enveloping thin perichondrium, continues to proliferate adding cartilage layer upon layer. Cross sections of such a body, after a prolonged existence free in the joint, disclose an irregular lamellation. The joint chemistry appears to dictate whether or not calcification will occur in the exposed layer of cartilage. The lamellations represent layers of non-calcified cartilage interspersed with irregular and often incomplete layers of calcified cartilage. Abortive attempts at bone formation may appear in scattered patches. The central area of a chondroma usually is degenerated and necrotic, presumably from inadequate nutrition.

If a free osteochondroma subsequently reattaches itself to the synovial membrane and thereby receives a blood supply, vessels will penetrate to the necrotic bone in the core to deliver cells and minerals that slowly replace the dead bone and marrow with viable elements (creeping substitution).

The formation of free joint bodies by the crowding out of cartilage fragments (epiarticular ecchondroses) from cartilage proliferation, lobulation, and infolding has already been described.

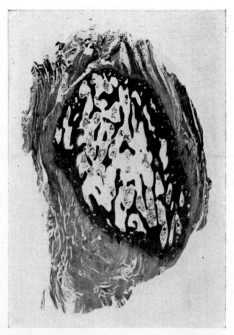

FIGURE 180. Joint body, entirely ossified, removed from the joint capsule of a knee joint.

Fractured-off marginal osteophytes represent a frequent source of arthritic joint bodies. Osteophytes, often bulbous and insecurely attached, fracture off by minor traumata. Once the osteophyte is free in the joint, its bone and marrow elements die; if a pedicle is retained all elements may survive. The fracture surface soon becomes covered by a fibrous and fibro-cartilaginous layer which creeps out like a pannus from the borders of the cartilage surface. The cartilage element may proliferate as in osteochondromata.

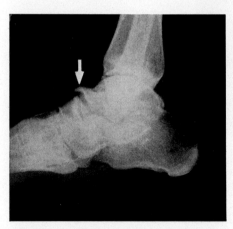

FIGURE 181. Osteoarthritis of the astragaloscaphoid joint with a large osteophyte projecting from the astragalar head (arrow).

ROENTGENOGRAPHIC
CORRELATION

EARLY STAGE: The roentgenogram usually is entirely negative in the early stage of osteo-arthritis. Since the early changes are limited to the superficial layers of the articular cartilage they cannot be expected to be reflected by the roentgen-ray.

MODERATELY ADVANCED STAGE: In this stage the wearing away of the articular cartilage is reflected by a narrowed cartilage space. Beginning marginal osteophyte formation is indicated by the sharpening of joint margins. In the knee joint the tibial spines become pointed and drawn out. A beginning increase in density may be noted in the articular cortices at sites of maximum stress.

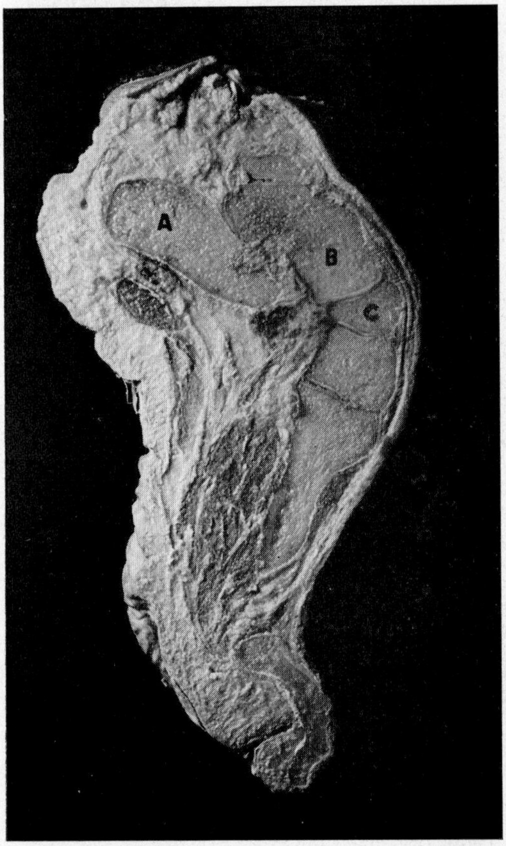

ADVANCED STAGE: In the advanced stage all of the classical signs of osteo-arthritis materialize. These of course include marginal osteophytes, narrowed cartilage space, subchondral cysts, eburnation of articular cortices and at times subluxation, and a thickened joint capsule.

OSTEO-ARTHRITIS OF THE SPINE

The only true articulations in the spine are the intervertebral facet joints, the costovertebral joints, and the sacro-iliac joints. Responses of the vertebral bodies to intervertebral disc degeneration frequently are referred to as osteo-arthritis. As a matter of fact the pathogenesis of the disc and vertebral body changes is similar to that of osteo-arthritis.

FIGURE 182. Early osteoarthritic changes in the joints of an extreme talipes equinus. Patient was a male, age 18. The abnormal stresses led to areas of degeneration in the cartilage of most of the tarsal joints. *A*. Os calcis. *B*. Astragalus. *C*. Scaphoid.

Degenerative changes in the spine may be localized or generalized. When localized to one or two discs and vertebral bodies, a traumatic factor usually has set the degenerative changes in motion. Specifically, a nucleus pulposus may have been disloged from its normal position. to protrude or rupture into a vertebral body or the vertebral canal (Fig. 19).

Degeneration in intervertebral discs leads to the formation of marginal osteophytes on adjacent vertebral bodies. Narrowing of the disc and impairment of its resiliency are believed to stimulate the formation of marginal osteophytes. Narrowed discs lead to malalignment and malposition of the intervertebral joints, thereby altering the

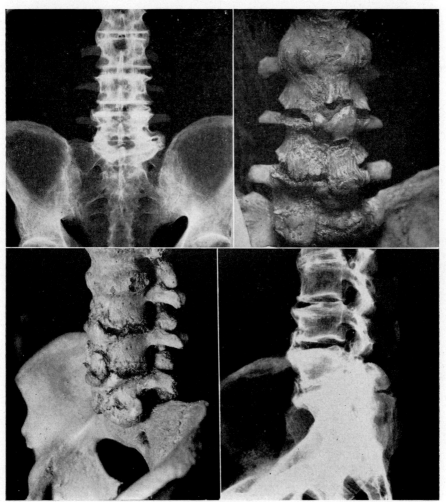

FIGURE 183. Osteoarthritic changes in a lumbar spine. A. *(Above)* Antero-posterior view of the dried specimen and the roentgenogram. B. *(Below)* Lateral view.

joint mechanism. Microtraumata are incurred with movements of the joint, and in time this adds up to degenerative changes. Wedging, such as from a fractured vertebra or osteomalacia, also alters the intervertebral joints.

Marginal osteophytes of adjacent vertebral bodies may become so large that they impinge. Impingement may be followed by fusion, (Fig. 183), this being the only place in the body where fellow marginal osteophytes of osteo-arthritis unite. To see the ultimate in marginal osteo-

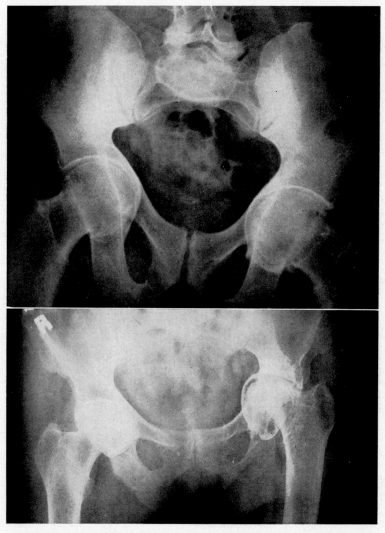

FIGURE 184. A. *(Above)* Otto-Krobak pelvis in a female, age 40. Bilateral acetabular protrusion of congenital origin. Osteoarthritis has led to narrowed cartilage space and beginning marginal osteophyte formation. B. *(Below)* Unilateral acetabular protrusion.

phyte formation in the spine, one has only to examine the grotesque marginal outgrowths in a Charcot spine.

While it is not rare in degenerative arthritis to see vertebral bodies become bridged through osteophyte formations, there is never the flowing or "icing" ossification of the anterior and posterior longitudinal ligaments as seen in the "Bamboo" spine of rheumatoid arthritis.

Otto Pelvis *(Arthrokatadysis)*

Although intrapelvic protrusion cannot be said to be caused by osteo-arthritis, it can be stated that every case develops degenerative hip joint changes sooner or later (Fig. 184). The deep acetabulum produces a mechanical impediment to normal mobility of the femoral head,

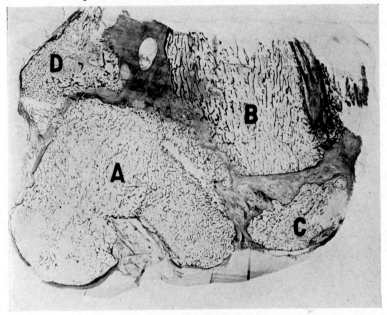

FIGURE 185. Post-traumatic ankylosing arthritis of the ankle joint. The astragalus, *A*, is subluxated medially on the tibia, *B*, and has carried with it the external malleolus, *C*, and pushed ahead of it the internal malleolus, *B*. All fragments are ankylosed by dense fibrous tissue (see Figure 160).

thereby creating the micro-traumata that lead to early cartilage degeneration.

In most cases, as in the case shown in figure 184, the involvement is bilateral and presumably congenital in origin. Unilateral cases have been reported in which the acetabular protrusion was secondary to a disease in the joint. In the case reported by Saupe the protrusion was secondary to a pyogenic infection.

Clinical Correlation

The senescent type of osteo-arthritis develops over a period of many years, and this frequently is true also of the traumatic type where micro-traumata are the source of the degenerative changes. But in cases of severe trauma, as from fractures or severe internal derangements, the degenerative arthritis may become far advanced in a priod as short as two or three years. Many such instances were seen during the World Wars and often were the result of severe knee injuries with cruciate ligament ruptures.

The joints most frequently involved by osteo-arthritis are the hips, knees, intervertebral, shoulders, and distal interphalangeal joint of fingers (Heberden's nodes).

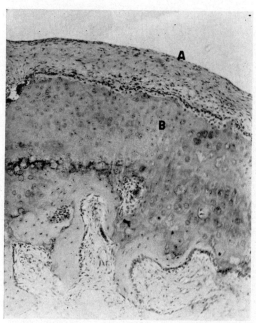

FIGURE 186. Post-traumatic ankylosing arthritis. A fibrous tissue pannus, *A,* is absorbing the articular cartilage, *B*. Fibrous tissue fills the subchondral marrow spaces. Inflammatory cells are characteristically absent. Section is from the head of the humerus.

Pain and muscle spasm frequently can be attributed to excessive use of the joint. In osteo-arthritis the joint has diminished tolerance and endurance, but if activity is restricted to the amount that the joint can accept gracefully then symptoms remain at a minimum. Minor excesses appear to be cumulative and, if persisted in, eventually precipitate an episode of pain and muscle spasm.

Restricted mobility in osteo-arthritis is due to marginal osteophytes, capsular contractures, muscle spasm, and alterations in contour of the articular surfaces.

Ligaments of an osteo-arthritic joint are more susceptible to sprain than are ligaments of a normal joint. The arthritic must perform heavy work with a measure of deliberation. A quick movement may take a heavy toll.

POST-TRAUMATIC ANKYLOSING ARTHRITIS

In discussing traumatic osteo-arthritis no mention was made of the extremely traumatized joint that terminates in fibrous or bony ankylosis. This was a purposeful omission since osteo-arthritis can develop only in a joint in which motion is preserved. The pathologic changes and pathogenesis of post-traumatic ankylosing arthritis are in many ways entirely separate and distinct from other forms of arthritis (Figs. 185-191).

ETIOLOGY

As the name implies, the principal cause is trauma, but not minor trauma, for it takes a severe injury to establish the events that lead to an ankylosis. Such injuries are by no means rare. Severe fractures that communicate with a joint by one to several fracture lines head the list of causes. Comminution of an articular cortex and its cartilage cov-

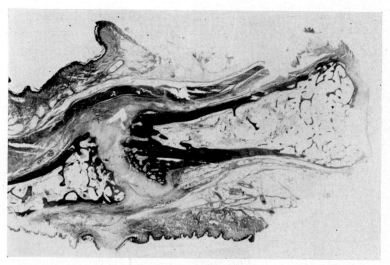

FIGURE 187. Post-traumatic ankylosing arthritis of the metacarpo-phalangeal joint of the right thumb representing the end-result of an unreduced fracture of the metacarpal head. Articular cartilage has been entirely replaced by fibrous tissue.

ering usually spells ankylosis. Severe compression fractures that telescope joints often lead to ankylosing traumatic arthritis. Falls from great heights inflict such injuries on the mid-tarsal, subastragaloid, ankle, knee and hip joints. Dislocation and extensive tearing of the ligaments has led to a post-traumatic ankylosing arthritis. Compound joint fractures and dislocations are particularly susceptible to ankylosis, even without secondary infection. Below deck explosions produced this form of arthritis in the joints of sailors standing on the deck.

PATHOLOGIC CHANGES AND PATHOGENESIS

Directly following a severe joint injury there is hemorrhage, often profuse, and productive of pronounced joint distention. A portion of the hemorrhage organizes and the remainder is absorbed. Granulation tissue appears at sites of capsular and ligamentous tears, and also from the subchondral marrow spaces whenever fracture crevices open up the joint surfaces. Granulation tissue pannus formations creep across the articular cartilage from origins in the synovial membrane at the perphery and from subchondral marrow. As is characteristic of such formations the articular cartilage is slowly absorbed. In severe cases most of the hyaline cartilage is lost, and with fibrous condensation of the granulation tissue, adjacent joint surfaces become frozen together by a mass of fibrous tissue. Subchondral marrow fibrosis occurs, and there is some resorption of articular cartilage from the marrow side, but it is not so active as in tuberculous and proliferative arthritis. Chondral and subchondral areas of aseptic necrosis are also a factor.

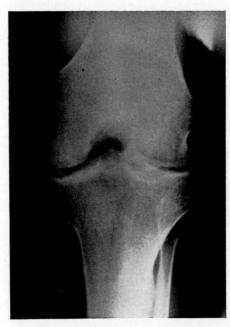

FIGURE 188. Post-traumatic ankylosing arthritis of the left knee joint in a 35 year old male. Nine years previously the left leg had caught in a revolving wagon wheel. No attempt was made to mobilize the knee. There were 10 degrees of painful motion and a 25 degree flexion contracture. A. Antero-posterior roentgenogram.

The synovial membrane usually becomes the site of anchorage for multiple powerful adhesions. Folds and pouches of the synovial lining become tightly knitted together.

Ossification of the fibrous tissue uniting the joint ends occurs in some instances and transforms the fibrous ankylosis to a bony ankylosis.

The duration of the period of immobilization of a severely traumatized joint plays an important part in the character of the end-result. Protracted immobilization, although at times mandatory, definitely favors the establishment of an ankylosis. In cases of hopeless destruction of a joint, a bony ankylosis is to be desired and striven for. A fibrous ankylosis may permit a few degrees of motion, which represents the degree of yield and play in the interposed adhesions. Such motion is seldom useful, and frequently painful. There are instances when protracted immobilization is contra-indicated and harmful. In such cases as comminuted elbow fractures, an ankylosis frequently can be prevented and an extremely useful range of motion preserved by instituting early elbow motion. Attention in such instances is focused upon preservation of motion, not upon achieving perfect healing of the fractures. Pannus formations and other adhesions across the joint line are prevented from uniting by joint movement.

There are times when an injured joint becomes involved in an ankylosing arthritis because the joint lesions coexist with other nearby injuries. An excellent example of this is seen when a knee injury and a fractured femur are incurred on the same side. Existing alone the knee injury in all probability would have healed with a good range of motion, but, coexisting with a fractured femur, the enforced immobilization leaves the knee with a fibrous ankylosis. The incidence of this

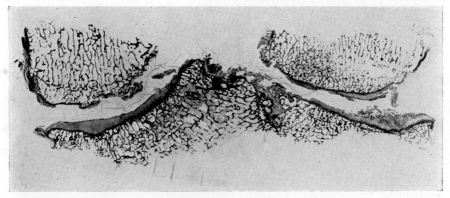

FIGURE 188. *(Continued)* B. Histologic sections of specimens obtained from an arthrodesis of the knee. Tibial condyles below and femoral condyles above.

unfortunate complication diminishes when the fullest possible opportunity is taken to exercise actively all lower extremity muscles during the healing period of the fracture. Traction methods of treating the fracture offer a better opportunity for an exercise regime than does envelopment of the extremity in a plaster cast. In some individuals, immobilization is capable of producing serious joint changes leading to permanent capsular damage, without there having been an injury. Aseptic inflammation and even a fibrous ankylosis may be observed. In many cases the immobilization may be more damaging to the joints than the trauma.

HEMOPHILIAC ARTHRITIS

Hemophilia is a disease of males transmitted by females. Cases of hemophilia that develop hemarthroses and eventually hemophiliac arthritis usually have their onset during middle and late childhood.

Periodical hemarthrosis occurs principally in the knees (Fig. 191), hips or elbows, following trauma, or at times without trauma. There is a tendency for hemophilia to improve during adulthood, but, if a given

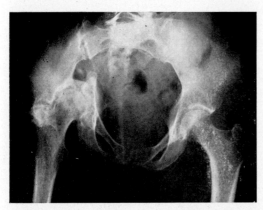

joint such as the knee has repeatedly filled up with blood, the damage done usually leads to arthritic changes and to symptoms that persist throughout the patient's life. An arthrotomy or even an aspiration is profoundly contraindicated, and, if carried out by error, could cost the patient his life.

FIGURE 189. Post-traumatic ankylosing arthritis of the right hip in a 54 year old female. The fractures were from an auto accident.

PATHOLOGIC ANATOMY

The joint changes in hemophiliac arthritis will be presented under the headings: (1) The joint capsule; (2) The articular cartilage; and, (3) The subchondral bone.

The Joint Capsule

During an acute episode the unchecked hemorrhage tremendously distends the joint capsule. One of Ely's patients described such a joint as being "swelled up like a balloon." Blood in a joint frequently can be identified in the roentgenogram, the blood being considerably more radio-opaque than synovial fluid.

The synovial membrane becomes stained a yellow-red, and later a brown-red from blood pigments. Iron and other blood ele-

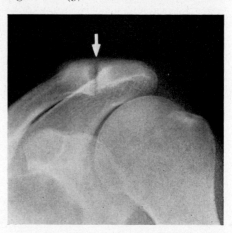

FIGURE 190. Post-traumatic ankylosing arthritis of the left acromioclavicular joint in a 42 year old male. Joint changes followed a fall on the lateral aspect of the left shoulder.

ments are deposited in and beneath the membrane. It was Freund's belief that these deposits were responsible for the increased roentgenographic visualization of the joint capsule in hemophilia. With repeated episodes of hemarthrosis the joint capsule becomes hyperplastic, the synovial villi enlarging and multiplying. In the beginning the capsule returns to normal after a period of hemarthrosis, but later the changes become permanent.

The Articular Cartilage

No visible changes occur in the cartilage during early episodes except the yellowish staining associated with joint hemorrhage from any cause. After a series of episodes there appears to be an interference with cartilage nutrition and metabolism. This may be explained by displacement of synovial fluid by blood, thus robbing the cartilage of its principal source of nourishment.

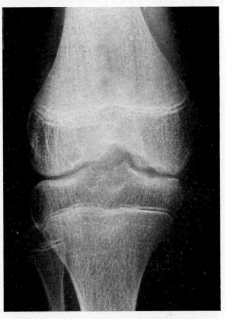

Degenerative changes eventually take place in the cartilage, and a narrowed cartilage space may develop from a wearing off of the cartilage. Areas of erosion are described, and they are not limited to weight-bearing areas. Fibrous ankylosis and deformation sometimes characterize longstanding cases.

The Subchondral Bone

No bone changes are seen at the outset but in time, if there is enforced disuse, the bone becomes porotic. *Subchondral cysts are a prominent feature of hemophilic arthritis.* It is Key's opinion that the cysts originate from localized

FIGURE 191. Hemophiliac arthritis of the right knee joint in a 15 year old boy. Since the age of five there had been repeated episodes of hemorrhages in both knees and the right elbow.

hemorrhages in the porotic cancellous subchondral bone. Aseptic necrosis of the bony trabeculae inclosed in the hematoma is followed by resorption of the trabeculae, which in the roentgenogram gives the appearance of a bone cyst. Subchondral cysts are small, seldom exceeding one centimeter in diameter, and are more frequently multiple than single. Hematoma cysts have been known to occur in other parts of the skeleton, as described by Furfota.

Marginal notching of the bone at capsular attachments is a rather common observation. In older individuals in whom joint function has been preserved, marginal osteophytes develop as part of the secondary osteo-arthritis which accrues in response to the many injuries inflicted upon the cartilage by the episodes of hemarthrosis.

RHEUMATOID ARTHRITIS

Rheumatoid arthritis is a destructive, non-exudative, chronic, poly-articular arthritis of undetermined etiology, characterized by diffuse and focal collections of lymphocytes and plasma cells in a proliferating, pannus-forming capsule. The disease is most common during the second and third decades but occurs occasionally in children and in the elderly. Whereas the majority of cases of osteo-arthritis develop after the age of forty, most cases of rheumatoid arthritis occur before the age of forty. Approximately twice as many women have the disease as men. Joints of the hands and feet are involved the most frequently. Other joints commonly affected include the wrists, knees, elbows, ankles, hips, spine, and temporo-mandibular. The onset may be sudden and febrile, or insidious and afebrile.

TERMINOLOGY

For almost every term designating osteo-arthritis there is a fellow term for rheumatoid arthritis. In the Garrods' terminology it is rheumatoid arthritis, the term that is the most widely used at the present time. Virchow termed it ankylosing arthritis, and Charcot, progressive chronic articular rheumatism. In this country Goldthwait referred to it as atrophic arthritis; Ely, as type I arthritis, and Nichols and Richardson, as proliferative arthritis. Until such a time as the mysteries of the etiology are unveiled we will be forced to base our terminology upon the dominant clinical, pathologic, or roentgenologic change.

TYPES

Clinically, the disease may manifest itself in a variety of ways, but it is doubtful whether one is justified in speaking of the several different types referred to by many observers. In a report of the British Medical Association, primary and secondary types were described: Primary, when no focal or general infection is present with which to associate the etiology of the arthritis, and secondary, when there is an associated focal or general infection.

Since Still's description of rheumatoid arthritis as he observed it in childhood, many have preferred to think of the disease in children as a separate entity. From the pathologist's viewpoint this is not justified since the joint pathology is not essentially different from that observed in rheumatoid arthritis of adults.

Just how and where to fit rheumatic fever into the picture with rheumatoid arthritis has been the subject of numerous investigations. It is generally agreed that no essential difference exists in the joint lesions. Clinically, the differentiation is based principally upon the status of the heart. Heart lesions are a consistent part of acute rheumatic fever; whereas in rheumatoid arthritis the heart seldom presents any evidence of involvement. It was formerly believed that subcutaneous nodules afforded diagnostic evidence of rheumatic fever. If sought for, such nodules will frequently be found associated with rheumatoid arthritis.

Two classifications, based upon the dominant pathological and anatomical alterations, deserve mention. Nichols and Richardson classified the joint changes into the following five types: serous, ulcerating, formative, fungating, and ankylosing. Of course, many combinations occur, and the same joint may represent one type during an early stage and other types during later stages, or several types at once. Less satisfactory is the Strangeway classification: capsular, adhesive dry, rarifying, villous, and infective. Such subdivisions as these have been virtually abandoned.

ETIOLOGY

Although innumerable theories have been proposed to explain the etiology of rheumatoid arthritis, not one has as yet been proved. Few subjects have been more extensively investigated than this distressing form of arthritis. Several investigators have seemed to approach very close to a solution, and have made important contributions, which in time may light up the path that will lead us out of the darkness of this subject. *The present investigations of adrenal cortex and pituitary hormones (Compound E and A.C.T.H.) are indeed promising!*

The very multiplicity of the etiologic theories being discussed today tells us the many sides from which the subject is being investigated. The following theories are widely discussed and investigated.

Infectious Theory

"Most of the evidence presented to date suggests that rheumatoid arthritis is at least in part an infectious disease" (Comroe). Until recently this was the most widely accepted theory, and it stated that infection may involve joints by one or more of three methods: first, through direct inoculation by blood-borne organisms; second, by blood-borne toxins originating at a remote focus of infection; and third, by developing a sensitization to an organism which promotes allergic responses in joint tissues that are manifest as arthritis.

It has been established by repeated experiments that immune bodies, agglutinins to certain strains of streptococci in particular, are present in the serum of patients with proliferative arthritis in a considerably higher incidence than they are in normal individuals (Angevine). Tests of skin sensitization to streptococci by Davidson and Goldie showed 75% positive reactions in chronic arthritic and 25% positive in non-arthritic individuals. These authors suggested that if the streptococcus was not the actual cause of the disease it certainly must play an important part in the process.

The significance of focal sepsis in arthritis has been the subject of much controversy and conflicting data. Statistical evidence is at hand to prove both pros and cons. Steindler, in an authentic study of a large series of cases, made the following statistical deductions: "the response in 15% of cases in arthritis of Type I, and 8.1% in cases of Type II approaches, we believe, the lower limit of frequency of definite and lasting responses to removal of foci."

Organisms have not been cultured with any significant consistency from either the blood stream or joints. Clausen, Small and numerous other investigators have been able to isolate several organisms, but, again, the interpretation of their findings remains clothed in speculation.

The explanation of rheumatoid arthritis on the basis of an allergic manifestation has a flare of popularity every now and again. Such observers as Zinsser and Freiberg have popularized this theory. Vigorous opposition to this conception has arisen; premature interpretation and inadequate evidence is claimed.

Metabolic Disturbances

This theory includes at least two phases: (1) Disordered, intestinal function from deficiency in such items as vitamins, proteins, and sulphur; (2) Food allergy and inability to digest carbohydrates adequately. In this country Pemberton has led the proponents of this theory. Nothing conclusive has been achieved.

Endocrine Imbalance

Various endocrine states are believed to contribute to the development of chronic arthritis. Menopausal arthritis is attributed to endocrine abnormalities. The adrenal cortex hormones may hold the key that will unlock the door to both the etiology and therapy of rheumatoid arthritis.

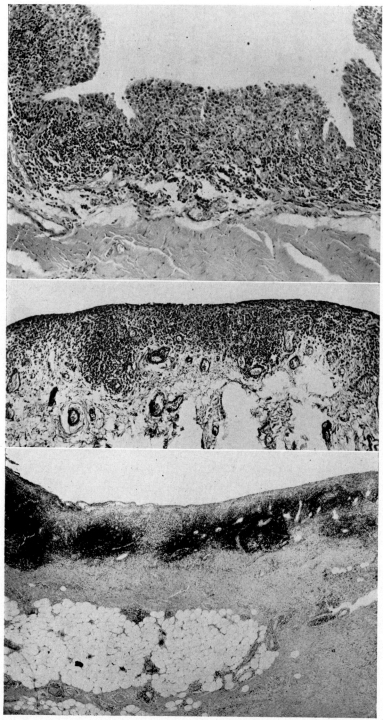

FIGURE 192. Diffuse and focal accumulations of lymphocytes and plasma cells in the synovial membrane and subsynovia.

Neurogenic Theory

Leriche and Policard have based their performance of sympathec-
tomies in rheumatoid arthritis on the belief that the disease is caused
or aggravated by vasoconstriction arising from an overstimulated
sympathetic system. Their results, and those of others, leave much to
be desired.

Circulatory Theory

It has been shown recently that in rheumatoid arthritis the capillary
bed of the involved joints is partially obliterated, and that an ischemia

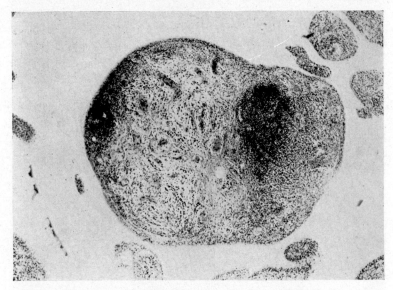

FIGURE 193. Round cell leucocytes in a synovial villus.

is frequently the result. The cause of these circulatory deficiencies and
the part they play in arthritis is unknown.

Precipitating Etiologic Factors

The following are definitely believed to be significant: overexposure
to inclement weather, mental and physical strain, general and focal
infections, inherited predisposition, constipation, and acute injuries.

PATHOLOGIC CHANGES AND PATHOGENESIS

Early Stage

Rheumatoid arthritis, like almost all other diseases of joints with
the exception of osteoarthritis, has its primary lesion in the synovial
membrane. The responses called forth by the etiologic factor (whatever

it may be) are chronic and inflammatory in nature. The synovial changes are ushered in by an active hyperemia. In the earliest stages the disease is a synovitis and later becomes an arthritis when the articular and subchondral marrow present their responses. Along with the synovial hyperemia comes edema, and a moderate increase in synovial fluid. In more acute and florid cases the synovial membrane may bulge into the joint to overlay the periphery of the articular surfaces. Hyperplasia of all capsular elements soon manifests itself. The synovialis may increase from a single cell layer to a great many cell layers. Syno-vial villi enlarge by edema and hyperplasia, and their increase in size is most con-spicuous opposite the joint line.

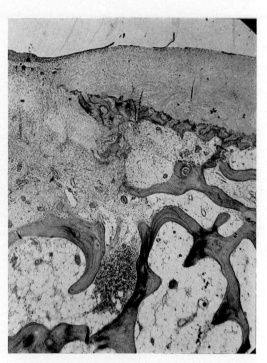

FIGURE 194. Rheumatoid arthritis: subchondral fibrous tissue destroying the articular cortex.

One of the most promi-nent and significant of the microscopic manifestations of proliferative arthritis is the appearance of diffuse and focal collections of round cell leucocytes, con-sisting mainly of lympho-cytes and plasma cells (Fig. 192). A variable number of polynucleated leucocytes may also appear. Allison and Ghormley have emphasized the importance of these round cells as a diagnostic criterion. Most significant is the tendency for the cells to concentrate at numerous points in the subsynovia to form follicles. Ghormley and Deacon have demonstrated by differential staining that the foci of round cells are not perivascular. These investigators believe that the round cells concentrate in response to some stimulus similar to that which prompts the formation of tubercles.

Synchronous with or following the capsular responses, the subchondral marrow undergoes some highly significant alterations. Granulation tissue grows in to replace the normal subchondral marrow elements, and rather quickly condenses to form fibrous tissue. Diffuse infiltration and focal collections of round cells are characteristic features of the marrow response. Also in the subchondral marrow response, osteoclasts accumulate and wage an attack on the articular cortex. After multiple perforation of this structure the attack is carried on

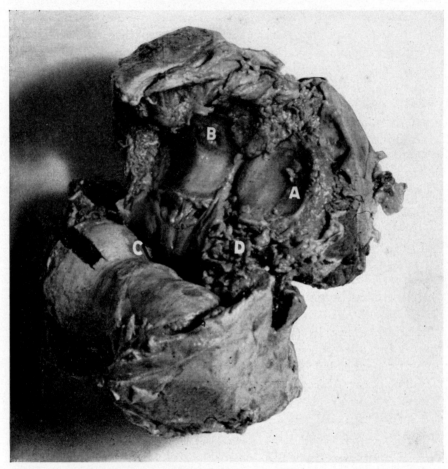

FIGURE 196. Rheumatoid arthritis of the elbow joint. *A*. Pannus creeping over the head of the radius. *B*. Olecranon pannus. *C*. Denuded area of articular cartilage lower humerus. *D*. Hyperplastic synovia.

against the cartilage, beginning with the zone of provisory calcification.

Osteoporosis appears early in rheumatoid arthritis. Some observers believe it results entirely from the inforced immobilization. Others believe that the inflammatory process is a prominent factor.

Moderately Advanced Stage

One of the most significant and serious manifestations of rheumatoid

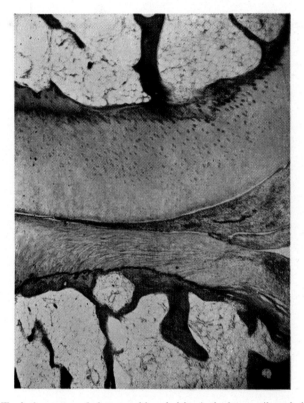

FIGURE 195. Typical pannus of rheumatoid arthritis. Articular cartilage is being absorbed.

arthritis are the pannus formations over the articular surfaces. Pannus formations originate in parts of the synovial membrane bordering the articular cartilage, and first appear as tongues of granulation tissue, creeping from the periphery toward the center of the joint surfaces. Occasionally a pannus meets and fuses with its fellow from the opposite side. De-

pending upon its age and maturity a pannus may vary in character from young, highly vascular granulation tissue to mature, dense, practically avascular fibrous tissue. Chondroclasts and fibroblasts originating in the pannus may actively absorb the subjacent cartilage. This chondroclastic activity may be very pronounced, or practically nil, depending upon the status of the disease. The proliferative response of cartilage is usually insignificant.

The pannus, like the joint capsule presents diffuse and focal collections of round cells. Occasionally a pannus destroys very little cartilage but fuses adjacent cartilage surfaces to produce a fibrous ankylosis. If motion is continued the pannus may not produce adhesions, but may remain smooth and transform to fibro-cartilage. Cartilage, and even bone formation, in a pannus is not rare. Tim-

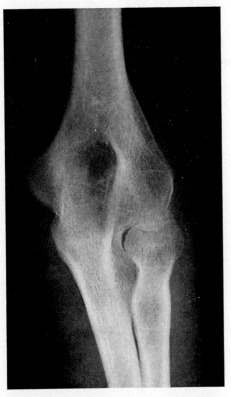

FIGURE 197. Bony ankylosis of the humero-olecranon joint from a previous rheumatoid arthritis. Motion was preserved in the radio-humeral and radio-ulnar joints, probably as a result of persistent pro and supination.

brell Fisher believes a pannus is nature's attempt to repair damaged cartilage; therefore, he recommends that motion be continued to the greatest possible degree to prevent adhesions and assist nature in forming new articular surfaces.

Nichols and Richardson called attention to proliferative activity in the gliding layer of the cartilage, and referred to it as a perichondrium. Cases were observed where such a perichondrium played a more active part than the pannus, and became the site of cartilage and bone formation. In recent years several investigators, including Allison and

Ghormley, have denied that the perichondrium plays any important part in proliferative arthritis. There appears to be insufficient evidence to warrant classifying the gliding layer of the articular cartilage as a perichondrium.

The subchondral marrow fibrosis with its chondroclastic activity continues to absorb the deep layers of cartilage. Subchondral elements may destroy the deep layers of cartilage more rapidly than the pannus destroys the superficial layers.

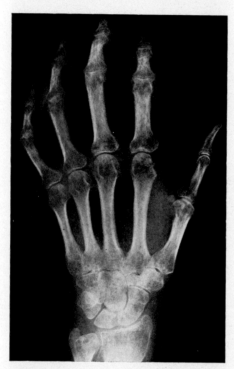

FIGURE 198. Active rheumatoid arthritis of the left hand. Principle involvement is in the proximal interphalangeal joints of the fingers.

Profound capsular thickening is the accomplishment of cellular proliferation in both the stratum fibrosum and stratum synoviale. The synovial villosity varies with the character of the capsular reaction; in some instances the villi become bulbous, develop an endarteritis obliterans in the pedicle arteries, become necrotic, and drop into the joint as free rice-like bodies (Fig. 199).

Advanced Stage

The disease process may become quiescent during early or moderately advanced stages, or continue to an advanced stage and ankylosis. Fisher has well described the advancing cartilage destruction. "Eventually the invading tide of vascular connective tissue of subchondral marrow spaces meets and merges with that derived from the synovial pannus." Fibrous ankylosis is thus produced and may or may not include persisting islands of articular cartilage. In most instances the fibrous ankylosis becomes trabecularized by fibrous bone to form a bony ankylosis. Pain is then forever dismissed unless, perchance, the patient gambles on an arthroplasty and loses.

Since rheumatoid arthritis is a systemic disease, changes in structures other than joints can be expected. Proliferative and inflammatory changes occur in lymph nodes, the spleen, muscles, nerves, pericardium and pleura.

Subcutaneous and Paraneuritic Nodules

Although subcutaneous nodules appear frequently in both rheumatoid arthritis and rheumatic fever, there are several important differences in the nodules of these two conditions. Whereas the nodules in

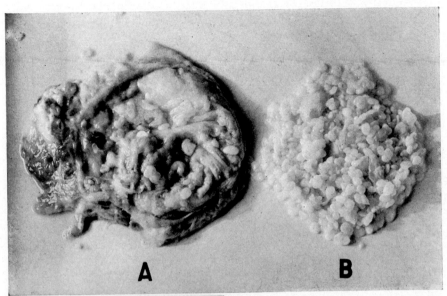

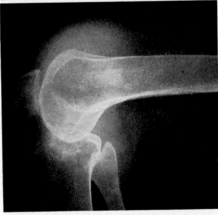

FIGURE 199. Rheumatoid arthritis of the knee joint with rice body formation. A. Synovial membrane (from a synovectomy). B. Rice bodies. C. *(Left)* Roentgenogram.

rheumatoid arthritis persist for many months, the nodules in rheumatic fever last only days or weeks and tend to appear in crops. The arthritic nodule usually has a necrotic center, minimal leucytic infiltration, appears in smaller numbers, and develops principally in older adults. Rheumatic fever nodules are more numerous, occur in younger patients, have more leucocytic infiltration and seldom a necrotic center.

Both types of nodules are distributed principally around the bony prominences of the body.

Freund found nodules in muscles, similar to the subcutaneous nodules. The muscle nodules were consistently present and were located alongside nerve fibers, prompting Freund to designate them as paraneuritic nodules. More nodules were found in early active cases than in late cases. Much of the muscle pain in rheumatoid arthritis is attributed to these nodules.

ROENTGENOLOGIC CORRELATION

Osteoporosis develops rapidly in an active case of rheumatoid arthritis and becomes most advanced in bones neighboring involved joints. Both the factor of disuse, and the inflammatory hyperemia appear to be responsible for the bone atrophy. Roentgenologists often refer to advanced osteoporosis in rheumatoid arthritis as ground glass atrophy. Bony trabeculae become of such thin caliber that their pattern is not visualized on the roentgenogram; this accounts for the homogeneous, ground glass appearance.

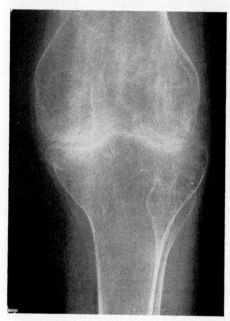

FIGURE 200. Advanced rheumatoid arthritis of the left knee joint. Loss of cartilage space, loss of articular cortices, concentric atrophy of the fibula, and ground glass atrophy of the tibia are all in evidence.

Narrowing of the cartilage space is due to resorption of the cartilage by pannus formations (Fig. 194), and not to wear and tear as in osteoarthritis, nor to lysis as in pyogenic arthritis.

Loss of definition of the articular cortex is observed relatively early in severe cases and is the work of the osteoclastic granulation and fibrous tissues that form in the subchondral marrow spaces. However, loss of the articular cortex is spotty and does not usually progress as rapidly as it does in tuberculous arthritis. Some degree of narrowing of the cartilage space ordinarily precedes defective definition of the articular cortex.

Marginal erosion not unlike that frequently seen in tuberculous arthritis may characterize rheumatoid arthritis, and is due to marginal tufts or bulbs of granulation tissue protruding into the notches.

The tremendously thickened joint capsule and the fusiform shape of the joint are readily visualized in the roentgenogram. Part of the capsular thickening is due to edema, part to an extensive fibrous tissue proliferation, and the remainder to a synovial membrane many cell-layers thick. Distention of the joint by increased synovial fluid occurs but is not the rule.

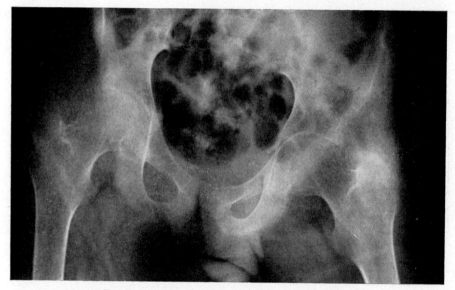

FIGURE 201. Rheumatoid arthritis of the hip joints.

A bony ankylosis can be clearly visualized roentgenographically, (Fig. 197), whereas a fibrous ankylosis must be assumed. When the cartilage space is narrow, the articular cortex faded, the bone porotic and the capsule thick, a fibrous ankylosis may be assumed to exist.

Subluxation in rheumatoid arthritis is not uncommon, and results from muscle spasm, flexion contracture, and the friable softened joint line tissues. Correction of flexion contractures by mechanical devices is another source of subluxations.

The Spine

Most characteristic of vertebral changes is the ossification of anterior and posterior longitudinal ligaments to create the "bamboo" spine that is so clearly portrayed roentgenographically (Fig. 202 & 203). When motion in the spine prevents uninterrupted ossification of the liga-

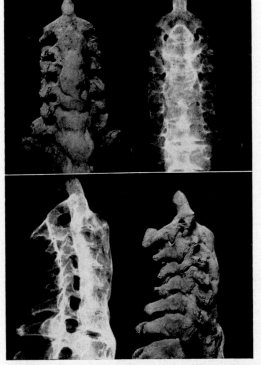

FIGURE 202. Rheumatoid arthritis with bony anky-losis in a dried specimen of a cervical spine. A. *(Above)* Front view of the specimen and roentgeno-gram. B. *(Below)* Lateral view.

ments, there may be margi-nal outgrowths resembling the marginal osteophytes of osteo-arthritis. However the marginal ossification in rheumatoid arthritis is prin-cipally from metaplasia of fibrous tissue; whereas, in osteo-arthritis, most margi-nal bone formations arise from enchondral ossifica-tion. Bony, or fibrous, anky-losis in the intervertebral, sacro-iliac, and costoverte-bral joints occurs whenever there is severe protracted spine involvement in rheu-matoid arthritis, and the pathogenesis is the same for all other true joints. Spine involvement frequently be-gins in the sacro-iliac joints, and there may be fibrous or bony ankylosis of these joints prior to any other skeletal change visible by roentgenogram. *In their pathologic anatomy there are no essential differences between Marie-Strumpel arthritis and rheumatoid arthritis.*

CLINICAL CORRELATION

The clinical picture dur-ing a febrile period with its high sedementation rate, leucocytosis, fever of 100 to 104 degrees, tachycardia, malaise, lymphadenopathy, and hot swollen joints is a clear-cut picture of inflam-mation. Spontaneous remis-

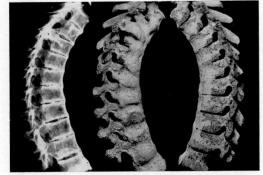

FIGURE 203. Bamboo dorsal spine. Diffuse bony ankylosis from rheumatoid arthritis. Lateral roent-genogram, and lateral photos of the dried specimen.

sions are the rule, but the course of the disease is treacherous and un-predictable.

Pain in involved joints come principally from involvement of the sensitive synovial membrane. Later, pain can come from a fibrous ankylosis.

Systematic active joint motion, as tolerated, helps prevent muscle atrophy, improves circulation, and may prevent ankylosis. Unwarranted, protracted immobilization is a standing invitation to ankylosis. It cannot be claimed, of course, that ankylosis is always preventable, but it is an unfortunate fact that many joints are needlessly sacrificed for want of proper and persistent active exercises.

Muscle spasm and gravity tend to cause ankyloses to take place with the involved joints in unsatisfactory positions. Unprotected and unexercised joints tend to develop flexion contractures; this is particularly evident in the knees, hips, and dorsal spine. A joint capsule allowed to remain in a contracted state for a long period may develop irreversible changes that prevent subsequent stretching and rehabilitation. Fibrous tissue proliferating in the capsule during rheumatoid arthritis is responsible for much of the restricted capsular mobility. Adhesions between folds and pouches of synovial membrane, as well as between articular surfaces, gain a secure foothold during protracted immobilization. The prevention of contractures requires a constant vigil.

REFERENCES

OSTEO-ARTHRITIS

ADAMS, R.: *Treatise on Rheumatic Gout or Chronic Arthritis.* Churchill J. London, 1857.

ALLISON, N. and GHORMLEY, R. K.: *Diagnosis in Joint Disease.* William Wood & Co., New York, 1931.

BAUER, W. and BENNETT, G. A.: *J. Bone & Joint Surg., 18*:1, 1936.

BENNETT, G. A., BAUER, W. and MATTOCK, S. J.: *Am. J. Path., 3*:5, 1932.

BENNETT, G. A., WAINE, H. and BAUER, W.: The Commonwealth Fund, N. Y. 1942.

CHARCOT, J. M.: *Clinical Lectures on Senile and Chronic diseases.* The New Sydenham Soc. London, 1881.

ECKNER, A.: *Arch. f. physical Heilk, 2*:235, 1843.

ELY, L. W.: *Inflammation in Bones and Joints.* J. B. Lippincott Co., Philadelphia, 1923.

ERDHEIM, J.: *Virchow's Arch f. path. Anat., 281*:197, 1931.

FISHER, A. G. T.: *Chronic (Non-tuberculous) arthritis.* The Macmillan Co., New York, 1929.

GARROD, A. B.: *The Nature and Treatment of Gout and Rheumatic Gout.* Walton & Maberly, London, 1859.

GARROD, A. E.: *Treatise on Rheumatism and Rheumatoid Arthritis.* C. Griffin & Co., London, 1890.

GOLDTHWAIT, J. E.: *Boston M. & Surg. J., 151*:529, 1904.

HEBERDEN, WM.: *Commentaries on the History and Cure of Diseases.* T. Payne, London, 1802.

HEINE, I.: *Virchows Arch. f. path. Anat., 260*:521, 1926.

KEEFER, C. S.: *M. Clin. N. Am., 18*:947, 1935.

KEY, J. A.: *J. Lab. & Clin. Med., 15*:1145, 1930. *J. Bone & Joint Surg., 11*:705, 1929.

KLING, D. H.: *Am. J. M. Sc., 197*:358, 1939.

KNAGGS, R. L.: *Diseases of Bone*. Wm. Wood & Co., New York, 1926.
NICHOLS, E. H. and RICHARDSON, F. L.: *J. Med. Res., 21*:149, 1909.
POMMER, G.: *Mikroskopische Befunde bei Arthritis Deformans*. Wien, 1913.
POMMER, G.: Die Funktionelle Theorie der Arthritis. Deformans. *Arch. f. orthop. &*
Unfall-Chir. Bd. 17, 1920.
SMITH, R. W.: *Dublin J. Med. & Chem. Sc., 6*:205, 1835.
VIRCHOW, R.: *Virchows Arch. f. path. Anat., 4*:261, 1852.
WEICHSELBAUMM, A.: *Virchow's Arch. f. path. Anat., 55*:217, 1872.

HOMOPHILIA ARTHRITIS

DOUB, H. P.: *Radiology, 24*:391, 1935.
FREUND, E.: *Virchows Arch. f. path. Anat., 256*:158, 1925.
FURFOTA, E.: *Röntgenpraxis, 3*:399, 1931.
GOCHT, H.: *Arch. f. klin, Chir., 59*:482, 1899.
KAY, J. A.: *Ann. Surg., 95*:198, 1932.
McDONALD, E. J. and LOZNER, E. L.: *Am. J. Roentgenol., 49*:405, 1943.

OTTO-KROBAK PELVIS

MAROTTOLI, O. R.: *Ann. de Chir. 6*:4, 1940.
POMERANZ, M. M.: *J. Bone & Joint Surg., 14*:663, 1932.
SAUPE, E.: *Fortschr. a. d. Geb. d. Röntgenstrahlen, 37*:1, 1928.

RHEUMATOID ARTHRITIS

ANGEVINE, D. M., ROTHBARD, S., and CECIL, R. L.: *J. A. M. A., 115*:2112, 1940.
BAUER, W.: *Ann. Int. Med., 19*:117, 1943.
BILLINGS, F.: *Focal Infection*. Appleton & Co., New York, 1916.
British Committee on Chronic Rheumatic diseases. The Macmillan Co., New York,
1936.
CECIL, R. L. and ANGEVINE, D. M.: *Ann. Int. Med., 12*:577, 1938.
CLAWSON, F. J. and WETHERBY, M.: *Ann. Int. Med., 5*:1447, 1932.
COMROE, B. I.: *Arthritis and Allied Conditions*. 3rd ed. Lea & Febiger, Philadelphia,
1944.
DAWSON, M. H., OLMSTEAD, M. and BOOTS, R. H.: *J. Immunology, 23*:205, 1932.
DOUB, H. P.: *Radiology, 24*:391, 1935.
FORKNER, C. E., SHANDS, A. R. and POSTON, M. A.: *Arch. Int. Med., 42*:675, 1928.
FREUND, E.: *Ann. Rheumat. Dis., 3*:336, 1943; *J. A. M. A., 115*:2210, 1940.
FREUND, H. A.: *Am. J. Path., 18*:865, 1942.
GHORMLEY, R. K. and DEACON, A. E.: *Am. J. Roentgenol., 35*:740, 1936.
GIBSON, A.: *J. Bone & Joint Surg., 10*:747, 1928.
HADJOPOULOS and BURBANK: *J. Bone & Joint Surg., 14*:471, 1932.
HENCH, P. S.: *Ann. Int. Med., 10*:754, 1936.
HOLBROOK, W. P. and HILL, D. F.: *Southwest Med., 21*:161, 1937.
KEEFER, C. S.: *New England J. Med., 213*:644, 1935.
KINSELLA, R. A.: *J. A. M. A., 101*:345, 1933.
KLING, D. H.: *The Synovial Membrane and the Synovial Fluid*. Los Angeles Med.
Press, 1938.
PEMBERTON, R.: *Arthritis and Rheumatoid Condition*. Lea & Febiger, Philadelphia,
1930.
PORTIS, R. B.: *Am. J. Dis. Child., 55*:1000, 1938.
SHANDS, A. R.: *South. M. J., 23*:818, 1930.
STILL, G. F.: *Common Disorders and Diseases of Childhood*, 2nd Ed. Henry Frowde,
London, 1912.
STEINDLER, A.: *Proc. Am. A. Study and Control of Rheum. Dis*. Cleveland, Ohio,
June 11, 1934.
STRANGEWAYS, T. S. P.: *Tr. Med. Soc. London, 42*:12, 1919.
SWIFT, H. F.: *J. A. M. A., 115*:2113, 1940.
YOUNG and MACMAHONS *J. Bone & Joint Surg., 17*:151, 1935.
ZINSSER, H.: *Bull. New York Acad. Med., 4*:351, 1928.

CHAPTER VII

Neuro-Arthropathies

Contents

Mitchel in 1831 published the original description of neuropathic arthropathies. He reported arthropathies associated with spinal cord lesions from tuberculous spondylitis, and attributed the joint changes to a disturbance of the trophic centers in the spinal cord. It remained for Charcot in 1868 to present the first detailed account of the subject and show the frequent association with tabes dorsalis. According to Shands the first description of arthropathies in syringomyelia was by Schultze and Kahler in 1888. Schlesinger in 1902 reported 150 cases of syringomyelia and emphasized the predominant involvement of upper extremity joints. In 1863 Packard described the arthropathic changes in the knee and foot of a patient in which the sciatic nerve was impinged by a tumor.

ETIOLOGY

Approximately 90 percent of the neuro-arthropathies are related to tabes; the other ten percent are principally from syringomyelia with rare cases caused by a variety of brain, cord, and peripheral nerve lesions. A classification based on etiologic factors has been outlined by Shands:

1. Tabes dosalis
2. Syringomyelia
3. Following lesions of the peripheral nerves
   a. Injury
   b. Peripheral neuritis
   c. Leprosy

4. Following lesions of the spinal cord
  a. Injury
  b. Congenital malformations
    (1) Spina bifida vera
  c. Tumors
  d. Tuberculosis of the spine
  e. Acute myelitis
  f. Anterior poliomyelitis

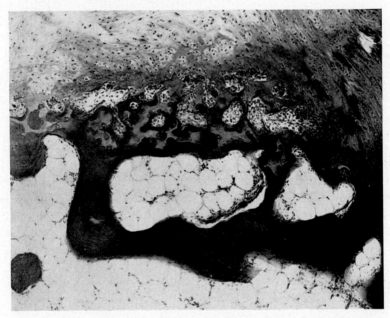

FIGURE 204. Tabetic arthropathy: Histologic section from the periphery of a femoral condyle. Reactivated enchondral ossification is replacing the deeper aspect of the cartilage.

  g. Progressive (central) muscular atrophy
    (1) Aran-Duchenne type
    (2) Spastic type (amyotrophic lateral sclerosis)
5. Following lesions of the cerebrum
  a. Dementia paralytica
  b. Hemiplegia following cerebral hemorrhage

Because of their extreme importance as etiologic factors, tabes and syringomyelia were given separate headings in place of listing them with the spinal cord lesions.

Charcot was of the opinion that the joint changes followed damage to "trophic centers" in the spinal cord or degeneration of peripheral nerves. Trauma to the analgesic joints was believed by some of the early investigators to play a part, but it was not until 1917, when Eloesser reported the results of his cat experiments, that the role of trauma

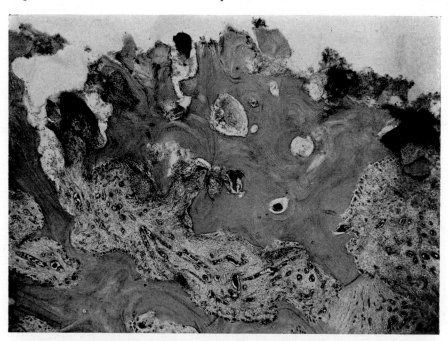

FIGURE 205. Tabetic arthropathy: A section from the tibial plateau of an atrophic tabetic arthropathy. Articular cartilage and cortex are lost and the exposed bony trabeculae are being ground off by joint motion.

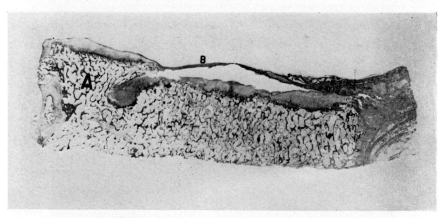

FIGURE 206. Tabetic arthropathy: A frontal section taken near the periphery of a lateral tibial condyle. *A* shows elevated lateral margin of condyle from reactivated enchondral ossification. *B* is a pannus covering the periphery of the condyle. (Elevation of pannus occurred during preparation of section.)

became clear. Eloesser showed that section of the posterior roots alone did not cause joint changes, but section of the posterior roots plus traumatic insults to an analgesic joint did lead to the development of a typical neuro-arthropathy. Continued function in an analgesic joint leads inevitably to joint trauma, and it is the reactions of the joint to

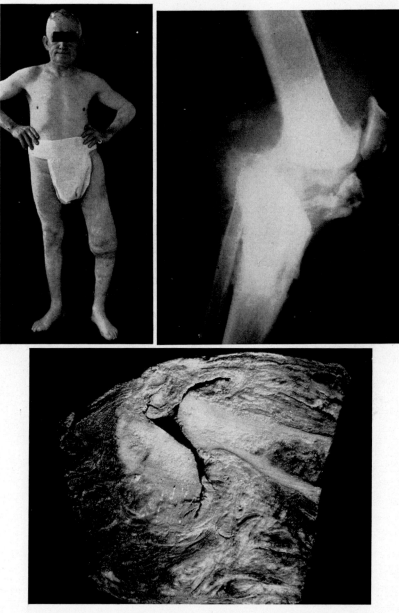

FIGURE 207. Tabetic arthropathy left knee. A. *(Left)* Photo of patient. B. *(Right)* Lateral roentgenogram. C. *(Below)* Sagital section of amputation specimen. (A pyogenic infection of the knee developed a few weeks after the photo, A, was taken, and an amputation became necessary as a life saving measure.)

the multiple injuries that creates the arthropathy. The existence of trophic centers is doubted.

That there is much in common between the changes in a Charcot joint and an osteo-arthritic joint has long been understood. Both entities represent responses of joints to multiple traumata, and both show degeneration of articular cartilage.

As a rule, the more stresses and friction to which a joint is subjected after its sensation is lost, the more rapidly will the arthropathy develop. This accounts for the more rapid changes in the lower extremity arthropathies with their weight - bearing stresses, than is observed in the upper extremity arthropathies.

GROSS PATHOLOGY AND PATHOGENESIS

CAPSULAR CHANGES

A thickened, hyperplastic joint capsule develops relatively early in an arthropathy. This is caused by the repeated and frequently prolonged episodes of synovial effusion and hemarthrosis. Clusters of synovial villi form around the joint line and not infrequently become pinched. As the arthropathy advances, the capsule becomes thick, bulky and stretched, holding a considerable quantity of fluid. Rupture of the capsule with

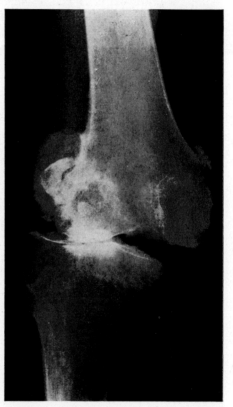

FIGURE 208. Tabetic arthropathy of the right knee showing a subluxation of the tibia on the femur and a lateral dislocation of the patella.

extension of the synovial fluid into neighboring fascial planes is not rare. The author once treated a tabetic arthropathy of the knee in which the entire anterior aspect of the thigh had become filled with synovial fluid.

Hypermobility of the joint, the most important clinical symptom, results from the stretching and rupture of the joint ligaments. Subluxations and dislocations become possible through the yielding of the ligamentous apparatus.

Heterotopic cartilage, and bone, sooner or later forms in the joint capsule. Such formations may be small or massive, single or multiple.

When multiple, some of the formations usually hang by pedicles into the joint or become separated from their pedicles to roam the joint as free bodies.

Another remarkable capsular alteration is seen in the form of migration of the capsular attachments. As the articular cartilage and underlying bone are worn away, the capsule may be forced to shift its bony attachment proximally or distally for several centimeters in order to continue to inclose the bone ends. In the ankle joint, migration of the capsule distally to the scaphoid or beyond may cause the astragalus to lose all of its capsular anchorages and become a free body inclosed in the arthropathy.

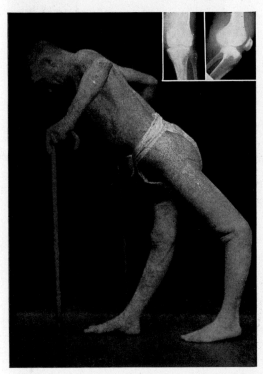

FIGURE 209. Tabetic arthropathy of the left knee with recurvatum deformity. The need for a brace is striking.

CARTILAGE CHANGES

Degenerative changes that take place in the articular cartilage during the early stages of an arthropathy are similar to those of osteoarthritis. However, the sequence of events that leads to a wearing away of the articular cartilage proceeds much more rapidly in an arthropathy. Unlike osteoarthritis, the arthropathies develop active pannus formations over portions of the articular cartilage not subjected to pressure and friction. A pannus may creep out from the synovial membrane at several points in the periphery, or sprout from underlying marrow spaces through fissures and fractures in the joint surface.

BONE CHANGES

Bone underlying the articular cartilage may be rapidly exposed, or the process may consume several years. When the process is rapid, the subchondral bone accomplishes but little toward adapting itself for serving as an articular surface. When the process is slow, the articular

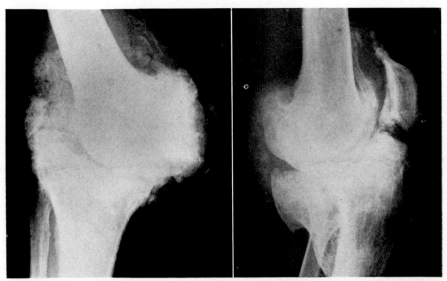

FIGURE 210. Hypertrophic tabetic arthropathy of the knee. A. *(Left)* Antero-posterior roentgenogram. B. *(Right)* Lateral roentgenogram.

cortex becomes sclerotic just as it does in osteo-arthritis. In the arthro-pathies the area of sclerosis may become wide and extremely dense. It

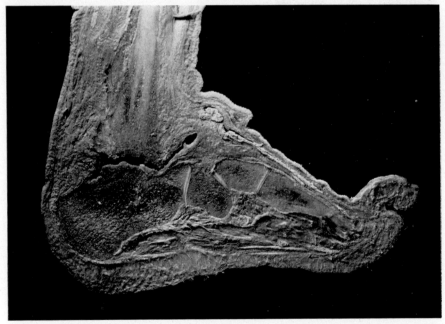

FIGURE 211. Tabetic arthropathy of the ankle. The astragalus was destroyed except for a small fragment that existed as a free body. Amputation was made necessary by an uncontrollable pyogenic infection. This patient was a 31 year old male who had bilateral Charcot ankles.

is not unusual for one of the component bone ends of a joint to become sclerotic and the other, porotic. This is seen in the hip joint where the acetabulum often becomes sclerotic and the femoral head, porotic. The softened femoral head may be completely ground off by the pressure and friction of motion against the dense and roughened acetabulum. Fragmentation of the bone ends is seen grossly as multiple fissures and minute fractures. Considerable debris consisting of bone sand and necrotic granulation tissue may lie on the articular surface and at the periphery.

Marginal exostoses often form in an arthropathy and do so through reactivated enchondral ossification just as in osteoarthritis. The arthropathic osteophyte is liable to become enormous and have heavy supporting buttresses. In the hip an osteophyte may project from the acetabular margin and resemble a bony shelf of the type constructed surgically in congenital luxations of the hip. In many arthropathies the marginal exostoses are broken off or worn off as the bone ends are ground down. This is another source of free bodies in arthropathies.

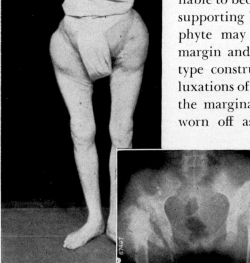

FIGURE 212. Bilateral hip arthopathies: Photo of patient, female age 50; symptoms in right hip two years and in left hip 15 months. Antero-posterior roentgenogram (insert).

FRACTURES

Both pathologic and spontaneous fractures occur in the arthropathies. Pathologic fractures result from osteoporosis and usually represent compression fractures of the bone ends, the tibial condyles being a good example. Spontaneous fractures are the response to the combination of a loss of the protective influence of pain sensation, and poorly coördinated, weakened musculature. Fractures heal normally if properly immobilized. Since immobilization is more difficult when there is analgesia of the fracture area, the healing time generally is delayed.

Periosteal bone formation is occasionally seen near the joint in an arthropathy and appears related to periosteal tears and hemorrhages.

Para-articular Changes

Hetertopic bone formation in neighboring muscles and fascia may be associated with an arthropathy (Fig. 215). Massive deposits of fibrous bone develop in such structures as the gluteal muscles and fascia lata.

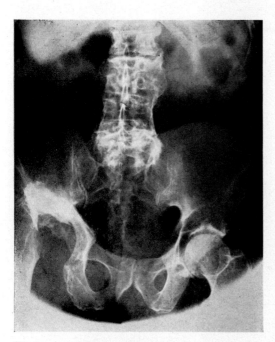

FIGURE 213. Tabetic arthropathy of the right hip and the lumbar spine.

Bone, forming in muscles, represents myositis ossificans and may form large spur-like bony projections. Fibrous bone is gradually replaced by mature lamellar bone.

MICROSCOPIC PATHOLOGY

Capsule

The increased thickness of the capsule is the manifestation of active fibroblastic proliferation, edema, and proliferation of synovial cells. Signs of trauma in the form of organizing and absorbing hemorrhage, scar tissue, and discoloration from blood pigments generally are in evidence.

Chondromata form in the joint capsule and ossify by cartilage replacement as previously described. Areas of diffuse ossification through metaplasia may also involve the capsule.

Cartilage

With degeneration of the matricial binding substance, the collagenous fibers are exposed, giving the picture of fibrillation. Flaking off of the gliding layer exposes the underlying radially arranged collagen bundles. The softened cartilage wears off first in those areas where the articular surfaces are in contact. In the non-contacting areas, granulation tissue in the form of a pannus grows over the articular cartilage. Soon the pannus matures into cellular fibrous tissue, and all the while, ot course, it actively absorbs the hyaline articular cartilage to which it is intimately attached (Fig. 206). No doubt the pannus formations are called forth by the substantial traumata inflicted upon all of the joint structures. The histologic appearance of an arthropathic pannus suggests that it is similar to the pannus of ankylosing traumatic arthritis. In both instances diffuse or focal collections of leucocytes are absent. Theoretically, there probably are arthropathies (the rapidly disintegrating type) that would undergo bony ankylosis if they were completely immobilized, and no doubt the picture would be that of post-traumatic ankylosing arthritis. This theoretical concept does not apply to advanced arthropathies with extensive osteosclerosis; in fact, this type has not often fused, even after an arthrodesing operation.

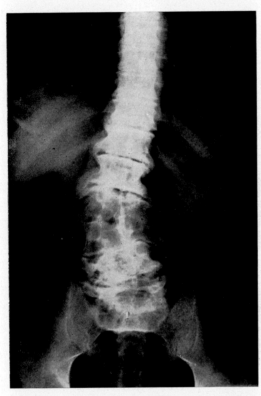

FIGURE 214. Spinal arthropathy with enormous marginal osteophytes. This patient was a male age 48 who also had a Charcot knee, the roentgenogram of which is shown in Figure 208.

BONE

Enchondral ossification adjacent to the articular cortex becomes reactivated relatively early. The articular cortex is perforated at numerous points by tonguelike inroads of marrow elements. Replacement of deep layers of articular cartilage by cancellous bone proceeds until the cartilage is replaced, or worn off. At the periphery this process gives rise to marginal osteophytes. Both the enchondral line and the osteophytes become irregular and bizarre, a condition which is in keeping with this entity.

When the cartilage is lost and the subchondral bone is becoming increasingly sclerotic, active new bone formation is seen. Large numbers of osteoblasts cover the bony trabeculae. After layer upon layer of new bone is applied, the cancellous bone gradually transforms to dense compact bone with typical haversian systems.

When the cartilage is lost without the underlying bone having become sclerotic, the exposed marrow spaces near the surface become filled with fibrous tissue or debris. Microscopic fractures are numerous. The marrow becomes hyperemic and osteoclasia is active, giving rise to further osteoporosis and rendering the bone more vulnerable to the grinding action of joint motion (Fig. 205).

ROENTGENOLOGIC CORRELATION

Arthropathies vary widely in the density of the component bones, and the extent of marginal and heterotopic bone formations. Two types of arthropathies have long been described: (1) Atrophic, and (2) Hypertrophic. In the roentgenogram of the *atrophic type* there are few, if any, marginal bone formations; the bone is of normal density or is porotic, and capsular and paraosseous bone formation is minimal or entirely absent. This is the rapidly destructive type, the type in which bone ends are speedily ground off if joint motion is permitted. Osteoabsorption and an active hyperemia are predominant. Bone formation is physiologically impossible so long as the trauma and hyperemia are unchecked.

Hypertrophic arthropathies are characterized by

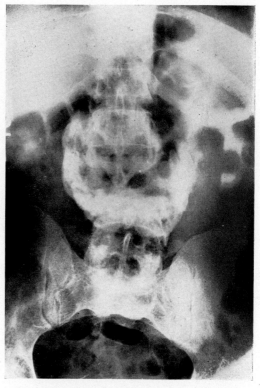

FIGURE 215. Tabetic spinal arthropathy in a 40 year old male showing massive para spinal heterotopic bone formation.

moderate to vast capsular and paraosseous bone formations, enormous marginal osteophytes, and sclerosis of the bone ends. Bone formation is the keynote. Brailsford observed an atrophic type of arthropathy that later transformed into the hypertrophic type, and contends that the two types represent stages in the same arthropathy.

In the hip joint, as has been mentioned, the acetabulum may become sclerotic and the femoral head porotic, thus showing characteristics of both types. After the femoral head is ground off, dislocation generally occurs, following which the acetabular sclerosis disappears. In other cases the acetabulum deepens and dislocation does not take place.

Knee joint arthropathies are almost as frequent as all other arthropathies combined. Deformation usually occurs early and becomes severe. A distorted relationship of the femoral to the tibial condyles may be one of the first roentgenographic signs of an arthropathy (Fig. 209).

In the ankle joint the astragalus disintegrates extensively and may even disappear (Fig. 211). Lateral or medial subluxation or dislocation

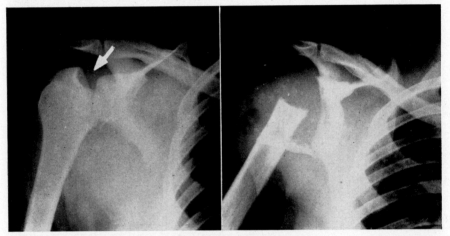

FIGURE 216. Syringomyelic arthropathy of the right shoulder in a 35 year old female. B. *(Right)* Taken eight months after A.

is observed in advanced stages creating an arthropathic talipes varus or valgus.

Spinal arthropathies, like all other arthropathies, are vividly portrayed in the roentgenogram. Involvement of the lumbar spine is the rule, when caused by tabes; and involvement of the dorsal spine is the rule when syringomyelia underlies the cord changes. Scoliosis or kyphosis develop as a consequence of compression fractures, subluxations, and destruction through "grinding." Grotesque marginal spurs and paraosseous bone formations are commonplace (Figs. 214 and 215). In some cases the massive marginal osteophytes projecting from adjacent vertebral bodies fuse and fix that portion of the spine.

Shoulder and elbow joint involvement leads to flail joints. Flailness, however, does not become incompatible with continued function, as it sometimes does in the weight bearing joints. Marginal osteophytes form invariably. Neither rapid destruction nor extensive osteosclerosis are as prominent in the upper extremity arthropathies as they are in those of the lower extremity.

CLINICAL CORRELATION

An arthropathy develops in approximately 5 percent of the cases of tabes, and in about 25 percent of the cases of syringomyelia. Approximately 80 percent of tabetic arthropathies involve lower extremity joints, whereas an equally high percentage of syringomyelic arthropathies involve upper extremity joints.

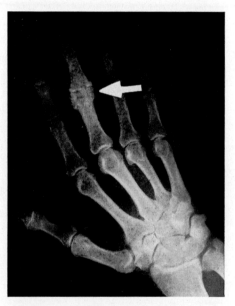

Steindler, Williams, and Puig reviewed 214 arthropathies in 134 patients, all of which were due to tabes "with the exception of one or two." In 57 percent of these cases the joint symptoms were the first symptoms of which the patient complained. A sudden joint effusion is the most frequent initial symptom and generally is the response to a sprain, sprain-fracture, or joint fracture. In two of the author's cases a fractured patella ushered in a tabetic arthropathy of the knee.

Braces are the usual treatment for lower extremity and spinal arthropathies. Braces not only stabilize the joint, but, in the case of the tuber-bearing braces used

FIGURE 217. Tabetic arthropathy of the proximal interphalangeal joint of the right middle finger (arrow). Patient was a male age 45, who also had an arthropathy of both knees, the right shoulder, and the left first metatarso-phalangeal joint.

for the lower extremity, the brace also relieves the weight-bearing stresses borne by the arthropathy. Protection of an arthropathy greatly diminishes the traumatic factor, thus slowing down the process of disintegration.

Arthrodesing operations have been employed in scattered instances for arthropathies of the ankle, knee, hips and spine. In several knee joint arthropathies, satisfactory end-results are reported in the literature of this subject. Steindler, Williams and Puig reported four successful fusions out of six cases. Of the two failures, one developed a fibrous ankylosis, and the other continued to disintegrate, it being an advanced arthropathy. Cleveland and Smith reported having done Hibb's fusions on four knee joint arthropathies, of which three developed a solid bony ankylosis, and one failed. The failure was in an advanced case. Soto-Hall has recommended a two stage procedure for fusing arthropathies. In the first stage, multiple drill holes are made through the bone ends to interrupt the zone of sclerosis; in the second stage, a conventional arthrodesis is performed.

PYOGENIC ARTHRITIS IN ARTHROPATHIES

It is not rare for a pyogenic infection to involve an arthropathy. Organisms gain entrance to the joint either from the blood stream or from an overlying ulcer perforating into the joint. Suppuration in an arthropathy is very much feared since control of the infection has been unsuccessful in the majority of instances. In serious pyogenic infections of extremity arthropathies an amputation usually has been necessary. In the 214 arthropathic joints of the Steindler, Williams, and Puig series, ten developed a pyogenic infection and eight of the ten came to amputation. With present day antibiotics, future statistics should show a lower incidence of amputation.

REFERENCES

BRAILSFORD, J. F.: *Radiology of Bones and Joints.* Williams and Wilkins Co., Baltimore, 1944.

CHARCOT, J. M.: Sur quelques arthropathies qui paraissant d'ependre d'une lesion du cerveau on de la moelle epiniere. *Arch de physiol, norm. et. path., 1*:161, 1868.

CLEVELAND, M. and SMITH, A. DeF.: Fusion of the knee joint in cases of Charcot disease, *J. Bones & Joint Surg., 13*:4, 1931.

ELOESSER, L.: On the nature of neuropathic joints. *Ann. Surg., 66*:201, 1917.

KERNWEIN, G. and LYONS, W. F.: Neuroarthropathy of the ankle joint from complete severance of the sciatic nerve. *Ann. Surg., 115*:267, 1942.

KING, E. J. S.: On some aspects of the pathology of hypertrophic Charcot's joints. *Brit. J. Surg., 18*:113, 1931.

DELORIMER, A. A.: *The Arthropathies.* The Year Book Pub. Co., Chicago, 1943.

MITCHEL, J. K.: On a new practice in acute and chronic rheumatism. *Am. J. M. Sc., 8*:55, 1831.

POTTER, H. E.: X-ray findings in neuropathic joints. *J. Nerv. & Ment. Dis., 45*:449, 1917.

POTTS, W. J.: Pathology of Charcot joints. *Am. J. Surg., 86*:596, 1927.

RIDLON, J. and BERKHEISER, E. J.: Neuropathic arthropathies, Charcot's spines. *J. A. M. A., 79*:1467, 1922.

SCHLESINGER, H.: *Die Syringomyelia,* 2nd Ed. Leipsig, 1902.

SCHULTZE, F. and KAHLER, O.: Quoted from Shands, A. R., *Arch. Surg., 20*:614, 1930.

SHANDS, A. R.: Neuropathies of the bones and joints. *Arch. Surg., 20*:614, 1930.

SOTO-HALL, R.: Fusion in Charcot joints of the knee. A new technique for arthrodesis. *Ann. Surg., 108*:124, 1938.

STEINDLER, A.: Tabetic arthropathies. *J. A. M. A., 96*:250, 1931.

STEINDLER, A., WILLIAMS, L. A., and PUIG, J.: Tabetic arthropathies *Urolog. & Cut. Rev., 46*:633, 1942.

CHAPTER VIII

Skeletal Manifestations of Metabolic Disorders

Contents

Metabolic disorders manifest by conspicuous skeletal changes include rickets, osteomalacia, scurvy and gout.

RICKETS

Historical

In the first classical description of this disease in 1850, Glisson gave it the name rachitis. The term rickets which previously had been used to cover many of the deforming diseases of children was, after Glisson, limited to the rachitis syndrome. The origin of the words rickets and rachitis is said to have been from the Anglo-Saxon word "wrickken," meaning to twist.

Following Glisson's observations, little of importance was contributed to the subject until near the middle of the nineteenth century, when Trousseau recognized the similarity of rickets to osteomalacia, and also noticed the value of cod liver oil in its treatment. However, cod liver oil and other fish oils had been used empirically for some time. Pommer published the first complete microscopic description and pathogenesis of the disease in humans in 1875. Shortly after the turn of the century, Schmorl gave a very complete description of the gross and microscopic pictures during both the active and healing stages. Erdheim did some exhaustive and accurate work on experimental rickets, employing the rat in most of his work. Palm demonstrated the part that sunlight could play in rickets, as early as 1890. Findlay, in 1909, produced experimental rickets, which he believed due to lack of exercise on the part of his experimental animals.

It was not until 1918 that Mellanby described rickets as definitely a deficiency disease. Since this time there has been a steady stream of both clinical and experimental contributions. Rickets and osteomalacia have come to be among the most clearly understood of all disease entities. Park, in 1921 and 1923, was first to give us unassailable experimental evidence of the role of vitamin D. At this time, Pappenheimer, McCollum, and Hess also made important contributions. Standardization of cod liver oil biologically on the basis of its vitamin D content soon followed. The work done in the past few years in further purifying and concentrating vitamin D is too familiar to require review.

Age Distribution

All ages and stages of human life are susceptible to malacic bone diseases. During the growing years the entity is termed rickets; after growth ceases, it is osteomalacia. Although such earlier writers on the subject as Virchow believed them to be two entirely different diseases, more recent observers have proved that they are the same disease occurring at different age periods.

Until recently, the existence of foetal rickets was denied, even by such capable investigators as Schmorl. In 1930, Maxwell, working in China, reported two cases of foetal rickets in babies born of mothers suffering from prolonged untreated osteomalacia. This same author, with Hu and Turnbull, reported another case in a baby from the same type of mother in 1932. This report was complete in every detail, leaving no doubt as to the existence of foetal rickets.

Infantile rickets is by far the most common type, developing between

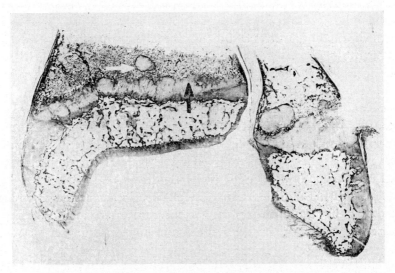

FIGURE 218. Active rickets in late childhood. Histologic section of the lower tibia and fibula showing widened irregular epiphyseal plates. Photomicrographs of areas at arrow points are Figures 219 and 220.

the ages of six weeks and three years. Late rickets, or rachitis tarda, is rare except under circumstances of famine such as has occurred in Europe and Asia after the World Wars. Famine causes many cases of so-called famine or starvation rickets. There is no basis for doubting that rickets may occur at any time during the growing period.

PHYSIOLOGY

When there is a disturbance of calcium metabolism, the skeleton is the loser. In rickets and osteomalacia the calcium and phosphorous are inadequately absorbed from the gastro-intestinal tract as a consequence of insufficient vitamin D intake. In idiopathic steatorrhea coeliac disease and sprue, the inadequate mineral absorption is the outcome of impaired fat absorption and episodes of diarrhea. The fat combines with the calcium and phosphorous to form soaps which are lost in the faeces.

Thus the skeleton must be robbed of its minerals in order to maintain proper levels of calcium and phosphorous in the blood. Since additional parathormone is required to mobilize the needed calcium from the skeleton, a secondary, or compensatory parathyroid gland hyperplasia develops.

In infantile rickets the serum calcium remains normal or at most only slightly decreased. A slight to moderate decrease of serum phosphorus is common. Blood phosphatase is nearly always slightly elevated, and occasionally it is moderately elevated.

In another group of entities absorption of minerals is unimpaired, but the normal quantities of blood minerals are insufficient to meet the pathologically increased demand. In chronic interstitial nephritis, additional calcium is needed by the kidneys for bases. In primary hyperparathyroidism it is the excessive secretion of parathormone that wastes the calcium and causes its excretion. Acidosis, particularly the ketosis of diabetes mellitus, appears to utilize part of the skeletal calcium as a base to diminish excessive acidity. In hyperthyroidism and basophilism, excessive calcium is mobilized from the skeletal storehouse, but the exact mechanism underlying it is not clear.

The following outline, though incomplete, is suggested as an aid in visualizing the relationship of the various etiologic factors to the skeletal disease they create during altered calcium metabolism:

SKELETAL DISEASES RESULTING FROM ALTERATIONS OF CALCIUM METABOLISM

Alteration of Calcium Metabolism	*Etiology*	*Skeletal Disease*
Inadequate absorption of calcium from the gastrointestinal tract.	1. Deficiency of Vitamin D.	1. Rickets in children and osteomalacia in adults.
	2. Intestinal diseases, idiopathic steatorrhoea, chronic coeliac disease, sprue and certain gastro-intestinal malignancies.	2. Coeliac rickets in children and osteomalacia in adults.
	3. Deficiency of calcium and phosphorus in diet.	3. Rickets or osteomalacia.
Excessive mobilization of skeletal calcium.	1. Chronic kidney disease.	1. Renal rickets.
	2. Primary hyperparathyroidism (Parathyroid adenoma or primary hyperplasia).	2. Generalized osteitis fibrosa. (von Recklinghausen's disease.)

RENAL RICKETS

The mechanism by which chronic kidney disease causes rickets is complex and confusing. Several of its features, however, are fairly well

understood and deserve review. The damaged kidneys become unable to
excrete the phosphates necessary for the production of urinary ammonia.
Bases must then be secured elsewhere in order to neutralize the acid ions
(sulfate, chloride) excreted by the kidneys. The only storehouse of bases
in the body is the skeletal system; therefore, through an increased secretion of parathormone, calcium to serve as a base is mobilized from the
bones and carried to the kidneys by the blood stream. A physiological

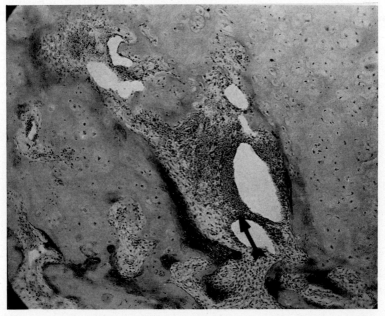

FIGURE 219. Active stage of rickets. Area opposite the point of the black arrow, Figure 218,
shows the accumulation of cartilage at the enchondral line, loss of the zone of provisory
calcification, loss of column arrangement of cells, and a deep chondroclastic inroad into
the epiphyseal plate (arrow).

acid-base balance is restored but at the expense of the skeleton. Mitchel
described another mechanism of calcium loss in renal rickets. His studies
led him to believe that part of the excessive phosphates accumulating in
the blood stream are excreted into the intestinal tract where they combine with calcium to form an insoluble calcium salt that cannot be
absorbed, so is lost in the faeces.

The majority of cases of chronic kidney disease that lead to skeletal
changes make their appearance during childhood, generally in late
childhood (Fig. 236). Growth is disturbed, giving rise to dwarfing that
has been termed renal dwarfism. Changes develop in epiphyses and
metaphyses (Fig. 235) similar to those in vitamin D deficiency rickets.
In both renal and vitamin D deficiency rickets, the generalized skeletal

deossification and osteoid apposition are similar. Some observers have contended that osteoid apposition is less active in renal rickets. Renal rickets causes a generalized fibrous osteitis (Albright).

Hyperphosphatemia is a characteristic of renal rickets, and represents, of course, a retention of inorganic phosphate in the blood. Blood calcium levels are correspondingly lowered, upsetting the normal calcium-phosphorus balance. Only the secondary parathyroid hyperplasia with its increased secretion of parathormone keeps the serum calcium level above the tetany stage. In many cases the serum calcium level is only slightly higher than the serum phosphorus.

PATHOLOGIC ANATOMY AND PATHOGENESIS

Active Stage

Epiphyseal plate: To acquire a clear understanding of the pathogenesis of rickets it is essential to know the histology of enchondral ossification. This was described in detail in Chapter I. Recall that the zone of preparatory or provisory calcification is invaded by capillaries and cells from the adjacent marrow spaces. The deepest cartilage cell lacunae are opened up, the chondrocytes released, and the projecting bar of calcified matrix made a nucleus for the formation of a primary bony trabeculum. After the bar of calcified cartilage is severed, it exists for some time as an "island" in the center of the bony trabeculum. The epiphyseal plate cartilage, with its cell columns separated by bars and plates of cartilage matrix, is divided into a zone of mother cells, a zone of proliferation, a zone of resting cells, and a zone of preparatory calcification. Erdheim made meticulous measurements of these zones in experimental rickets, and found little change in width or histologic structure of any of the zones except the zone of preparatory calcification. It is in this zone that the profound changes appear in both human and experimental rickets.

In severe cases there may be a complete cessation of calcification. Normal orderly enchondral ossification then fails to occur, since it is dependent upon the zone of calcified cartilage. Proliferation of the epiphyseal cartilage, although retarded, steadily continues, giving an ever widening zone that was meant to be only the narrow band of preparatory calcification (Fig. 219). The bizarre picture that develops at the epiphysis in florid cases is not surprising. The cartilage cell columns may grow to such lengths as to contain ten or twenty times their normal number of cells. The column formation is lost, especially in the deeper aspects. The extent of the changes and the width to which the cartilage may grow depend upon the rate of growth of the individual. If growth is slowed by any cause, such as a poor state of health, the epiphyseal changes become less flamboyant. Likewise in the epiphyses, whose growth is normally slow, changes are less striking (Fig. 230).

Although enchondral ossification may cease in severe rickets, one sometimes sees a distorted and disorderly type of cartilage invasion, found only in severe rickets. Chondroclastic cells from the adjacent marrow spaces may here and there make "tongue-like inroads" into the

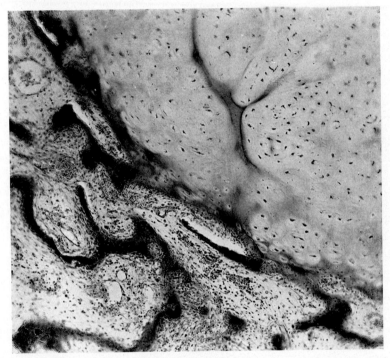

FIGURE 220. Active rickets. Metaphyseal island of non-calcified cartilage surrounded by osteoid (area opposite point of white arrow, Figure 218).

cartilage. Osteoid is then deposited along these paths. In this process large islands of non-calcified cartilage may become isolated from the main mass and become surrounded by osteoid (Fig. 220). Some observers believe they have seen direct metaplasia of cartilage to osteoid at the periphery of these islands.

Metaphysis and Diaphysis

Conspicuous changes take place in the metaphysis and diaphysis. It must be understood that rachitic changes occur throughout the osseous system and not just at the epiphyses. Active osteoid apposition occurs throughout the metaphyses, often giving large, bizarre shaped trabeculae. which often join to form a subchondral plate. These trabeculae assume no purposeful or orderly arrangement. They do not respect the longitudinal orientation that normally characterizes primary metaphyseal trabeculae. Other trabeculae are formed around nuclei of uncalcified cartilage, which sit like islands in their centers; still other trabeculae are built upon the porotic remains of mature calcified trabeculae that existed previous to the onset of the rickets. In the latter a striking con-

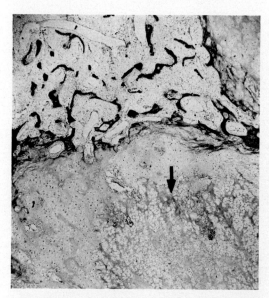

trast exists, with hematoxylin and eosin stain, between the pink of the osteoid and the red or bluishred of the mature calcified bone. If the rickets has been active for a considerable time, thick layers of osteoid (Fig. 221) are laid down upon the old porotic bony trabeculae throughout the skeleton. At the same time the compact bone reveals varying amounts of osteoid in the walls of the haversian systems.

FIGURE 222. Early in the healing stage of rickets. Showing beginning reformation of the zone of calcified cartilage in the epiphyseal plate. Note that the new zone of calcification (arrow) is not at the metaphyseal junction but inside the epiphyseal plate.

Haversian osteoid apposition may, in severe cases, become disorderly, losing a static arrangement. A layer of osteoid often appears subperiosteally and subendosteally. The globular, fusiform enlargements seen in children at such places as the wrists and costochondral junction of ribs (rachitic rosary) are due to an exuberant growth of osteoid perichondrally. The process really represents an osteoid extension from the metaphyseal cortex over the epiphyseal cartilage.

Cupping of the metaphysis (Fig. 225), which is so often of diagnostic significance in roentgen interpretation, appears to result from the persistence of enchondral ossification peripherally after it has greatly slowed or ceased in the central aspect of the epiphyseal plate. Thus more cartilage is replaced by new bone peripherally than centrally, giving rise to a cupping of the metaphysis even in foetal rickets.

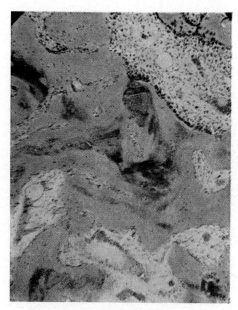

FIGURE 221. Active rickets. Only the central portion of the trabeculae is bone, the remainder is osteoid.

Fibrosis and hyperemia of the marrow are seen rather frequently in metaphyses, and consistently appear at such sites of unusual mechanical traumatic irritation as fractures. Otherwise marrow fibrosis is not a prominent feature of rickets. This is in contrast to the profoundly extensive marrow fibrosis of generalized osteitis fibrosa.

Healing Stage

BEGINNING HEALING is observed microscopically very soon after the inauguration of an adequate antirachitic regime. Experimental rickets in rats has disclosed microscopic evidence of healing within twenty-four

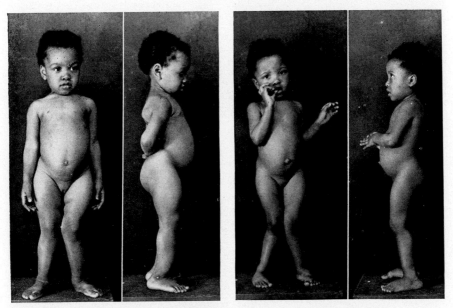

FIGURE 223. Rachitic deformities in the lower extremities of twins. Their diet had been high in calories and minerals but very low in vitamin D.

hours after carefully regulated administration of cod liver oil or its vitamin D principle. Pappenheimer found calcification throughout the zone of preparatory calcification of rat ribs, after five to seven days of antirachitic therapy. According to Harris the healing process in human rickets does not appear microscopically for at least ten days even under the most favorable conditions.

The first evidence of healing is seen as scattered and irregular patches of matricial calcification within the widened zone of provisory calcification (Fig. 222). Simultaneously, a process of resorption begins in the epiphyseal plate and in the adjacent excessive osteoid deposits. Osteoclasts may become numerous. The healing process has much to accomplish in restoring orderly enchondral ossification in such a disturbed and distorted epiphysis and metaphysis. As healing progresses, calcium salts are deposited in those osteoid trabeculae that are to be utilized and

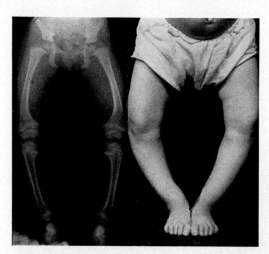

not absorbed. In many of the osteoid trabeculae the mere process of calcification transforms them to mature lamellar bone. Other osteoid that has developed on the basis of fibrous tissue forms primitive fibrous bone simply by calcification.

WELL ESTABLISHED HEALING is marked by the reestablishment of matricial calcification in the zone of preparatory calcification. The contour of the zone may still be jagged and broken, but even so, growth by enchondral ossification is resumed. The osteoid laid down around the bars of calcified matrix at the enchondral

FIGURE 224. Rachitic genu varum (Bowlegs).

line promptly becomes calcified to form bone. At this stage the epiphyseal plate is still wide, but it is rapidly trimmed down toward normal dimensions. Metaphyseal trabeculae begin to assume their normal static orientation. A reduction in size may be observed in such globular enlargements as the rachitic rosary. Fibrosis, wherever present in the marrow, begins to be replaced by fatty and hematogenous elements. Roentgenograms disclose a diminishing malacia.

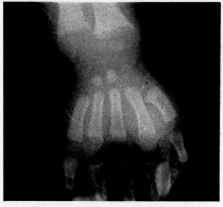

FIGURE 225. Active infantile rickets. Roentgenogram showing metaphyseal widening and cupping of the lower radius and ulna.

ADVANCED HEALING may be said to have been reached when in the epiphyseal plate the cartilage cell columns have an approximately normal number of cells, and a well formed zone of calcified cartilage. Extensive calcification of osteoid may be observed, together with reorientation of the trabeculae and haversian canals in the axis of the lines of stress.

COMPLETED HEALING finds the epiphyseal plate grossly and histologically normal except for irregularities in contour (Fig. 232). All osteoid

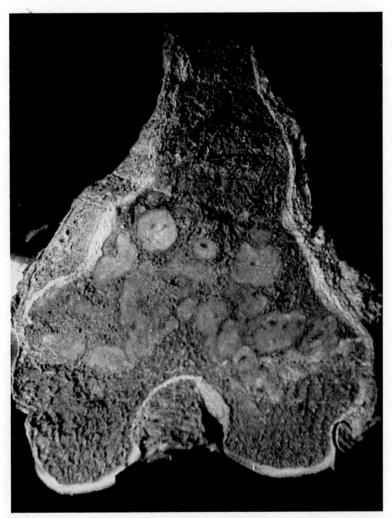

FIGURE 226. Rachitis tarda of long duration. The lower femoral epiphyseal plate is broken up into multiple cartilage islands. A. Gross specimen.

calcifies. The osteomalacia disappears, and the bones assume their normal density. The rachitic rosary, together with the wrist and skull enlargements, usually do not entirely disappear. Mild or moderate bowing in the extremities often undergoes spontaneous correction.

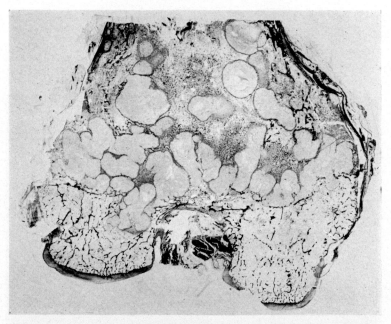

FIGURE 226. *(Continued)* B. Histologic section.

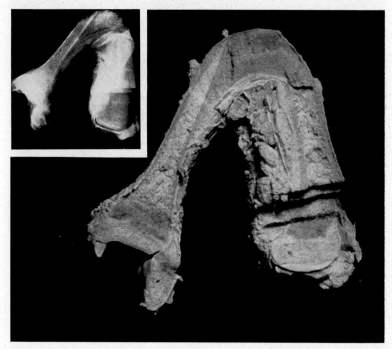

FIGURE 227. Far advanced rickets. Patient died of starvation in Austria after World War I. A. Healed fracture of the left tibia. The distal one-half of the tibia is doubled back upon the proximal one-half.

ROENTGENOLOGIC CORRELATION

During rickets the roentgenograms clearly and accurately reflect both the diagnosis and the stage of the disease.

EPIPHYSEAL CHANGES include retarded growth in the ossified portion of the epiphysis, and loss of definition. In severe cases growth may cease

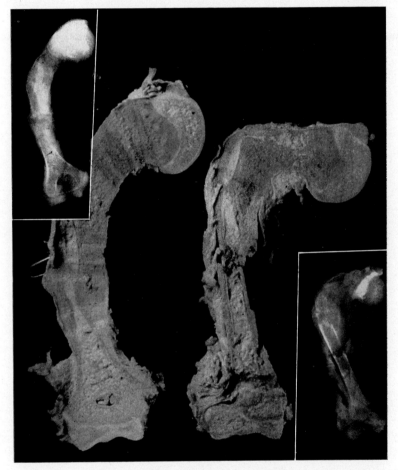

FIGURE 227. *(Continued)* B. Sectioned humeri (Frontal sections).

until vitamin D again becomes available to the epiphyses. Thickening of the epiphyseal plate, which is the most important single change, represents the accumulation of non-calcified cartilage. The chondrocytes pile up through activity of the zone of proliferation, unaccompanied by the cartilage replacement process of enchondral ossification. The thickness of any specific epiphyseal plate in rickets is in direct

proportion to the rate of growth normally existing in the plate, together
with the severity and duration of the disease. In protracted cases of
vitamin D deficiency, the lower femoral and upper tibial epiphyseal
plates become extremely wide and irregular (Fig. 229). In the roentgenogram the narrow transverse white line that represents the line of
provisory calcification becomes broken up, and in severe rickets it entirely disappears. Its reappearance is an indication that healing has been
established.

Cupping of epiphyses can be clearly seen in the roentgenogram and

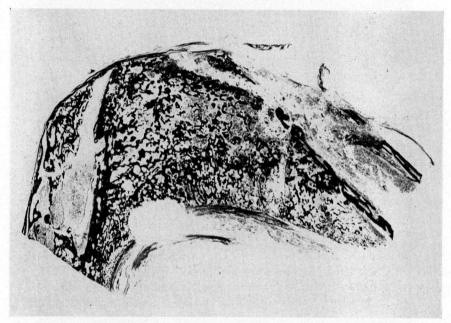

FIGURE 228. Histologic section of the healed tibial fracture shown in Figure 227 A.
Disoriented osteoid trabeculae fill the space between the tibial fragments and represent
the site and cause of the angulation.

may persist for considerable time after healing is complete. Widening
of the epiphyseo-metaphyseal junction and an outward flaring of the
metaphyseal cortices produces what has been aptly called "trumpeting"
(Fig. 224).

THE BONE CHANGES, as seen in the roentgenogram, present various
degrees of osteomalacia. Since the transverse or secondary trabeculae are
absorbed more rapidly than the longitudinal or primary trabeculae,
the latter become relatively more prominent in the roentgenogram and
explain the "coarse trabeculation" so often mentioned by roentgenologists. "Coarse trabeculation" characterizes all forms of bone porosis and

is not pathognomonic of rickets and osteomalacia. In far advanced stages even the calcified portion of the longitudinal trabeculae may become thin or almost entirely absorbed, giving the metaphyses and epiphyses a homogenous appearance in the roentgenogram.

Cortices lose much of their sharp definition in rickets, partly from the osteoporosis and partly from osteoid deposited in haversian systems and on trabecular surfaces. In their softened state, the long bones, as well as many of the short and flat bones, bend into a variety of abnormal contours. Bowing occurs in long bones with the convexity of the curve laterally (as in bow legs), medially (as in knock knees), or anteriorly. Cortices become wider on the concave side in response to the need for mechanical reinforcement, in keeping with Wolff's law. No bones are immune from deformation. Even skull bones may bend, particularly in the occipital region (craniotabes). Deformation of the skull also takes place through the deposition of osteoid on the outer table in the parietal and frontal regions (bosses). During healing, part of this osteoid is absorbed, but part of it ossifies and remains permanently as a monument to the rickets.

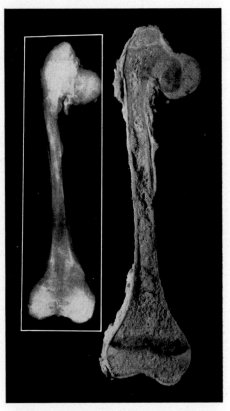

FIGURE 229. Rachitis tarda advanced. Frontal section of the right femur showing diffuse osteoporosis, coxa vara, and pronounced widening of the epiphyseal plates. The insert is an antero-posterior roentgenogram of the specimen.

In renal rickets the skull, particularly the outer table, develops what Camp calls a "fine granular osteoporosis." In renal rickets the skull porosis (malacia) is finely granular; in hyperparathyroidism it is coarsely granular; and in Paget's disease it is woolly.

CLINICAL CORRELATION

Medical students, and young physicians who have come into medicine during the vitamin era frequently need to be reminded that it is only

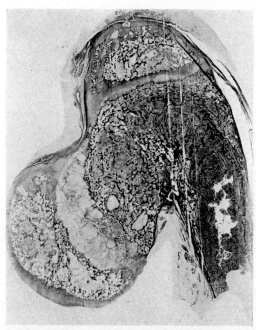

FIGURE 230. Histologic section of the upper portion of the femur shown in Figure 229. The epiphyseal plate of the capital epiphysis is much wider than the epiphyseal plate for the greater trochanter. This is in keeping with the rule in rickets that epiphyseal plates at sites of the most rapid growth show the most pronounced changes.

in recent years that we have had a clear appreciation of the role vitamin D plays in rickets and osteomalacia. As late as 1929 Hess stated in Cecil's textbook of Medicine: "The time is not ripe to appraise accurately the role of vitamins in the etiology of rickets." And in 1931 Osgood and Allison wrote: "There are then two factors in the cause of rickets which are: radiant energy and diet factor x." The radiant energy referred to proved to be ultra violet light. Sunlight or artificial ultra violet rays act upon sterols in the skin to produce vitamin D. Thus we may secure vitamin D both through the diet and through ultra violet irradiation.

Phosphorus deficiencies in the diet are of greater consequences in the production of rickets than calcium deficiencies. Prior to the discovery of vitamins, phosphorus frequently was administered in rickets and usually with benefit. Phemister, Millar, and Bonar stated in 1921: "Clearly, phosphorus and also cod liver oil in some way restore the power of normal ossification which is temporarily lost."

The response to vitamin D therapy may be delayed

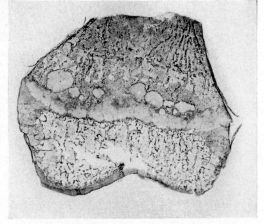

FIGURE 231. Histologic section of the lower portion of the femur shown in Figure 229.

when there has developed a substantial secondary hyperplasia of the parathyroid glands. The temporarily persisting excessive secretion of parathormone protracts the generalized skeletal malacia.

Deformities

Deformation of long bones in infancy should receive conservative

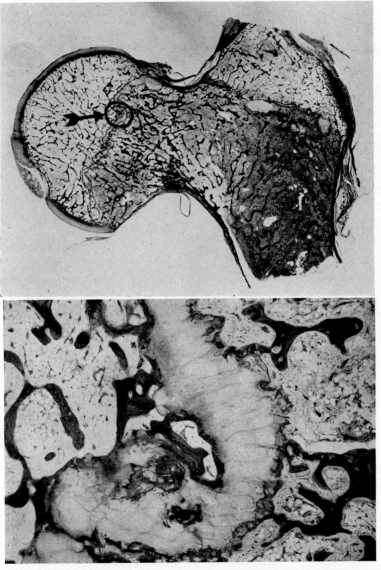

FIGURE 232. Rachitis tarda. Advanced healing as indicated by well established enchondral ossification. The kinks seen in the epiphyseal plate are typical of those frequently seen in healing rickets. A. *(Above)* Histological section of upper femur. B. *(Below)* Photomicrograph of the segment of epiphyseal plate enclosed in circle on Figure 232A.

orthopedic therapy. Even rather pronounced varus or valgus deviations of the tibia and femur tend to improve, and may even disappear with the advent of healing of the rickets, and continued growth. Osteotomies are not done as frequently now as formerly. Wolff's law generally takes better care of the bent bones of infants and young children than surgery of osteoclasis. Braces and osteotomies are now reserved for severe cases in which the deformity has not yielded to the test of time.

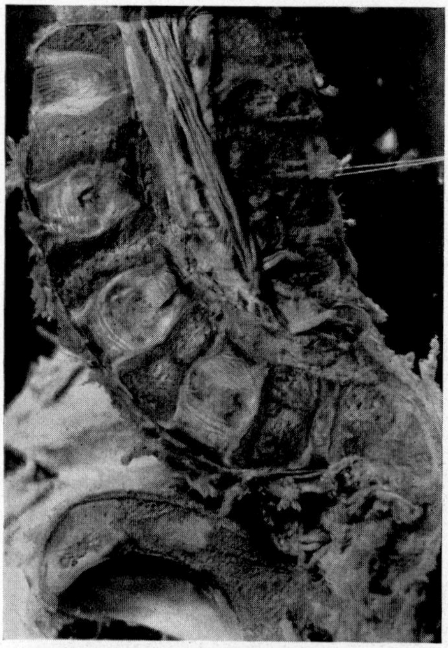

FIGURE 233. Advanced rickets as shown in a sagital section of the lumbar spine. The vertebral bodies were too soft even to resist the thirty pounds of intrinsic pressure in the intervertebral discs. As a result the discs have expanded until they are now wider than the compressed vertebral bodies.

OSTEOMALACIA

Osteomalacia is the rickets of the adult; it has the same etiology, and its pathology is similar except for the growth factor. This concept of osteomalacia is of relatively recent origin. Virchow taught that rickets and osteomalacia were totally different diseases. He believed that in rickets the bone in the process of formation failed to calcify, whereas the bone in osteomalacia, being already formed and calcified, lost its calcium by "a leaching action of the blood." Virchow watched the effect of hydrochloric acid upon bone specimens and believed a similar decalcifying action took place in the body from acid that was said to be in the blood and tissue. Cohnheim's classical treatise of 1889 was the first to refute Virchow's theory. Previously Virchow had been unchallenged in spite of Trausseau's early observations that cod liver oil had a curative influence on both rickets and osteomalacia. McCrudden, in 1908, emphasized and elaborated Cohnheim's precepts. Many of our present concepts of osteomalacia originated with McCrudden. Schmorl and Looser also helped uproot the dichotomy concept of rickets and osteomalacia.

THEORIES ON ETIOLOGY

Von Recklinghausen taught that osteomalacia was the response of a vasomotor irritation which produced a hyperemia that, in turn, caused a "washing out" of skeletal calcium salts through hyperacidity, said probably to be the result of an excess of lactic acid in the blood. Conclusive experimental evidence long ago disproved this theory.

In 1894, Fehling reported good results in the treatment of puerperal osteomalacia from oophorectomy. It was believed that an excessive internal ovarian secretion caused a sympathetic system paralysis which, through the associated hyperemia, produced skeletal decalcification. This theory received wide acceptance and oophorectomy became a commonly practiced therapeutic measure. No ovarian lesion or hyper-secretion has ever been identified. The reported improvement following removal of the ovaries is attributed principally to the general supportive measures such as a balanced hospital diet used in conjunction with the operation. Of course, the prevention of further pregnancies was often beneficial. If the osteomalacia is unsuccessfully treated, succeeding pregnancies progressively accentuate the skeletal deossification and deformities.

Osteomalacia is a deficiency disease. It is caused by a deficiency of vitamin D with or without a calcium deficiency in the diet. McCrudden was the first to demonstrate the existence of a deficiency of assimilable calcium in the blood stream. He showed that

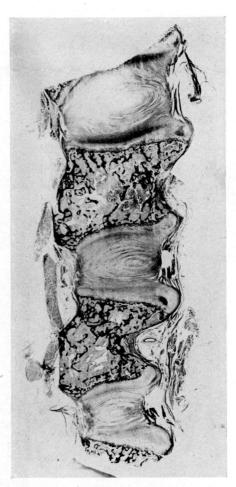

FIGURE 234. Histologic section taken from the proximal portion of the spine specimen shown in Figure 233.

the catabolic changes had progressed satisfactorily and that osteoid had formed during anabolism, but that for some reason, not discovered for years later, the calcium mobilized during catabolism did not become available to the newly formed osteoid. McCrudden carefully analyzed the body excretions and emphasized the fact that much of the calcium which should have been employed in ossification was lost in the feces. The part played by vitamin D in calcium metabolism has been described in the discussion of rickets, and need not be repeated.

Physiological Chemistry

The blood calcium and phosphorus usually are slightly lowered but

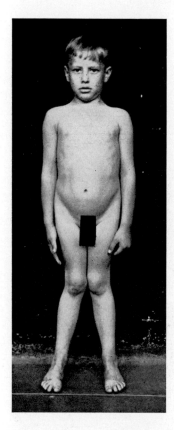
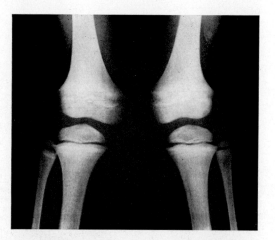
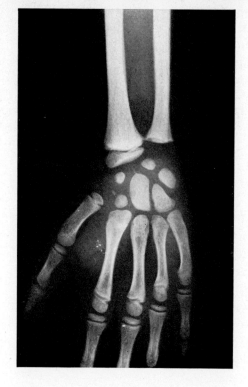

Figure 235. Renal rickets. A. (Left) Photo of patient showing genu valgum. B. (Right) Antero-posterior roentgenogram of knees. C. (Below) Antero-posterior roentgenogram of the right wrist.

may be entirely normal. In severe cases, particularly of the puerperal type, the blood calcium may drop to the tetany level. Phosphatase activity may also be normal but generally is slightly to moderately elevated, especially in the healing stage. Urine calcium and phosphorus frequently are normal; if abnormal, they are usually low. The fecal calcium content is almost always increased, often to a extremely high degree.

Types of Osteomalacia (*Locke's Classification*)

Puerperal

This is the type most frequently observed (Fig. 238). Symptoms appear during the last trimester of pregnancy. The disease develops during the latter part of pregnancy because during the last three months calcification is most active in the foetal skeleton. Women with puerperal osteomalacia have in their diet a deficiency of vitamin D, and often also of calcium. Before pregnancy they may have scarcely maintained their calcium balance; then when they begin sharing their calcium and vitamin D with the foetus, a deficiency is established that becomes manifest in the mother's skeleton as osteomalacia. Symptoms may steadily progress during the latter part of the pregnancy;

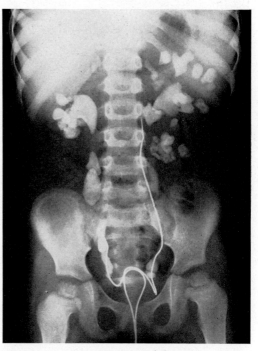

FIGURE 236. Renal rickets. Roentgenogram showing multiple renal stones.

the pelvic deformity occasionally becomes so extreme as to preclude a normal delivery. When the pregnancy terminates symptoms gradually improve, since the foetal demands have ceased. However, if the infant nurses the breast, the drain of the mother's calcium and vitamin D continues, since lactation makes heavy demands for these substances.

Many osteomalacic mothers experience one pregnancy after another. The skeletal changes just begin to come under control when another pregnancy produces an exacerbation. Each pregnancy leaves the skeleton more deformed. In this type of osteomalacia the pelvis is the site of the earliest and most pronounced changes; in severe cases the entire skeleton may become deformed. Cases have been observed where the lower lumbar vertebrae and sacrum have telescoped down into the pelvis. The acetabulae, through weight-bearing, may intrude so deeply into the pelvis that their inner walls almost touch (Fig. 242). When this extreme deformity occurs, the pubic rami protrudes forward like a horn. The vertebral column may become involved in grotesque scoliotic and kyphotic curvatures. Vertebral body compression is the rule and often attains an extreme degree.

It is not unusual for the sternum to assume the pigeon breast type of deformity. Long bones become bent and crumpled. In such extreme cases the patient becomes bed fast and frequently dies. The mortality rate for osteomalacia in localities where it is endemic has reached 90 percent. Although occasional instances of this stage of osteomalacia are seen in all parts of the world, it is most common in parts of India and China, where the women have severely deficient diets and often are deprived of adequate light and exercise. In India many Mohammedan women who live under the Purdah custom (Purdah is the Islamic word for curtain) keep

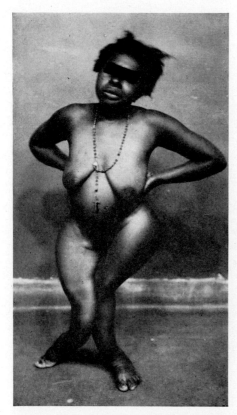

FIGURE 238. Osteomalacia. Age 25. Patient bore six children in seven years and it was during this period that the lower extremities became deformed. Eight osteotomies were required to straighten the femora and tibiae.

FIGURE 239. Osteomalacia. A. *(Left)* Frontal section of the distal one-third of the femur. Trabeculae are like threads and cortices like paper; marrow is fatty and gellatinous. This is a striking combination of far advanced osteoporosis and osteomalacia. B. *(Below)* Histologic section of the lower portion of specimen. Articular cortex of the femoral condyles is of microscopic dimensions, but has osteoid seams. C. *(Right)* Photomicrograph of the segment of cortex in the square marked on B.

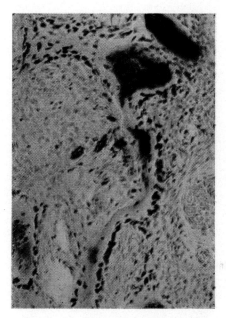

FIGURE 237. Photomicrograph of osteo-malacic trabeculae to show the wide osteoid seams.

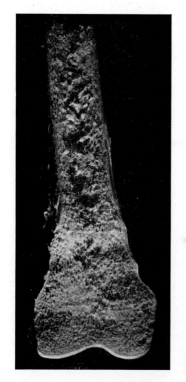
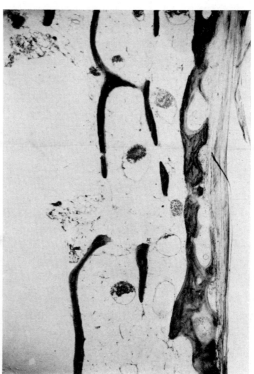
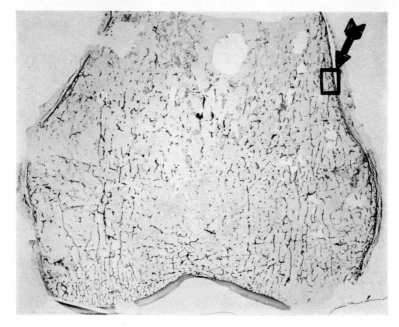

their faces and bodies heavily covered and remain indoors most of the day. They usually marry before the age of fourteen, frequently before menstruation begins; after marriage they live in seclusion, never being seen except by their husbands and brothers. Prolonged periods of lactation are practiced, two years or even more being common. It certainly is not remarkable that these women develop malacic skeletons.

Non-puerperal

This type occurs in parts of India, China and Japan, and is seen principally in women who remain indoors, and at the same time on diets deficient in vitamin D and minerals. In China this disease is seen among middle class women, and in India among the upper classes. Snapper has pointed out that the poorer class women in China and India work in the fields or on boats and receive enough sunshine to spare them from osteomalacia.

Hunger Osteomalacia or Osteopathy

As the name implies, this form is due to dietary insufficiencies. A notable outbreak of hunger osteomalacia and rickets occurred in Central Europe, especially Austria and parts of Germany, after the first World War. The majority of the cases were among the middle-aged, the elderly, and adolescent boys (Figs. 239 to 242) living in the poorer districts. A prolonged moderate quantitative and qualitative dietary deficiency is required for the development of hunger osteopathy; a brief period of severe food deprivation does not produce this syndrome. This form of the disease is usually more chronic and less deforming than the puerperal type. The deformities are more diffusely distributed over the skeleton, and there is no preference for the pelvis.

Senile Osteomalacia

Many observers believe this form of skeletal malacia is not a true member of this group. McCrudden was of the opinion that the osteoporosis of senility was due to a retarded process of anabolism. We know that all tissues during senility become deficient in their regenerative powers, whereas the catabolic process remains active and even accelerated. It is on this basis that most senile cases are explained, rather than on the basis of a vitamin D and calcium deficiency. Hypogonadal function is a factor in many cases. Senile osteoporosis is a more accurate term than senile osteomalacia.

Juvenile Osteomalacia

Some classifications include the cases of vitamin D deficiency observed during puberty as osteomalacia. In this study these cases are classified under rickets as rachitis tarda. This is proper since most of the epiphyses of the long bones are still growing and develop characteristic rachitic changes.

Chronic Steatorrhea Osteomalacia

Diseases that disturb fat absorption appear also to cause a loss of much of the vitamin D ingested (Fig. 245). Miyakawa and Stearns emphasized that in steatorrhea a considerable quantity of the fat soluble vitamins is excreted with the fat in the faeces.

Osteomalacia in Animals and Fowls

Numerous animals and fowls develop the typical skeletal changes of osteomalacia. This condition has been developed in experimental animals by feeding a deficient diet. In White's observations on zoological animals (Philadelphia Zoo), the primates constituted 50 percent of the animals affected by osteomalacia. Among fowls, doves were the most frequently affected. Occasionally the beak of a fowl would become too soft to be used in picking up food. Steenbock's observations in 1912 on a cow and a goat are classical. Osteomalacia is said to be common among cattle in Central Europe, especially after dry, hot seasons.

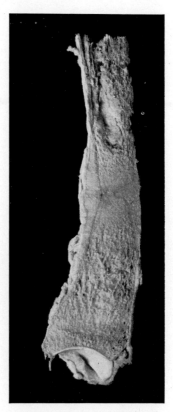

FIGURE 240. Osteomalacia: sagittal section of the lower tibia. A crumpling type of fracture in the middle of the specimen is enveloped in periosteal callus (see Figure 151 B.).

Pathologic Anatomy and Pathogenesis

Early Stage

A progressive bone malacia becomes evident early in the disease. Multinucleated giant cell osteoclasts may be seen but there are not nearly so many of these cells as are found in most cases of von Recklinghausen's osteitis fibrosa. The skeletal deossification usually is much more rapid in the latter than in osteomalacia. As the process continues, the cortices gradually become narrower and the medullary canals, wider. Haversian canals enlarge, and much of the compact bone is transformed to cancellous. Osteoblastic activity continues with the formation of osteoid, layer upon layer, on the surfaces of the old and porotic trabeculae, and in the enlarged haversian canals (Fig. 237). Persisting osteoid seams stand out as one of the most characteristic signs of malacic bone disease.

Osteoid formation in rickets is most active at the metaphyses and in the outer layers of diaphyseal cortex. In osteomalacia the process is diffused throughout the bones. Osteoid layers observed on the old trabeculae were believed by Virchow to represent, not newly applied layers, but layers of the old bone that had been decalcified. No attempt

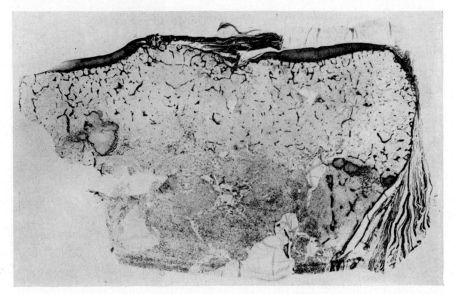

FIGURE 241. Osteomalacia: histologic section of the upper tibia of a young adult. Islands of cartilage are the remains of the epiphyseal plate.

is made by the cambium layer to form periosteal osteoid, with the exception of sites of periosteal injury or irritation such as fractures. Fractures and deformities during early stages of the disease are not common.

Advanced Stage

As the pathologic process advances, several other changes appear. Pronounced generalized skeletal malacia and osteoporosis become manifest. In some parts of the skeleton there is an abundance of osteoid; in other parts there is a paucity of osteoid. Von Recklinghausen and Freund have demonstrated that osteoid forms in response to stresses and strains, and is nature's attempt to reinforce sites of maximum mechanical stress. Therefore, the sites of ligamentous and muscular attachments, and areas of bone subjected to shearing, torsion or bending stresses, become sites of more abundant osteoid apposition. In such areas bits of the old bone, stained dark red, stand out with striking contrast in the center of the pink osteoid masses. A thin envelope of fibrous connective tissue forms around many of the trabeculae. The marrow frequently becomes fibrous at sites of mechanical irritation and may give rise to fibrous osteoid trabeculae. Part of the fatty marrow may be replaced by myelogenous marrow. Hyperemia and edema of marrow is the rule. Areas of hemorrhage are common, and in those areas phagocytes may be seen removing the blood pigment. Grossly the marrow appears yellow, dark red, or brown.

Far Advanced Stage

In areas where osteoid formation has been active the bones often appear wax-like, and can be readily sliced with a sharp knife. Such areas become involved in grotesque deformities. Other bones reveal little osteoid, but are involved by a profound osteoporosis. The cortex is like parchment, and is so thin that microscopically it may contain no

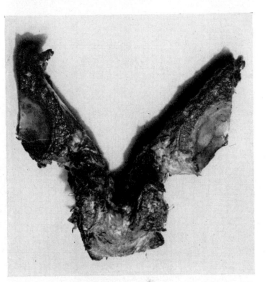

FIGURE 242. Osteomalacia: specimen from the pelvis showing a portion of the acetabulae and the pubic rami. Weight bearing has bent the rami and caused the acetabulae to intrude into the pelvic canal.

haversian systems. The trabecular system of the cancellous bone resembles a spider web stretched between the paper-thin cortical walls (Fig. 239). The marrow is usually fatty, or gelatinous. Fatty cysts, filled with an oily debris are common, and appear to be localized in areas of fat necrosis. Kaufman has aptly described the long bones in this far advanced stage as "membranous tubes filled with a soft pulpy mass."

Fractures usually are multiple and mostly of a crumpling type, depending upon the amount of osteoid present. An abundant callus formation is the rule; this is especially true of the external (periosteal) callus (Fig. 240). Calcification does not make its appearance until the healing stage of the disease is established.

Healing Stage

Calcification of part of the osteoid, resorption of excess osteoid, and re-establishment of normally constructed cancellous and compact bone occur in much the same manner as in rickets.

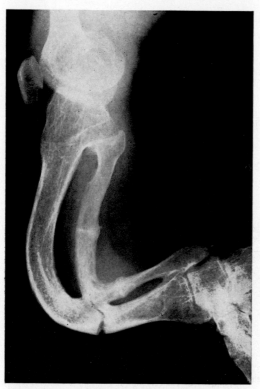

FIGURE 243. Osteomalacia: male age 47. Frequent gastro-intestinal upsets and vomiting since early childhood. Deformities of all extremities began during childhood (rickets) and continued to increase during adult life (osteomalacia). Lateral roentgenogram of the right tibia and fibula. Looser's zone of transformation appears at the junction of the middle and lower thirds. A similar deformity is sometimes seen in osteogenesis imperfecta.

ROENTGENOLOGIC CORRELATION

The roentgenogram serves a dual purpose in osteomalacia. In diagnosis few entities are more clearly portrayed radiographically than osteomalacia. And during the period of therapy, if the roentgenograms are taken by identical technique each time, they serve to record the rate of skeletal reossification. In early stages osteomalacia cannot be differentiated from osteoporosis. Secondary transverse trabeculae disappear, giving a coarse reticular appearance to the cancellous bone. Cortices soon become narrowed, for in osteomalacia the diaphyses become involved early in the disease.

Deformities may slowly increase until extreme and even grotesque contours are incurred (Fig. 243).

Narrow transverse defects (Umbauzonen) in the long bones are frequent in osteomalacia; they were first described by Looser. He contended that they represented zones in which the bone was absorbed and replaced by osteoid. Some authorities have contended that Looser's zones are fractures; others, that they are pseudofractures. Displacement of fragments does not take place. Looser zones of transformation are most in evidence on the convex side of bowing in long bones (Fig. 243).

While cyst-like areas in the bones are not common in osteomalacia they do occur, and generally are small and multiple (Fig. 244B).

CLINICAL CORRELATION

The deformities of osteomalacia present many difficult orthopedic problems. There are occasions where multiple osteotomies are required to straighten a bent tibia or femur. A patient with untreated osteomalacia should be carefully protected by braces or bed rest from incurring further skeletal deformation.

Joint symptoms accrue from collapse of the articular cortex. The trabecular system underlying the articular cortex may become so weakened by deossification that compression fractures develop, thus altering the joint contours and leading to limited mobility and degenerative changes in the articular cartilage. Even when there is no direct insult to the joints in osteomalacia there eventually may be osteo-arthritic changes on the basis of altered joint mechanics from curvatures of the long bones and spine.

Tetany is a frequent complication of osteomalacia in China, according to Snapper, but is said to be relatively rare in the osteomalacia of India.

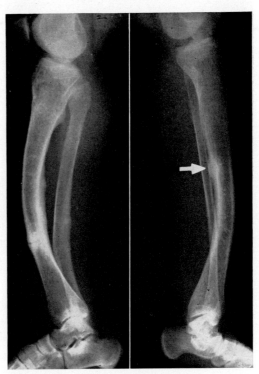

FIGURE 244. Mild osteomalacia in a female age 21. A. Lateral roentgenogram of tibiae. The Looser zone (arrows) is anterior on the right and posterior on the left.

SCURVY

Scurvy has long been recognized: Hippocrates observed it among soldiers; it occurred among the 13th Century Crusaders; and during the 15th and 16th Centuries it decimated the sailors making long voyages with the great explorers.

It was not until 1753 that James Lind revealed the remarkable curative power of lemon juice. By the end of the 18th Century the British Admiralty had eliminated scurvy from its sea-going personnel by the routine use of lemon and lime juice during all long voyages.

In 1859 Möller described cases of scurvy in Germany, but erroneously called them acute rickets. During this same period Thomas Smith referred to cases of scurvy in England as hemorrhagic periostitis. Sir Thomas Barlow's classical description of 31 cases in 1883 clearly established scurvy as an entity separate from other types of dietary deficiency. Infantile and adult forms were then conceded to be the same disease. Except for a brief period during World War I in Central Europe and Russia, there have been relatively few cases of adult scurvy reported during the past fifty years. However, Ireland is said by Hess to have numerous cases of adult scurvy whenever their potato crop fails. Infantile scurvy may still be seen in this country among babies fed on boiled or pasteurized milk, and denied fruit juices and fresh vegetables.

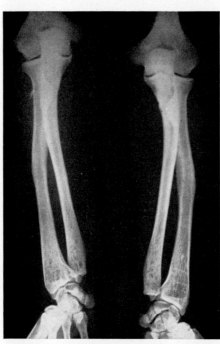

FIGURE 244. (Continued) Antero-posterior roentgenograms of forearms. In the distal one-half of the radii and ulnae there is coarse trabeculation and small circular zones of osseous resorption.

The Norwegian investigators, Holst and Frolich, demonstrated experimental scurvy in 1907. Hess described the pathology of scurvy in 1920, utilizing experimental animals for many of his observations. Without adequate vitamin C, guinea pigs and monkeys develop scurvy, but cows, rats, mice, and fowls do not need vitamin C in their diet. Ascorbic acid was isolated by Waugh and King in 1932. It has been established that the body has only a meager capacity for storing vitamin C; under optimum conditions, approximately a seven day supply can be stored.

PATHOLOGY AND PATHOGENESIS

Hojer, Wolback and others have noted that the bodily changes in avitaminosis C take place in cells and tissues of mesodermal origin.

There is an impairment of the cohesive property of the matricial substance of the connective tissues and endothelium. Capillary hemorrhages may appear in the mucous membranes and connective tissues throughout the body. The most common sites of hemorrhage in scurvy are the gums, conjunctivae, skin, intestines, bladder, kidneys, and beneath the periosteum.

Periosteum

Subperiosteal hemorrhage is said by Kato to be the most important single sign of scurvy. The periosteum becomes edematous and congested; the hemorrhage beneath it may be slight, or it may be so extensive as to give the hematoma the proportions of a large tumor. Coagulation of the subperiosteal blood occurs promptly and is followed by resorption or organization. Larger hematoma are organized and transformed to fibroblastic tissue. In complete scurvy little or no ossification takes

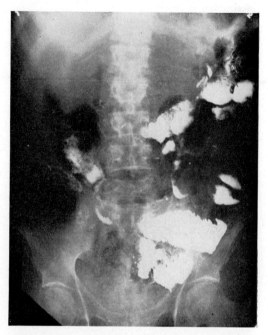

FIGURE 245. Osteomalacia in a male age 30. Malacia of the skeleton was from chronic idiopathic sprue of three years duration. Antero-posterior roentgenogram taken after a barium meal shows characteristic pooling of the barium.

place until treatment is established (Fig. 247). But if the avitaminosis C is only partial, the organized subperiosteal hematoma becomes well ossified previous to therapy (Fig. 246C). Fibrous bone forms in the same manner as in the formation of primary callus or an involucrum. During the healing process the periosteal bone is gradually resorbed.

Epiphyses and Metaphyses

Striking and frequently profound changes develop at epiphyseal lines and in the metaphyses during infantile scurvy. Enchondral ossification slows down, and in protracted avitaminosis C, growth ceases. Growth at enchondral lines ceases, not because of a paucity of calcium as in rickets, but because of a disturbance of osteo-apposition. Osteoblasts are inactive and fewer in number.

The zone of provisory calcification becomes broadened and irregular.

This manifestation is derived from the simple facts that the zone of proliferation continues to form new chondrocytes at the normal rate, and
calcification of the matrix in the zone of calcified cartilage continues
to take place in a normal manner. It is the third step in enchondral
ossification that does not proceed normally. The minute bars of calcified cartilage projecting into the metaphysis do not become nuclei for
new bony trabeculae; but instead, the calcified cartilage accumulates,
giving the widened zone known as the "white line" of Fraenkel.

In protracted scurvy epiphyseal plates lose the column arrangement

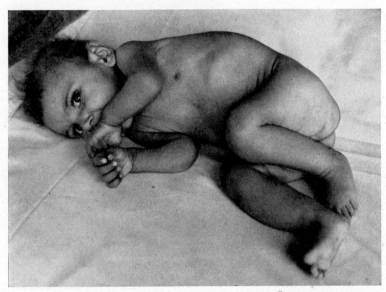

FIGURE 246. Acute infantile scurvy. A. Male age eight months. Had had symptoms for
two months. Posture and apprehensive expression are characteristic. Had never had fruit
juices in diet and was bottle fed after four days of age. Dramatic recovery followed vitamin C
therapy.

of their chondrocytes. In less severe scurvy a few poorly constructed
bony trabeculae form at the epiphyseo-metaphyseal junction, and are
characterized by the presence of large irregular central islands of calcified cartilage.

Hemorrhages characterize scorbutic metaphyses. The hyperemia
brought by organization, and resorption of the hematomata causes the
cancellous bone of the metaphyses to be greatly weakened through osteoclastic activity. Although all parts of the bones are deossified, the
process is most conspicuous in the metaphyses. In the roentgenogram
this fact is portrayed by a dark zone adjacent to the "white line" of the
epiphyseal plate (Fig. 246C), a zone referred to by Pelkan as the "scurvy

line." In infants and small children, epiphyses such as those of the upper tibia and lower femur are spherical or oval in shape, and have an enchondral line encircling their periphery. The zone of calcified cartilage in this enchondral line becomes widened and presents a fine irregularity. This widened encircling zone of calcified cartilage is referred to as "Wimbergers line" or "ringing of the epiphysis."

Because of the extreme porosis of the metaphyses, fractures occur at the epiphyseo-metaphyseal junction; generally such fractures are called epiphyseal separations. True epiphyseal separations do occur however, and take place in the zone of calcified cartilage. When treatment is established, normal enchondral ossification is rapidly restored.

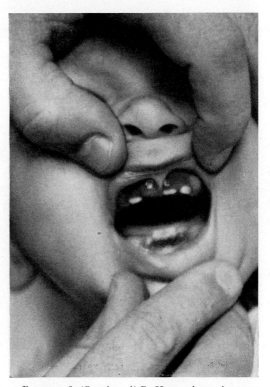

Marrow

Degenerative changes and hemorrhage appear in the metaphyseal marrow. In chronic cases there is gradual replacement of the myelogenous elements of the marrow with a cellular fibrous tissue. At this stage the metaphyseal marrow has been termed the "framework marrow" by Brower, and the "Gerustmark" by Schodel and Nauwerck. Scattered hemorrhages occur through the diaphyseal marrow and are absorbed or organized.

FIGURE 246. *(Continued)* B. Hemorrhages in gums are limited to areas where teeth have erupted.

Bone

The entire skeleton undergoes deossification, the principal cause of which is the enforced immobilization. An additional factor is the retardation or complete loss of osteogenesis. Osteoclasis (catabolism) proceeds at a normal or accellerated rate, whereas the deposition of new bone (anabolism) is at a standstill. In long standing severe cases the cortices become paper thin and the cancellous trabeculae become so fine that in the roentgenograms the bone has a ground-glass radiolucency. Pathological fractures are common, occurring through the metaphyses in infantile scurvy and through the diaphyses in the adult form.

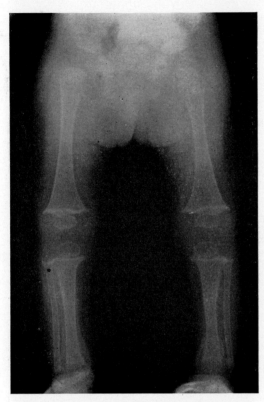

FIGURE 246. *(Continued)* C. Antero-posterior roentgenogram of lower extremities. Extensive sub-periosteal hematomas of tibia are ossifying.

Teeth and Gums

Howe, Hojer and Wolback have described the changes observed in the teeth and gums during both human and experimental scurvy. Because of the alveolar porosis the teeth may become loosened and lost through mastication of food. A brittleness also develops in teeth; in advanced stages the teeth may be snapped in two like a piece of chalk. Hemorrhages occur in the pulp, followed by degeneration vacuolization, and in some instances necrosis. Dentine formation ceases in complete scurvy but is rapidly restored with therapy. The enamel is not altered.

Bleeding, congested, edematous gums are a prominent symptom in scurvy (Fig. 246B). It is claimed that the gum changes take place only in the presence of erupted teeth.

Blood

A secondary anemia is the rule, together with a leucocytosis in which polymorphonuclear neurtrophils are increased. Ascorbic acid may be entirely absent from the blood and urine. One mg. percent or above is normal, 0.5 mg. percent is borderline and below 0.5 mg. percent usually means scurvy (McBride).

ROENTGENOLOGIC CORRELATION

Since biopsies are not indicated in scurvy we must lean heavily upon roentgenograms for both diagnosis and progress of healing. The roentgenogram is of particular value and interest in the infantile form. Kato has summarized the ten most important roentgenographic changes in infantile scurvy as follows:

1. Broadened, irregular, radio-opaque epiphyseal lines, the zone of provisory calcification representing the "white line" of Fraenkel.

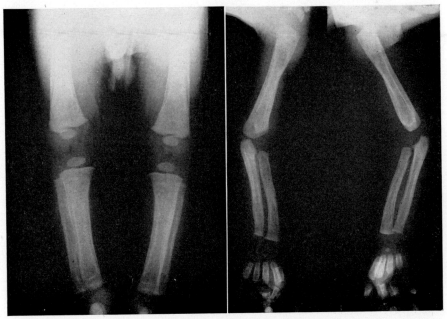

FIGURE 247. Infantile scurvy soon after therapy was instituted. The extensive sub-periosteal hematomata of all extremity long bones are well ossified. A. (Left) Roentgenograms of the lower extremities. B. (Right) Roentgenograms of the upper extremities.

2. A small bony spur (Pelkan spur) protruding from the lateral border of the epiphyseal line. Occasionally a similar spur protrudes medially.

3. A translucent zone of metaphyseal-rarefaction adjacent to the epiphyseal place. This zone has been termed the "scurvy line" by Pelkan, the "framework marrow" by Bromer and the "Gerustmark" by Schodel and Nauwerk. (The term "Trümmerfeld zone" is now little used because of the confusion arising from its being used to describe the "while line" by many German authors, and the "scurvy line" by several American investigators).

4. "Ringing of the epiphyses" or the Wimberger line. (This is the "white line" encircling the epiphysis proper.)

5. Ground-glass translucency of the bones.

6. Thinned cortices.
7. Subperiosteal hemorrhages with and without ossification.
8. Epiphyseal separation.
9. Costochondral and vertebral angulation of the ribs.
10. Subperiosteal and metaphyseal fractures.

CLINICAL CORRELATION

Very often the *severe pain in the legs* is the first definite symptom of scurvy. The pain, the exquisite tenderness, and the swelling are the direct result of the subperiosteal hemmorhage. Any movement causes severe pain and muscle spasm. The enforced immobilization is termed pseudo-paralysis.

SYMPTOMS OF SEVERE SCURVY, in addition to those in the legs, include cachexia; purple, swollen, bleeding gums; loose, brittle teeth; hemorrhages in the skin, intestines, bladder and eyes; elevated temperature up to 105 degrees; and apprehension. If avitaminosis C is not corrected, death occurs within a few months. Scurvy lowers resistance to infection. Pneumonia is the leading cause of death in complete scurvy.

Epiphyseal separations and metaphyseal fractures have their highest incidence in the upper tibia, lower femur, and upper humerus. After treatment is instituted, healing of the fracture or epiphyseal separation is rapid, and fortunately normal enchondral ossification is restored.

Extreme displacement of the epiphyses does not prevent resumption of growth and realignment of the bone. Scott reported a case in which the upper humeral epiphyses were displaced more than the diameter of the humerus, yet well aligned humeri finally were formed. Such cases emphasize the versatility of nature in rebuilding the skeleton of childhood.

COSTOCHONDRAL SEPARATIONS are seen in scurvy with the occasional result that the sternum displaces posteriorly. The anterior ends of the ribs shorn of their cartilage protrude forward and are readily palpable. Ribs protruding in this manner form what has been termed the "scorbutic rosary." In the "scorbutic rosary," the protruding ribs are sharp, whereas in the "rachitic rosary" the costochondral junctions are merely enlarged and rounded.

ADULT SCURVY

Except for the growth factor, adult scurvy is similar to the infantile form. The incidence of pathological fractures is high in adults, and the favored site is the diaphyses and not the metaphyses. Fractures are caused by the profound skeletal deossification.

Adult scurvy is most frequently observed among elderly men and women who live alone and prepare their own meals. This is known as "bachelor scurvy." In all forms of scurvy, approximately six months of deprivation are required before clinical symptoms become manifest. For every case with full blown scorbutus, many other cases remain subclinical and go unrecognized and untreated.

Foetal Scurvy

In 1935, Jackson and Park reported autopsy findings on a 16-day old infant that unquestionably had scurvy. Although the existence of scurvy of the new born cannot be denied, it is extremely rare.

The Healing Process

Few experiences in the practice of medicine are so gratifying as the response of a patient with scurvy to vitamin C therapy. Pain and tenderness are relieved and hemorrhages cease in 24 hours. Ossification of the subperiosteal hematomata proceeds rapidly. Once ossified, the entire deposit of periosteal bone is slowly removed. Enchondral ossification is resumed as already explained.

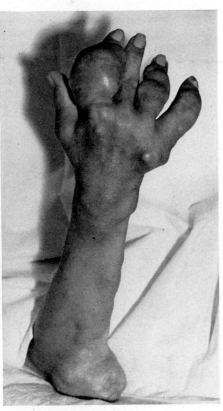

FIGURE 248. Gout: advanced involvement of the right upper extremity in a 43 year old male. Duration of symptoms, 15 years. Highest blood uric acid level was 7.4 mg. Average level over a period of several years was 5.6 mg.

Wound Healing

Lauman and Ingalls and many others have shown that subclinical vitamin C deficiency is relatively common, and may be manifest by a delay in the healing of wounds. A six months period of vitamin C deficiency has been found necessary by Lund and Crandon to create interference with wound repair. The response to asorbic acid therapy is dramatic.

Differential Diagnosis

Infantile scurvy may need to be differentiated from: (1) Rickets. (2)

Acute osteomyelitis. (3) Luetic osteochondritis, and (4) Osteogenesis imperfecta. In rickets there is more cupping of the metaphyses, but less periosteal bone and little or no zone of provisory calcification. Acute osteomyelitis is limited to one bone, whereas scurvy symptoms appear simultaneously in both legs, and frequently also in the upper extremities. Luetic osteochondritis is more common during the first three months of life, while scurvy is more common after the age of three months. In osteogenesis imperfecta, the fractures usually are diaphyseal; in infantile scurvy the fractures are metaphyseal.

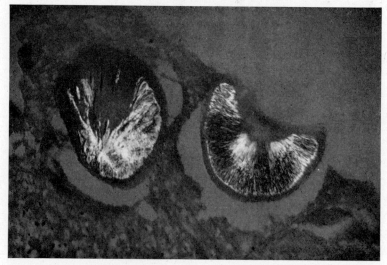

FIGURE 249. Gout: sodium biurate crystals photographed with polarized light x 280. (Courtesy, White Memorial Hospital, Los Angeles.)

GOUT

Gout has been recognized for centuries. Hipocrates was familiar with it, naming it podagra when it involved the foot, gonagra when localized in the knee, and cheiragra when it invaded the wrist. In spite of numerous investigations the etiology remains a mystery.

Most cases of gout occur in men past the age of thirty. In a review of 1484 cases in recent literature, McCracken, Owen and Pratt found that all were men except 98 or 6.6 percent. These authors reported 100 cases of their own of which 93 were acute and seven were chronic. The average age was 46.8 years.

Gout frequently is hereditary. In approximately half of the cases there is a family history of the disease (Comroe).

It has long been established that gout generally represents the response of a disturbed metabolism of uric acid. But what precipitates the metabolic disturbance and the acute attacks is not understood. It might be expected that a rise in blood uric acid would precipitate an acute episode, but Lichwitz has emphasized that this is not the case. As a rule there is no elevation of the blood uric acid during the initial attack. Later a hyperuricemia may appear and remain for several years without precipitating another acute episode. Factors responsible for the level of the blood uric acid are understood. Virtually all mammals with the exception of man destroy excessive uric acid through the action of the ferment uricase. In man, uric acid is the end product of purin metabolism, there being no synthesis of uric acid as there is in birds and reptiles.

PATHOLOGY

The most important lesions in gout are in the joints (gouty arthritis). White, chalk-like deposits of sodium biurate appear on the articular surfaces and resemble drops (gutta) of white paint. Similar tophi appear in the joint capsule and the other ligaments, as well as at the periphery of the articular cortices, and in the epiphyses. A low grade inflammatory reaction develops around the tophi, the picture representing a foreign body reaction, with edema, foreign body giant cells,

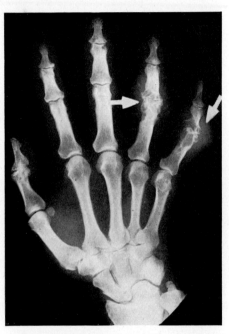

FIGURE 250. Gout: roentgenogram showing characteristic changes in the interphalangeal joints and phalanges (arrows).

lymphocytes and monocytes (Fig. 251). A narrow margin of necrosis often develops. A granulation tissue pannus may extend out from the synovial membrane over parts of the articular cartilage as a response to the presence of the crystal deposits in the cartilage. During acute attacks the joint fluid is moderately increased, is clear and contains a few sodium biurate crystals. In many cases the joint lesions rapidly heal, and the joint function returns to normal between acute episodes. In long standing cases with a history of numerous acute attacks, permanent damage may be done to the joint, resulting in continuous disability.

During acute attacks, the skin overlying an involved joint may become reddened and shiny, resembling a cellulitis. Occasionally such areas are erroneously incised. In gout the superficial veins become much more distended than in a cellulitis. When a tophus is superficial, the overlying skin may undergo trophic changes and ultimately ulcerate, a smear of the discharge usually revealing urate crystals.

Tophi

The deposits of sodium biurate vary from a millimeter to several centimeters in diameter, and when close to the surface of the skin the tophi appear white or yellowish. They occur most frequently in the cartilages of the ear and the joints, but may appear in such other structures as bone, periosteum, tendons, bursae, muscles, heart valves and fascia. Bone and joint tophi occur most often in the fingers and toes, the first metatarsophalangeal joint being the favorite site.

The formation of tophi is not related to the acute attacks. Neither does there appear to be any relation between the level of the blood uric acid and tophus formation.

Comroe pointed out that tophi are found in only 2 percent of cases during the initial attack. They are identified sometime during the course of the disease in about half of the cases.

Murexide or Weidels test—Crystals (Fig. 249) are readily recovered from a superficial tophus through the use of a needle. By preparing a smear of the urate crystals in a microscopic slide and applying first nitric acid and then ammonium hydroxide, one finds that the crystals take on a distinctive purple color.

ROENTGENOGRAPHIC CORRELATION

Joint changes of a character reflected in the roentgenogram occur in only about one third of the cases. Therefore the roentgen-ray must not be relied on regularly to corroborate the diagnosis. Marginal notching is seen in gout. The notches are small, as are the so-called cysts occasionally observed at the periphery of the articular cortex, and in the epiphyses (Fig. 250). Such notches and cysts are radiographically translucent since they represent deposits of urate crystals. The most frequent site at which radiographic changes are detected is the head of the first metatarsal, and the base of the phalanx opposite it.

Marginal defects are by no means pathognomonic of gout. Somewhat similar defects are observed in osteoarthritis, rheumatoid arthritis, and Boeck's sarcoid.

After tophi are of many years duration they may become infiltrated with calcium and thereafter are radio-opaque. This is particularly true of the large urate deposits that occasionally appear in olecranon and prepatellar bursae.

CLINICAL CORRELATION

Hench, Vanzant and Nomland stated that when an arthritis, acute or subacute, is associated with complete remissions it should be considered gout until proved otherwise. The dramatic onset of acute pain, swelling, redness, and exquisite tenderness of the involved joint is

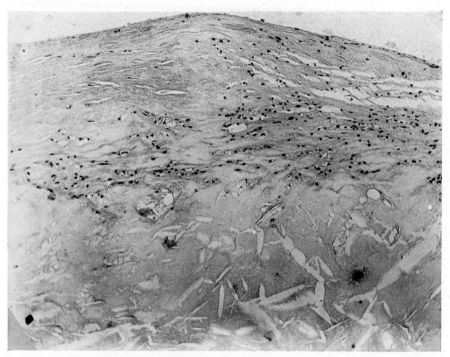

FIGURE 251. Gout: photomicrograph of a section taken through a small tophus. The deposit of urate crystals is shown in the lower one-half of the photo. (Courtesy, *U. S. Army Institute of Pathology*, Acc. No. 29227.)

truely impressive both to the victim and to his physician. Much of the pain is from vascular engorgement. Relief of pain by colchicum is said to result from the diminution of vascular tension. As has been mentioned, relief of joint symptoms is complete between acute episodes, until the tophi do sufficient permanent damage to set up secondary osteo-arthritic changes, or create massive soft tissue deposits (Fig. 248).

Sydenham in his masterful clinical description in the 17th century stated that gout affects "more rich men than poor, more wise men than simple." The disease appears to have a higher incidence among men who live well, but not wisely.

Factors capable of precipitating acute attacks include the following: (1) Trauma; (2) Surgical operations; (3) Debauches and excessive fatigue; (4) Ingestion of foods high in purines or to which the patient is allergic; and, (5) Lead poisoning.

Distribution

The incidence of involvement of the first metatarsal is given variously between 68 percent (McCracken, Owen, and Pratt) and 90 percent (Comroe). Other joints occasionally involved include those of the longitudinal arch of the foot, the finger joints, the ankle, wrist, knee, and elbow. While no joint is immune from gouty arthritis, involvement of the spine, hips and shoulders is rare.

Most cases of gout present only monoarticular lesions. However, there is a severe form of the disease that is polyarticular, and is associated with a relatively high fever, a leucocytosis, and an elevated sedimentation rate. An acute episode of this type may last for several weeks.

Serum uric acid in gout generally is elevated both during relapses and remissions and varies from 4.5 mg. per 100 c.c. of blood to as high as 25 mg. per 100 c.c. of blood (normal 1.0 to 4 mg. per 100 c.c. blood). it is well established that a hyperuricemia does not precipitate an acute attack of gout. Urates in large quantities have been injected into blood streams experimentally without precipitating acute symptoms. In uremia and eclampsia, blood uric acid is elevated, but gout never results.

Urine uric acid is normal or at most only slightly elevated.

REFERENCES

RICKETS

ASHCROFT, G. V.: Renal rickets. *J. Bone & Joint Surg.*, 8:279, 1926.

BROMER, R. S.: Rickets. *Am. J. Roentgenol.*, 30:582, 1933.

CAMP, J. D.: Roentgenologic changes in malacic diseases of bone. *Radiology*, 26:399, 1936.

CLARK, G. L. and MRGUDICK, J. N.: X-ray diffraction study of rachitic bone. *Am. J. Physiol.*, 108:74-79, 1934.

DODDS, G. S. and CAMERON, H. C.: Studies in experimental rickets in rats. *Am. J. Anat.*, 55:135, 1934; *Am. J. Path.*, 14:273, 1939; and 19:169, 1943.

FINDLAY, L.: Rickets, a historical note. *Glasgow M. J.*, 91:147, 1919.

FINDLAY, L., PATON, D. N., and SHARPE, J. S.: Studies in the metabolism of rickets. *Quart. J. Med.*, 14:352, 1920.

FREEMAN, S. and McLEAN, F. C.: Experimental rickets. *Arch. Path.*, 32:387, 1941.

FREUND, E.: Behavior of joint cartilage in late rickets. *Arch. Surg.*, 37:470, 1938.

HAMILTON, B. and SCHWARTZ, C.: Rickets and hyperparathyroidism. *Am. J. Dis. Child.*, 46:775, 1933.

HESS, A. F.: *Rickets Including Osteomalacia and Tetany.* Lea and Febiger, Philadelphia, 1929.

HESS, A. F.: *Cecil's Textbook of Medicine*, page 554. W. B. Saunders Co., Philadelphia, 1929.

KARSCHNER, R. G.: Rickets occurring late in chronic interstitial nephritis. Report of a case. *Am. J. Roentgenol., 18:*442, 1927.

McMASTER, P.: Cartilage inclusions in rachitic bones and their possible relation to cartilage tumors. *J. Bone & Joint Surg., 17:*373, 1935.

MAXWELL, J. P.: Osteomalacia and foetal rickets. *Brit. J. Radiol., 3:*375, 1930.

MAXWELL, J. P., HU, C. H., and TURNBULL, H. M.: Foetal rickets. *J. Path. & Bact., 35:*419, 1932.

MELLANBY, E.: The part played by an "accessory factor" in the production of experimental rickets. *J. Physiol., 52:*11, 1918.

MELLANBY, E.: An experimental investigation on rickets. *Lancet, 1:*407, 1919.

MITCHELL, A. G.: Consideration of the pathogenesis of renal rickets. *Acta Paediat., 11:*352, 1930.

PALM, T. A.: The geographical distribution and etiology of rickets. *Practitioner, 45:*270, 1890.

PAPPENHEIMER, A. M.: Anatomical changes accompanying healing experimental rat rickets under influence of cod liver oil or its active derivatives. *J. Exper. Med., 36:*335-356, 1922.

PARK, E. A.: Etiology of rickets. *Physiol. Rev., 3:*106, 1923.

PARSONS, L. G.: The bone changes occurring in renal and coeliac infantilism and their relationship to rickets. *Arch. Dis. Child., 2:*1, 1927.

PHEMISTER, D. B., MILLER, E. M., and BONAR, B. E.: The effects of phosphorus in rickets. *J. A. M. A., 76:*850, 1921.

POMMER, G.: *Untersuchungen uber Rachitis und Osteomalazie.* Leipzig, 1885.

SCHILLER, A. C. and STRUCH, H. D.: Tensile strength of healed rat tibiae. *Proc. Soc. Exper. Biol. & Med., 46:*198, 1941.

SCHMORL, G.: *Ergebn. d. inn. Med. u. Kinderh, 4:*403, 1909.

SIGNORELLI, J., HOSEN, H. and MILES, J. M.: Epiphyses in rickets. *J. Pediat., 7:*182, 1935.

SNAPPER, I.: *Medical Clinics on Bone Diseases.* Interscience Publishers Inc., New York, 1943.

STEARNS, G., JEANS, P. C. and VANDECAR, V.: The effect of vitamin D on linear growth in infancy. *J. Pediat., 9:*1, 1936.

TROUSSEAU, A.: *Lectures on Clinical Medicine.* New Sydenham Soc., London, 1872.

VOGT, E. C.: Renal rickets. *Am. J. Roentgenol., 30:*624, 1933.

OSTEOMALACIA

DALYELL, E. J. and CHICK, H.: Hunger-osteomalacia in Vienna, 1920. *Lancet, 2:*842, 1921.

DIECKMANN, W. J.: Osteomalacia in pregnancy. *Am. J. Obst. & Gynec., 23:*478, 1932.

GUNN, F. D. and NADLER, W. H.: Necropsy observations in man on osteomalacia. *Arch. Int. Med., 54:*145, 1934.

HODGES, P. C. and LEDOUX, A. C.: Osteomalacia and rickets. *Am. J. Roentgenol.,* pp. 590-595, Dec. 1933.

KAUFMANN, E. and REIMANN, S. P.: *Kaufmann's Pathology,* Vol. II. P. Blakiston's Son and Co., Philadelphia 1929.

KIENBOCK, R.: Osteomalacia, osteoporosis, osteopsathyrosis, and porotic kyphosis. *Fortschr. a.d. Geb. der Röntgenstrahlen, 62:*3, 1940.

KLEINBERG, S.: Senile osteomalacia., *Arch. Surg., 30:*30, 1935.

LOCKE, E. A.: Osteomalacia in *Oxford Medicine.* Oxford Univ. Press, 1927.

LOOSER, E.: Uber Spätrachitis und Osteomalacie. *Deutsche. Ztschr. f. Chir., 152:*210, 1920.

LOOSER, E.: Uber pathologische Formea von Infraktionen und callusbildningen bei Rachitis und Osteomalakie und anderen Knockenerkrankungen. *Zentralbl. f. Chir., 47:*1470, 1920.

McCRUDDEN, F. M.: Studies in bone metabolism and osteomalacia. *Arch. Int. Med., 5:*596-630, 1910.

MAXWELL, J. P.: Adult rickets, Further studies. *Proc. Roy. Soc. Med., 28:*265, 1935.

MAXWELL, J. P.: Osteomalacia in China. *China M. J., 38:*349, 1924.

MAXWELL, J. P.: Osteomalacia and foetal rickets. *Brit. J. Radiol., 3:*375, 1930.

MEULENGRACHT, E.: Osteomalacia of the spinal column in Denmark resulting from inadequate diet or diseases of the intestinal tract. *Wien. klin. Wchnschr.*, page 725, Aug. 4, 1939.

MIYAKAWA, G. and STEARNS, G.: Severe osteoporosis (or osteomalacia) associated with long-continued low-grade steatorrhoea. *J. Bone & Joint Surg.*, *24*:429, 1942.

RICHARDSON, E. P., AUB, J. C. and BAUER, W.: Parathyroidectomy in osteomalacia. *Ann. Surg.*, *90*:730, 1929.

ROSS, G. and ABBOTT, H.: The relation of the thyroid, the adrenals and the islands of Langerhans to malacic diseases of bone. *Am. J. Roentgenol.*, *30*:641, 1933.

STAPLETON, G.: Late rickets and osteomalacia in Delhi. *Lancet, I*:1119, 1925.

STEENBOCK, H. and HART, E. B.: The influence of function on the lime requirements of animals. *J. Biol. Chem.*, *14*:59, 1912.

STEENBOCK, H., HART, E. B., SELLS, M. T., and JONES, J. H.: The availability of calcium salts. *J. Biol. Chem.*, *56*:375, 1923.

STONE, E. L. A.: A brief review of the literature of osteomalacia with the report of a case. *Surg., Gynec. & Obst.*, *39*:599, 1924.

VAUGHN, K.: Osteomalacia (late rickets) studies. Clinical symptoms in relation to bone changes as shown by X-ray examination. *Indian J. Med. Research*, *17*:399, 1929-30.

WYATT, H. G.: Notes on osteomalacia in North China. *China M. J.*, *44*:1168, 1930.

ZACHO, A.: Osteoporosis and osteomalacia of the spinal column. *Acta orthop. Scandinav.*, *11*:3, 1940.

SCURVY

American Pediatric Society: Collective investigation on infantile scurvy in North America. *Arch. Pediat.*, *15*:481, 1898.

BARLOW, T.: On cases described as acute rickets. *Med. Chir. Tr.*, *66*:159, 1883.

HARRIS, H. A.: *Bone Growth in Health and Disease*. Oxford Press, 1933.

HESS, A. F.: Scurvy Past and Present. J. B. Lippincott, Philadelphia, 1920.

HOOER, J. A.: Studies in scurvy. *Acta Paediat.*, *3*:8, 1924.

HOLT, H. and FROLICH, T.: Ueber experimentallen Skorbut. *Ztschr. f. Hyg. u. Infektionskr.*, *72*:1, 1912.

HOWE, P. R.: The effect of scorbutic diet upon the teeth.

KATO, K.: A critique of the roentgen signs of infantile scurvy. *Radiology*, *18*:1096, 1932.

LAUMAN, T. H. and INGALLS, T. H.: Vitamin C deficiency and wound healing. *Ann. Surg.*, *105*:616, 1937.

PELKAN, K. F.: Roentgenogram in early scurvy. *Am. J. Dis. Child.*, *30*:174, 1925.

SCOTT, W.: Epiphyseal dislocations in scurvy. *J. Bone & Joint Surg.*, *23*:314, 1941.

WIMBERGER, H.: Die Spätdiagnose des Säulingsskorbuts. *Fortschr. a. d. Gel. d. Röngenstrahlen*, *32*:17, 1924.

WOLBACH, S. B.: Controlled formation of collagen and reticulum. *Am. J. Path.*, *9*:689, 1933.

WOLBACH, S. B. and HOWE, P. R.: Intercellular substance in experimental scorbutus. *Arch. Path. & Lab. Med.*, *1*:1, 1926.

GOUT

BUNIM, J. J. and McEWEN, C.: Tophus of the mitral valve in gout. *Arch. Path.*, *29*:700, 1940.

COMROE, B. I.: Arthritis and allied conditions, 3rd ed. Lea and Febiger, Philadelphia, 1944.

HENCH, P. S., VANZANT, F. R. and NOMLAND, R.: Basis for early differentiation of gout. *Tr. A. Am. Physicians*, *43*:217, 1928.

LICHTWITZ, L.: *Functional Pathology*, Grune and Stratton, New York, 1941.

McCLURE, C. and McCARTY, E.: Roentgenographic studies in gout. *Arch. Int., Med.*, *24*:563, 1919.

McCRACKEN, J. P., OWEN, P. S., and PRATT, J. H.: Gout: Still a forgotten disease. *J. A. M. A.*, *131*:367, 1946.

SMYTH, C. J. and FREYBERG, R. H.: A study of the hereditary nature of gout. *Ann. Int. Med.*, *16*:46, 1942.

SYDENHAM, T.: The Works of Thomas Sydenham, Vol. II: page 123. Sydenham Society, London, 1850.

TALBOT, J. H. and COOMBS, F. S.: Metabolic studies on patients with gout. *J. A. M. A.*, *110*:1977, 1938.

CHAPTER IX

Osteitis Fibrosa

(Fibrous Osteodystrophy)

Contents

As a matter of convenience and to clarify their differential diagnosis, the solitary bone cyst, fibrous dysplasia, and generalized osteitis fibrosa (hyperparathyroidism) will be discussed under the chapter heading of osteitis fibrosa. This is not a lasting arrangement since there is abundant evidence at hand to indicate that these entities are quite separate and independent.

THE SOLITARY BONE CYST

A typical solitary bone cyst is represented by a central, circumscribed, sharply defined, oval shaped, hollow defect in the metaphysis or diaphysis of a long tubular bone (Figs. 252 to 256). Such cysts are often referred to as localized osteitis fibrosa cystica. This probably is unwarranted, considering the wide differences in the pathologic and clinical manifestations of localized, regional, and generalized fibrous osteitis. Until the time comes when we have a better understanding of these conditions, it is practical to deal with them both pathologically and clinically as separate diseases. When the bony defect is solitary and of the character now to be described, it will be called a solitary cyst. The so-called regional, or unilateral, type, in which there generally are multiple defects filled with fibrous tissue and fibrous bone, will be referred to by Lichtenstein's term, fibrous dysplasia. Skeletal changes associated with primary hyperparathyroidism will be called generalized fibrous osteitis or osteitis fibrosa generalizata.

Age Incidence

Nearly all solitary bone cysts develop in childhood, the diagnosis being made in the majority of cases just prior to or during adolescence. In most of the 205 cases studied by Geschickter and Copeland the age was between 10 and 15 years. But instances in older adults and in infants are by no means rare. Several congenital solitary cysts have been reported in which a pseudarthrosis developed following a pathologic fracture. Compere and others have suggested that such cysts frequently are the underlying cause of congenital pseudarthroses.

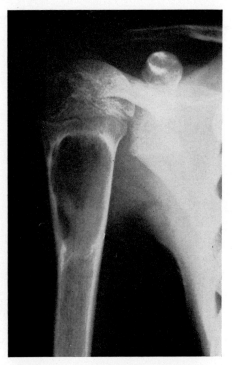

FIGURE 252. Solitary cyst of the upper humeral metaphysis. This cyst had a very thin, lining membrane, and the cyst was empty except for a few drops of serous fluid.

Distribution

Solitary bone cysts are rare outside of the long tubular bones. Most lesions in the short tubular bones that resemble solitary cysts in roentgenograms prove to be enchondromata. The humeral diaphysis and proximal metaphysis are the sites of approximately one-half of the cases. In the series of 19 cases reported by Jaffe and Lichtenstein, 9 were in the upper humerus. The next most frequent sites of involvement in the author's experience are the proximal aspect of the femur and the lower one third of the tibia.

Etiology

So long as the etiology remains unknown, there will continue to be an array of theories. A widely accepted theory is that of Pommer who believed that the solitary cyst is the end result of an intramedullary hematoma. With the increased pressure incident to a localized hemorrhage, osteoclasia becomes accelerated and a circumscribed area of bone is absorbed. This theory has been challenged on the basis of the rarity of solitary cysts in hemophilia where intramedullary hemorrhages are far more frequent than in normal individuals.

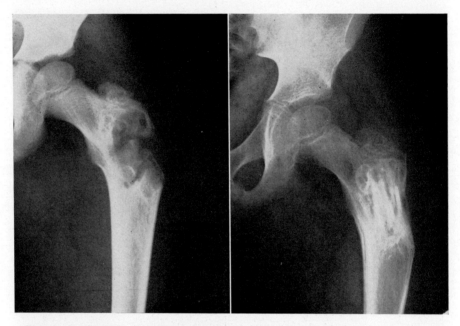

FIGURE 253. A. *(Left)* Solitary cyst and pathologic fracture of the trochanteric area. B. *(Right)* Four months after curetage and insertion of bone chips from the tibia.

Geschickter and Copeland support the belief that a solitary cyst is the healed stage of giant cell tumor. This theory has received little support as an explanation of typical solitary bone cysts, and this is not surprising since most giant cell tumors appear in an older age group and are located principally in epiphyses.

Jaffe and Lichtenstein explain the solitary cyst, and also fibrous dysplasia, as a local defect in bone growth and development.

Phemister and Gordon contend that the solitary bone cyst represents the healed end-stage of a localized, low grade pyogenic osteomyelitis.

Thus far the various etiologic theories have been of little practical value in our understanding and treatment of the solitary cyst.

Pathologic Anatomy

A single cavity (unicameral of Jaffe and Lichtenstein) characterizes the solitary cyst, and it is lined by a thin connective tissue membrane. The lining tissue is fibrous in character, usually avascular and varies from microscopic thickness to a well developed membrane (Fig. 256). In most instances the lining is almost invisible and very little tissue is secured even with a sharp curette. A few drops to several cubic centimeters of a thin, brown colored fluid is ordinarily found in the cyst cavity. When the cyst is explored following trauma or a pathological fracture, the fluid is usually blood stained and increased in amount; and the lining membrane is thickened and vascular.

Ridges often extend along the cyst wall but only seldom is there a partitioning into two or more cavities (multilocular or multicameral). Occasionally, following a pathological fracture, a fibrous curtain forms during the healing process and divides the cyst into two or more cavities.

There is a widespread belief that a fracture into a solitary bone cyst results in healing and filling of the cyst cavity. With small cysts there is an occasional instance of healing after a fracture, but the larger cysts do not heal even after sev-

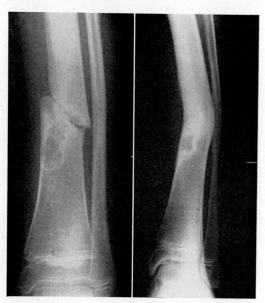

FIGURE 254. A. *(Left)* Pathologic fracture through the upper one-half of a solitary cyst in the tibia. B. *(Right)* Four and one-half months after the fracture showing obliteration of only the proximal one-half of the cyst. Fractures do not entirely obliterate bone cysts.

eral pathologic fractures. A large cyst may diminish in size but it does not disappear (Fig. 254). *Site of origin:* Virtually all solitary bone cysts begin in a metaphysis. There may be extension to the epiphyseal plate but no instances have been reported where the epiphyseal plate was perforated. When the cyst is enlarging it is in an active phase; when it ceases to enlarge it is said to be in a quiescent phase. With continued growth at the epiphyseo-metaphyseal junction, the cyst is left behind and may be located in the diaphysis by the time the epiphyseal plate ceases functioning. The age of the patient at the time the cyst appeared frequently can be estimated by the location of the cyst.

ROENTGENOLOGIC CORRELATION

The roentgenogram is extremely helpful in identifying the solitary bone cyst, but it must be emphasized that a positive differentiation from such conditions as a solitary xanthoma, a non-ossifying fibroma, a soli-

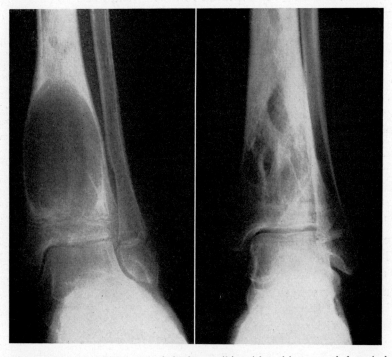

FIGURE 255. A. *(Left)* Solitary cyst of the lower tibia with a thin, expanded cortical wall. B. *(Right)* Two years after curetage and packing with bone chips. Ossification is not complete but is adequate.

tary enchondroma, or a monocentric fibrous dysplasia cannot always be made.

Overlying cortex is thinned and generally is expanded. Except at sites of pathological fractures, the cortex is sharply defined and intact. High ridges in the inner cortical wall of the cyst may, in the roentgenogram, give an appearance of multiloculation.

Blood Chemistry: No material alteration occurs in the serum calcium, phosphorus, and phosphatase.

CLINICAL CORRELATION

Diagnosis: The solitary cyst is diagnosed when a roentgenogram is taken in order to explain pain, moderate swelling, or a pathologic fracture. In the large series of Geschickter and Copeland, 45 percent were diagnosed at the advent of a pathologic fracture. Such fractures vary from an almost microscopic size to a breakup of the cortical wall similar to crushing an egg shell.

Therapy: Roentgen therapy is useless. Surgical therapy has been highly successful and consists of the curettage of the lining membrane and filling of the cavity with bone chips or a single bone graft. Bone from the iliac crest is particularly satisfactory for this purpose. Reossification is believed to be more complete and more dependable when the surgery is performed during a quiescent phase.

FIBROUS DYSPLASIA

This syndrome is described in medical literature under a multitude of different terms, which include osteodystrophia fibro-

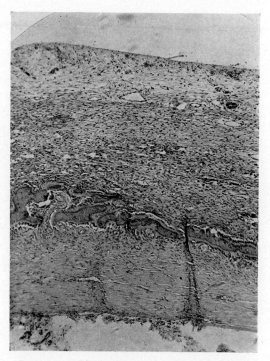

FIGURE 256. Photomicrograph of a lining membrane of a solitary cyst. Note the narrow zone of fibrous bone forming in the membrane.

sa unilateralis (Freund and Meffert), regional fibrocystic disease (Phemister), unilateral von Recklinghausen's disease, osteitis fibrosa disseminata, polyostotic osteitis fibrosa, fibrous dysplasia (Lichtenstein), and Albright's syndrome (Gorham). The term fibrous dysplasia was suggested by Lichtenstein after a study of biopsy material from eight cases. In his first paper (1938) he used the term polyostotic fibrous dysplasia. In a later paper (1942) in collaboration with Jaffe, the term was shortened to fibrous dysplasia, the reason being the discovery of several monostotic cases. Nine of their series of 23 cases were monostotic.

In 1937 Albright and his associates reported five cases of the more severe and disseminated form of fibrous dysplasia, and emphasized the triad of findings that characterize this form of the disease. (1. Disseminated fibrous osteitis, 2. areas of skin pigmentation, and 3. precocious puberty in females.) Since this time there have been numerous cases reported. In 1942 Gorham reviewed the literature and found reports of 51 cases. Of these cases 32 had the complete triad of Albright, and 19 were incomplete. In all probability, as the disease is more widely recognized and properly classified, there will be a preponderance of the less severe form. No doubt many cases of monostotic fibrous dysplasia are still being classified as solitary bone cysts, and the disseminated type as generalized osteitis fibrosa. Not a small number of parathyroid glands have been needlessly explored in instances where fibrous dysplasia was erroneously diagnosed as hyperparathyroidism.

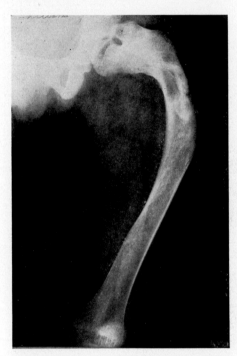

FIGURE 257. Fibrous dysplasia involving the left femur. The bowing and the attempted reinforcement of the medial cortex are characteristic.

ETIOLOGY

Nothing is known of the etiology. There is not the slightest evidence that the disease is caused by hyperparathyroidism. In none of the reported cases has there been significant deviation from normal of the serum calcium and phosphorus. And there have been no cases in which skeletal involvement was generalized, a condition that would be expected were the syndrome on an endocrine basis. Lichtenstein suggested that "the condition apparently results from perverted activity of the specific bone-forming mesenchyme."

PATHOLOGY

The areas of bone involvement that appear as cysts in the roentgenogram are filled with moderately dense, white or gray fibrous tissue thinly or thickly trabeculated with poorly calcified fibrous bone (Fig. 259). Areas of degeneration have been seen, but rarely a cyst.

Although vascularity varies, most of the fibrous tissue and fibrous bone contain few vessels. Anaplasia with its mitotic figures is not seen. The fibrous bone forms by direct metaplasia of the surrounding fibroblastic tissue. Trabeculae may be wide or narrow, and few or numerous. In some cases islands of calcified hyaline cartilage have been identified as in Telford's case. Inflammatory cells are absent. There is nothing in the histopathology to suggest that the process represents an inflammation. Osteoclasts are seen but are not nearly so numerous as they are in generalized osteitis fibrosa.

Overlying bony cortex becomes thin and tends to be expanded over areas of fibrous dysplasia (Fig. 258). Atrophy of involved bones exists only at sites of actual involvement. Diffuse involvement of the entire skeleton or an entire bone does not take place in fibrous dysplasia.

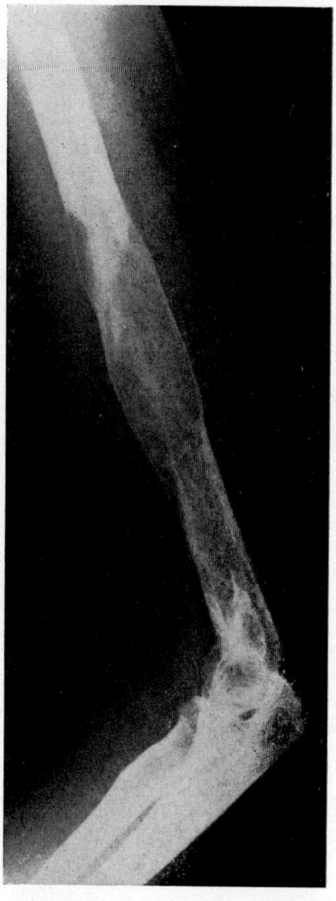

Distribution of Skeletal Lesions

Solitary lesions have been reported but in the great majority of cases the lesions are multiple. There is a decided tendency toward unilateral skeletal involvement. Long tubular bones have exhibited more lesions than have the short and the flat bones, and the lower extremities are more frequently involved than the upper. Skull and vertebral lesions are not infrequent. A given bone may possess a single circumscribed lesion or have multiple areas of involvement extending from end to end.

FIGURE 258. Fibrous dysplasia. Lateral roentgenogram of the left humerus.

Blood Chemistry

Serum calcium and phosphorus are normal, there being no disturbance of calcium metabolism. Serum phosphatase is slightly to moderately increased, presumably as a result of the accelerated osteoblastic activity.

ROENTGENOLOGIC CORRELATION

Since the fibrous bone in the fibrous tissue deposited at involved areas of the skeleton is incompletely calcified, the lesions tend to be radiolucent. It is for this reason that the erroneous diagnosis of multiple bone cysts is so often made. The structure of the bone is altered, and as a result of the inevitable mechanical weakening of the bone, bending and fractures are relatively common. Healing of fractures usually takes place but is slow. Reinforcement of the cortex takes place on the concave side of long bone bending deformities, but often is inadequate to stem the deformation.

Unquestionably many areas of fibrous dysplasia develop without leading to sufficient bone resorption to be reflected in the roentgenogram.

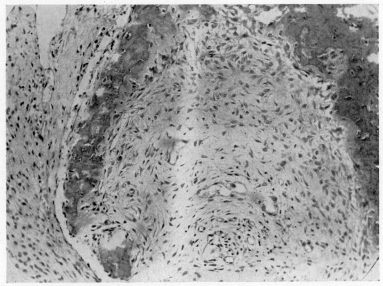

FIGURE 259. Fibrous dysplasia. Photomicrograph of the type of tissue that fills the areas of bone involvement. True cysts in fibrous dysplasia are rare, the cyst-like defects seen in roentgenograms are filled with fibrous tissue and fibrous bone.

CLINICAL CORRELATION

The disease usually becomes symptomatic during childhood, the majority of cases having been diagnosed near the age of adolescence. In Lichtenstein's cases the average age at the onset of symptoms was approximately ten years. The ratio of women to men in his series was three to one.

Since no deaths from fibrous dysplasia have been reported, the prognosis for life is excellent. Histological studies have come entirely from biopsies, and from Telford's amputated lower extremity.

Pain, moderate in character, frequently occurs from the skeletal lesions.

Deformities and pathological fractures usually accentuate the pain.

Precocious puberty occurs only in females and is a conspicuous symptom in the disseminated cases in which it appears. These cases generally are associated with areas of dark, usually amber, colored areas of skin pigmentation. Such areas have been found most often on the buttocks, back, thighs and neck.

The disease, beginning in childhood, presumably extends through-out life. Areas of bone in-volvement do not tend to heal and reossify. No effec-tive treatment is known. Roentgen therapy has not been mentioned in the ex-isting literature. Bone-grafts have been used in a few in-stances to stimulate reossifi-cation, and osteotomies have been carried out to correct deformities.

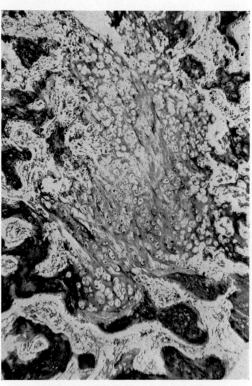

Differential Diagnosis: Fi-brous dysplasia must be dif-ferentiated from generalized osteitis fibrosa, neurofibro-matosis, xanthomata, and enchondromatosis. General-ized osteitis fibrosa with its blood chemistry changes, negative calcium balance, and generalized skeletal de-ossification, is not difficult to separate from fibrous dys-plasia. Neurofibromatosis

FIGURE 260. Photomicrograph of a field of carti-lage in fibrous dysplasia x 115. (Courtesy, *U. S. Army Institute of Pathology*, Acc. No. 117404.)

can be associated with central bone lesions, but they generally are small. Skin lesions of the two conditions bear only superficial resemblance. Ollier's disease, or enchondromatosis, usually produces localized growth disturbances. A biopsy should be resorted to whenever the diagnosis is in doubt, particularly when the bone lesions are enlarging.

GENERALIZED OSTEITIS FIBROSA
(Hyperparathyroidism)

HISTORICAL

Generalized osteitis fibrosa cystica was given the status of an entity

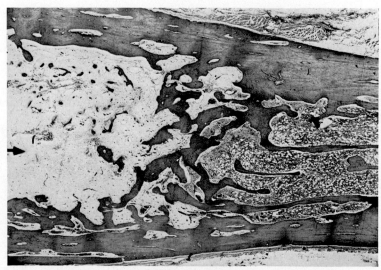

FIGURE 261. Fibrous dysplasia (arrow) involving a rib x 15.
(Courtesy, *U. S. Army Institute of Pathology*, Acc. No. 116461.)

by von Recklinghausen in 1891. At that time the disease was considered to be primary in the skeleton. Although Paget had given a classical

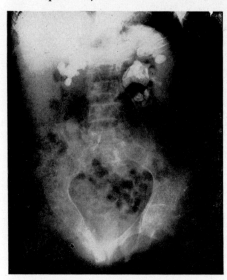

FIGURE 262. Generalized osteitis fibrosa in a female age 49. Symptoms for five years with bowing of lower extremities, pathologic fracture of right femur, dorsal kyphosis, and multiple radio-opaque renal calculi. Serum calcium 19.2 mg. Serum phosphorus 2.98 mg. Phosphatase 41.1 units (Bodansky). Parathyroid adenoma removed that measured 4½ x 2 x 2½ cm. Expired one week postoperatively from renal failure and tetany.

description of osteitis deformans in 1877, the two entities generally were considered to be variations of the same disease.

In 1904, Askanaza reported a case of von Recklinghausen's disease associated with a parathyroid tumor, and surmised a relationship. In 1913, he reported a second case. Erdheim, as far back as 1904, studied the parathyroids experimentally and announced their influence on calcium metabolism. It was his belief that the hyperplasia of these glands, observed in malacic diseases, was a compensatory reaction to enable the body to mobilize calcium from the skeleton in order to replace that lost in the urine and feces. Erdheim erroneously applied this concept to von Recklinghausen's disease. In 1925, Felix Mandl, a student of Erdheim, transplanted four parathyroid glands from a dying patient to the abdominal wall of a rather advanced case of generalized osteitis fibrosa.

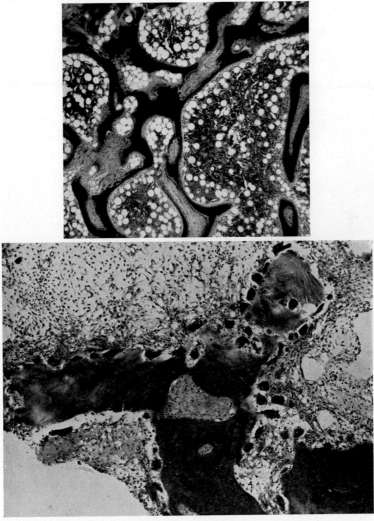

FIGURE 263. Early changes in generalized osteitis fibrosa. A. (*Above*) A dissecting osteitis is replacing the normal bony trabeculae. The normal marrow elements have not yet been replaced. B. (*Below*) Multinucleated osteoclasts in Howships lacunae.

This procedure should have benefited the patient had Erdheim's theory of compensatory hyperplasia been true. When the patient became worse Mandl not only removed the transplanted glands but also explored the patient's own parathyroids. A parathyroid tumor was found and removed. What followed made history. Fortunately, complete x-ray studies of the skeleton had been made pre-operatively. The post-operative roentgenograms taken at regular intervals disclosed a steady re-ossification of the skeleton. Clinical symptoms rapidly improved, the tide of calcium that was being lost in the urine was stemmed, and the serum calcium dropped to normal.

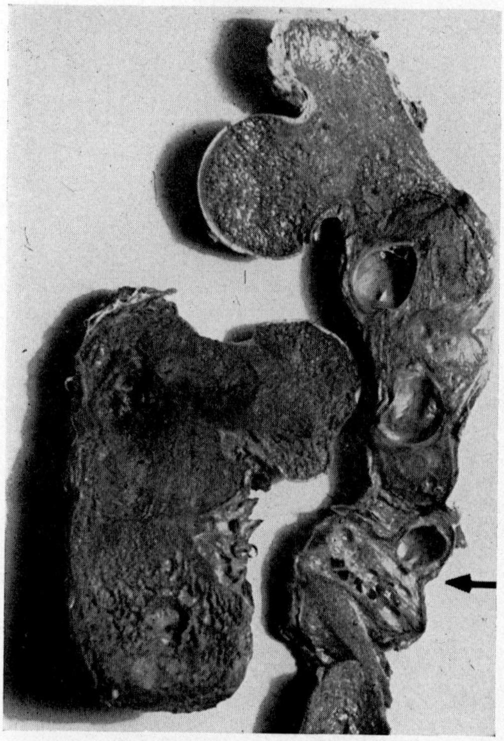

FIGURE 264. Femora from a patient that died from untreated hyperparathyroidism. The left femur shows multiple cysts through the diaphysis; the right femur (the shorter telescoped specimen) shows a large brown tumor involving the regions of the greater trochanter and femoral neck. Arrow points to cyst shown in Figure 265.

In this country, Hannon, Shorr, McClellan, and Du-Bois studied a case of hyper-parathyroidism, diagnosed by DuBois in 1926, and reported it in 1930. They recognized that the symptoms were similar to those produced by the excessive administration of parathyroid extract. After several fruitless explorations, a parathyroid adenoma was found in the upper mediastinum.

Another milestone was the discovery by Collip in 1925 of the active principle of the parathyroid gland secretion, a substance that has been termed parathormone.

Further confirmation of the role of parathormone in the production of generalized osteitis fibrosa came in 1930 when Jaffe, Bodansky and Blair reported results of guinea pig and dog experiments. Repeated injections of parathormone led to changes characteristic of generalized osteitis fibrosa.

THE PARATHYROIDS

That the parathyroid glands regulate the serum calcium level is well established. MacCallum and Voegtlin demonstrated in 1909 that removal of the parathyroid glands led to a profound drop in the blood calcium which ushered in tetany. Conversely an increase in parathyroid secretion leads to hypercalcemia. When inadequate calcium is absorbed from the intestinal tract as in Vitamin D deficiency, the parathyroids are called upon to rob calcium from the skeleton in order to maintain the serum calcium above the tetany stage. When protracted, this process is reflected in the skeleton as rickets or osteomalacia, and gives rise to a compensatory hyperplasia of the parathyroid glands. In an adenoma of a parathyroid gland, the excessive parathormone secreted into the blood stream continuously drains calcium from the bones; ultimately the skeletal response is generalized osteitis fibrosa.

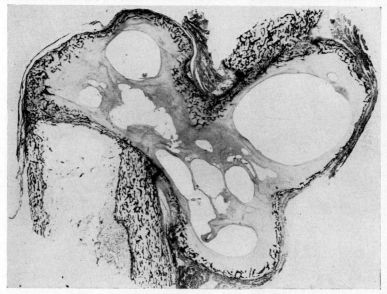

FIGURE 265. Multilocular cyst from the left femur shown in Figure 264. Overlying cortex is paper-thin. Cyst lining is dense, avascular fibrous tissue.

The mechanism through which parathormone mobilizes calcium from the bones is not understood. It is known that parathormone upsets the acid-base equilibrium to create an acidosis, which is a factor in facilitating osteoabsorption. Jaffe and his associates contend that parathormone produces decalcification by modifying the tissue fluids circulating around bone (halisteresis). Pommer held firm to his conviction that a stimulation of the osteoclasts was the basis of the accelerated resorption. Studies made by Albright and Ellsworth uncovered evidence that the initial action of parathormone is a lowering of the renal threshold for phosphorus. An elevated serum calcium is said simply to represent the response to a lowered serum phosphorus. The exact mechanism by which bone is absorbed, both under normal and abnormal circumstances, continues to elude us.

LABORATORY STUDIES

Among the most significant findings as indicated by laboratory procedures are hypercalcemia, hypophosphatemia, hypercalciuria, and increased phosphatase activity. The highest blood and urine calcium readings ever observed have been in cases of hyperparathyroidism. Serum calcium varies from slightly above normal (12 or 13 mg. per 100 c.c. blood) to more than 20 mg. per 100 c.c. blood. One of the highest serum calcium levels recorded was 23.5 mg.

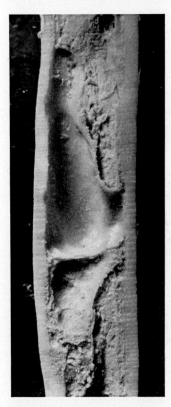

FIGURE 266. Monolocular cyst of a femur from a case of generalized osteitis fibrosa. The lining membrane is smooth and glistening.

The serum phosphorus frequently maintains a rather constant relationship to the serum calcium. As the calcium increases the phosphorus decreases; the converse is also true. When the serum calcium is elevated to the neighborhood of 20 mg., the phosphorus usually is around 2 mg. When serum calcium is 8 mg., the phosphorus may also be about 8 mg. Such levels as the latter are occasionally observed temporarily after parathyroidectomy and may be associated with tetany or impending tetany.

The urine consistently shows an increase in calcium, an increase that varies from two to ten times normal. Fecal calcium is increased but not to a remarkable degree.

In recent years the Bodansky and the Jenner-Kay tests for blood phosphatase activity have come into routine use. Tests for this enzyme in normal individuals are Bodansky 2-3 units, Jenner-Kay 4-10 units. Hyperparathyroidism is regularly associated with an increase in blood phosphatase activity. The increase generally ranges from 6 to 36 Bodansky units, and 15 to 100 Jenner-Kay units.

PATHOLOGIC ANATOMY

In the majority of cases a single adenoma, one to six centimeters in diameter, of one of the four parathyroid glands has represented the source of the excessive parathormone in primary hyperparathyroidism. In a small number of cases two adenomata have been found, and in a few other instances there has been no adenoma, but instead a diffuse hyperplasia of one or more of the glands.

In adenomata the pale, chief or principle cells predominate, the oxyphile cells appearing only in scattered groups. The cell uniformity seen in normal glands and in hyperplasia is not seen in an adenoma. Instead, there are areas of acinar formation interspersed with areas in which the cells form cords and patternless masses. The fibrous stroma

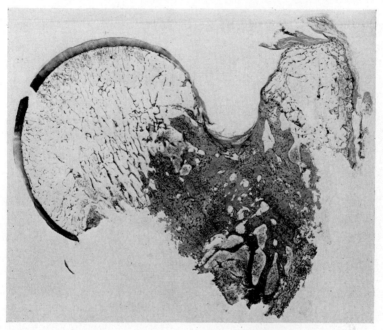

FIGURE 267. Fibrous osteitis of hyperparathyroidism. Histologic section of the upper femur showing fibrous replacement of normal marrow elements in the femoral neck and trochanteric region. This area could not be differentiated in the roentgenograms.

vascularity and cell structure tend to vary in different parts of the tumor. Areas of degeneration and small cyst formations are common.

In hyperplasia it is the clear cell that generally is predominant. A parathyroid gland may increase in size as much as a hundred times through diffuse hyperplasia.

Generalized osteitis fibrosa is characterized by many interesting alterations in the skeleton. At the outset let it be emphasized that this is a generalized skeletal disease. Many, or even all, of the bones may appear uninvolved grossly and roentgenographically, yet microscopically every portion of all bones presents evidence of the disease. In contrast to Paget's disease, von Recklinghausen's disease is not characterized by pathognomonic microscopic changes. However, a pathological diagnosis can definitely be made when adequate material is available for study. In most cases the diagnosis should be based not on microscopic slides alone but upon a combination of clinical, laboratory, roentgenographic, and pathologic anatomy evidence.

Bone Resorption

In the beginning the disease is characterized by diffuse deossification. This process may be slow or the most rapid ever observed. More often

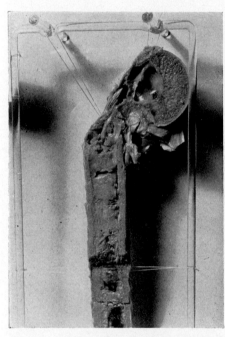

it is rapid, much more rapid than in simple calcium deprivation. Microscopically great numbers of multinucleated giant cell osteoclasts are seen lying in Howship's lacunae (Fig. 263B). These cells appear actively at work, playing a part in the mobilization of calcium. No other generalized skeletal disease is characterized by such vast armies of osteoclasts. It has been well established that the osteoclasts do not phagocytose calcium salts. How they absorb bone, if they do, is not known. It is Jaffe's opinion that the osteoclasts phagocytose bone matrix after the calcium has been withdrawn by halesteresis. Calcium is mobilized most readily in cancellous bone, presumably because there is more available surface on which osteoclasts may work. It has been demonstrated roentgen-

FIGURE 267. (*Continued*) A. Hemi-section of the right humerus of an advanced case of hyperparathyroidism. A pathological fracture exists in the surgical neck at the site of a large cyst.

ographically, and Jaffe and Bodansky have proved it experimentally, that in young bone resorption occurs most rapidly at sites of the most rapid growth. The haversian canals become larger and larger until the cortex is transformed from compact bone to cancellous bone. The process may advance until only a paper-thin outer shell of cortex remains. Bending deformities and pathologic fractures are the result of cortical deossification.

Osteoid Apposition

The picture is not exclusively osteoclasia; there is a minor osteoblastic phase. Osteoblasts may be seen overlying pink staining osteoid seams on trabecular surfaces and haversian canal walls. These osteoid

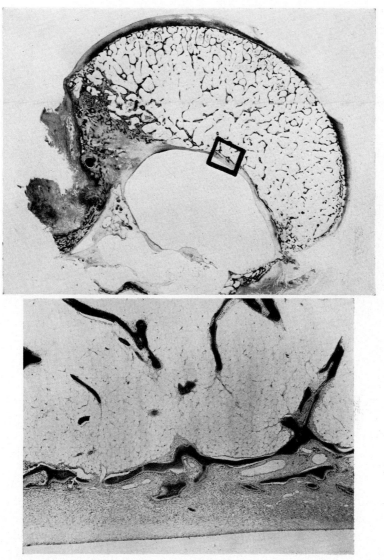

FIGURE 267. *(Continued)* B. *(Above)* Histological section of the head of the humerus in Figure 267A. C. *(Below)* Photomicrograph of square marked on B.

margins or "seams," except for being narrower, are similar to those seen in rickets and osteomalacia. Owing to the rapid loss of calcium, the osteoid may long remain in an uncalcified state. Osteoid apposition is most abundant at sites of distorted mechanical stresses such as pathologic fractures, and bending deformities. In these locations the excessive osteoid may be a reinforcing mechanism, even though it does not observe a static alignment.

Deformities

Deformities are most conspicuous in the long bones and in advanced stages may become grotesque (Fig. 264). The softened vertebral bodies often become compressed by the expanding intervertebral discs to form "codfish" vertebrae. Scoliosis and kyphosis are common, as is also herniation of the nucleus pulposus into vertebral bodies (Fig. 269). Rib and sternal bending deformities occur.

Skull Changes

The skull does not escape involvement. Skull cortices are replaced by cancellous bone to give the fuzzy granular appearance often seen roentgenographically. There may be a slight thickening of the calvarium and a loss of table differentiation.

Periosteal Bone

Periosteal bone formation is neither a consistent nor a prominent feature of generalized osteitis fibrosa. It may occur to a moderate degree at sites of pathologic fractures or bending deformities. It enveloped the phalanges and metacarpals in the case reported by Boyd, Milgram and Stearns. In that case the lace-like periosteal bone formation promptly disappeared after removal of the parathyroid adenoma.

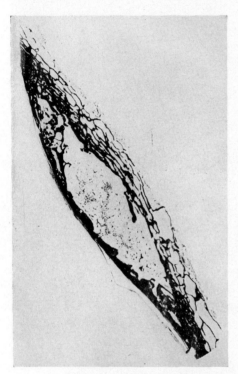

FIGURE 268. Histologic section of a femoral cortex cyst.

Marrow Changes

At the outset there is a pronounced increase in marrow vascularity. Granulation tissue then forms, fills marrow spaces, and transforms to young fibrous tissue. The exact etiology of the marrow fibrosis is

Almost all of the clinical symptoms arise from skeletal deossification, sodium deficiency, hypercalcemia, and hypercalciuria. Pathologic fractures and bone deformities are the rule in advanced cases. Bone pain and tenderness may become a prominent symptom especially over the long bones. Due to the hypercalcemia, both smooth and skeletal muscles become sluggish and weakened, being manifest clinically by malaise and constipation. Vomiting and abdominal pain may be prominent symptoms. The hypercalciuria excites a compensatory polydipsia and polyuria. If dehydration or inactivity occur, there is likely to be stone or sand formation in the genito-urinary tract (Fig. 262). Kidney stones occasionally become so large that they obstruct the kidney pelvis and lead to uremia. Not infrequently calcium salts deposit in many of the soft tissues of the body, particularly the lungs and kidneys (metastatic calcification).

Clinical manifestations depend upon the amount of parathormone secreted, and in turn upon the rate of calcium mobilization. Diet also plays a part since a low calcium diet aggravates the skeletal manifestations, and a high calcium diet tends to reduce the rate of calcium mobilization from the bones.

Prognosis

Without treatment a fatal termination can be expected after a few years. With surgical removal of the parathyroid adenoma, if removed before the patient is moribund or has suffered profound kidney damage, the prognosis for recovery is excellent.

Differential Diagnosis

Generalized osteitis fibrosa must at times be differentiated from osteomalcia, senile osteoporosis, Paget's disease, fibrous dysplasia, renal hyperparathyroidism, multiple myeloma, and carcinomatosis of the skeleton. It must be kept in mind that secondary (renal) hyperparathyroidism, associated with some types of congenital kidney lesions and certain nephritides, can lead to skeletal changes similar to those of primary hyperparathyroidism. The increased secretion of parathormone in secondary hyperparathyroidism is due to hyperplasia of part or all four of the parathyroid glands. In the secondary type resulting from renal damage, there is an acidosis, a high serum phosphorus (up to 10 mg.), normal or lowered serum calcium, and frequently stunted growth. The skeletal lesions are termed renal rickets when they develop during childhood.

Differentiation from osteomalacia and senile osteoporosis is not always easy, particularly when the hyperparathyroidism is in an early stage and produces only skeletal deossification. In a biopsy study there is more marrow fibrosis in generalized fibrous osteitis, and the osteoid seams are thinner than in osteomalacia. In simple osteoporosis there are neither osteoid seams nor a material degree of marrow fibrosis. Microscopic changes take place in the bones during primary hyperparathyroidism prior to gross and roentgenographic changes.

REFERENCES

GENERALIZED OSTEITIS FIBROSA (HYPERPARATHYROIDISM)

ALBRIGHT, F., BURNETT, C. H., COPE, O., and PARSONS, W.: Acute atrophy of bone (osteoporosis) simulating hyperparathyroidism. *J. Clin. Endocrinol., 1*:711, 1941.

ALBRIGHT, F. and ELLSWORTH, R.: A study on the physiology of the parathyroid gland. *J. Clin. Investigation, 7*:183, 1929.

ANDERSON, D. H. and SCHLESINGER, E. R.: Renal hyperparathyroidism with calcification of arteries in infancy. *Am. J. Dist. Child., 63*:102, 1942.

BALLIN, M.: Parathyroidism in reference to orthopedic surgery. *J. Bone & Joint Surg., 15*:120, 1933.

BALLIN, M. and MORSE, P.: Parathyroidism and parathyroidectomy. *Ann. Surg., 94*:592, 1931; *96*:649, 1932.

BARR, D. P., BULGER, H. A.: Hyperparathyroidism. *Am. J. M. Sc., 179*:449, 1930.

BODANSKY, H. L., BLAIR, J. E. and JAFFE, H. L.: Experimental hyperparathyroidism in guinea pigs leading to osteitis fibrosa. *J. Biol. Chem., 88*:629, 1930; *93*:543, 1931.

BOYD, J. D., MILGRAM, J. E. and STEARNS, G.: Clinical hyperparathyroidism. *J. A. M. A., 93*:684, 1929.

CASTLEMAN, B. and MALLORY, T. B.: The pathology of the parathyroid gland in hyperparathyroidism. A study of 25 cases. *Am. J. Path., 11*:1, 1935.

CHARNOCK, D. A.: Renal rickets. *J. Urol., 44*:850, 1940.

COLLIP, J. B.: The physiology of the parathyroid glands. *Canad. M. A. J., 24*:646, 1931.

COLLIP, J. B.: The extraction of a parathyroid hormone which will prevent or control parathyroid tetany and which regulates the level of blood calcium. *J. Biol. Chem., 63*:395, 1925.

COMPERE, E. L.: Bone changes in hyperparathyroidism. *Surg. Gnec. & Obst., 50*:783, 1930.

COMPERE, E. L.: Pathologic and biochemical changes in skeletal dystrophies. *Arch. Surg., 32*:232, 1936.

COMPERE, E. L.: The role of the parathyroid glands in diseases associated with demineralization of the skeleton. *J. Bone & Joint Surg., 15*:142, 1933.

DRAGSTEDT, L. R.: The physiology of the parathyroid glands. *Physiol. Rev., 7*:499, 1927.

FAIRBANK, H. A. T.: Some general diseases of the skeleton. *Brit. J. Surg., 15*:139, 1927.

HANNON, R. R., SHORR, E. McCLELLAN, W. S. and DuBOIS, E. F.: A case of osteitis fibrosa cystica with evidence of hyperactivity of the parathyroid bodies. *J. Clin. Investigation, 8*:215, 1930.

JAFFE, H. L., BODANSKY, A., and BLAIR, J. E.: The sites of decalcification and of bone lesions in experimental hyperparathyroidism. *Arch. Path., 12*:715, 1931.

JAFFE, H. L., BODANSKY, A., and BLAIR, J. E.: The influence of age and of duration of treatment on the production and repair of bone lesions in experimental hyperparathyroidism. *J. Exper. Med., 55*:139, 1932; *52*:669, 1930.

JAFFE, H. L.: Primary and secondary (renal) hyperparathyroidism. *S. Clin. N. Am., 22*:621, 1942.

McLEAN, F. C. and BLOOM, W.: Calcification and ossification. Mobilization of bone salt by parathyroid extract. *Arch. Path., 32*:315, 1941.

MANDL, F.: Therapeutischer Versuch bei einem Falle von Osteitis fibrosa generalizata mittels Extirpation eines Epithelkörperchentumors. *Zentralbl. f. Chir., 53*:260, 1926;*56*:1729, 1929.

MACCALLUM, W. G. and VOEGTLIN, C.: On the relation of tetany to the parathyroid glands and to calcium metabolism. *J. Exper. Med., 11*:118, 1909.

MOORE, R. A.: *A Textbook of Pathology.* W. B. Saunders, Philadelphia, 1944.

MORSE, P. F.: Parathyroidism; its pathologic and etiologic classification. *Am. J. Roentgenol., 30*:578, 1933.

PERLMAN, R. M.: Parathyropituitary syndrome. *Arch. Path., 38*:20, 1944.

POMMER, G.: *Untersuchungen über Osteomalasia und Rachitis.* F. C. W. Vogel, Leipzig, 1885.

POPE, A. and AUB, J. C.: Parathyroid glands and parathormone. *New England J. Med., 230*:698, 1944.

SMITH, E. E. and McLEAN, F. C.: Effect of hyperparathyroidism upon growth and chemical composition of bone. *Endocrinology, 23*:546, 1938.

THOMA, K. H.: A case of generalized osteitis fibrosa demonstrating the effect of hyperparathyroidism on tooth development. *Internat. J. Orthodontia, 22*:400, 1936.

VON RECKLINGHAUSEN, F.: *The fibröse oder deformierende Ostitis, die Osteomalacie und die osteoplastische Carcinose in ihren gegenseitigen Beziehungen.* Berlin, 1891.

VON RECKLINGHAUSEN, F.: *Festschrift Virchow zu seinen 71 Geburtstage.* G. Reiner, Berlin, 1891.

SOLITARY BONE CYSTS

BLOODGOOD, J. C.: Benign bone cysts, Osteitis fibrosa. *Am. J. Surg., 69*:345, 1919.

BREMER, J. L.: Osteitis fibrosa localizata. An experimental study. *Arch. Path., 32*:200, 1941.

COMPERE, E. L.: Localized osteitis fibrosa in the new-born and congenital pseudarthroses. *J. Bone & Joint Surg., 18*:513, 1936.

ELMSLIE, R. C.: Fibrocystic diseases of the bones. *Brit. J. Surg., 2*:17, 1914.

JAFFE, H. L. and LICHTENSTEIN, L.: Solitary unicameral bone cyst with emphasis on roentgen picture, pathologic appearance and pathogenesis. *Arch. Surg., 44*:1004, 1942.

PHEMISTER, D. B., and GORDON, J. E.: The etiology of solitary bone cyst. *J. A. M. A., 87*:1429, 1926.

PLATT, H.: Cysts of the long bones of the hand and foot. *Brit. J. Surg., 18*:20, 1930.

POMMER, G.: Zur Kenntnis der progressiven Hamatom und Phlegmasia veranderungen der Rohrenknocken. *Arch. f. orthop. u. Unfall-Chir., 17*:17, 1920.

VON MIKULICZ: Discussion of the case of Hans Haberer. *Centralbl. f. Chir., 31*:1323, 1914.

FIBROUS DYSPLASIA

ALBRIGHT, F., BUTLER, A. M., HAMPTON, A. O., and SMITH, P.: Syndrome characterized by osteitis fibrosa disseminata, area of pigmentation, and endocrine dysfunction with precocious puberty in females. Report of 5 cases. *New England J. Med., 216*:727, 1937.

FALCONER, M. A. and COPE, C. L.: Fibrous dysplasia of bone with endocrine disorders and cutaneous pigmentation (Albright's disease). *Quart. J. Med., 11*:121, 1942.

FREUND, E. and MEFFERT, C. B.: On the different forms of non-generalized fibrous osteodystrophy. *Surg., Gynec. & Obst., 62*:541, 1936.

GORHAM, L. W.: Albright's syndrome. *Clinics, 1*:358, 1942.

KNAGGS, R. L.: Osteitis fibrosa. *Brit. J. Surg., 10*:487, 1923.

LICHTENSTEIN, L.: Polyostotic fibrous dysplasia. *Arch. Surg., 36*:874, 1938.

LICHTENSTEIN, L. and JAFFE, H. L.: Fibrous dysplasia of bone. *Arch. Path., 33*:777, 1942.

TELFORD, E. D.: A case of osteitis fibrosa with formation of hyalin cartilage. *Brit. J. Surg., 18*:409, 1931.

CHAPTER X

Paget's Disease

(*Osteitis Deformans*)

Contents

HISTORICAL

For the classic clinical description and the term osteitis deformans, we are indebted to Sir James Paget's report of 1877. Since that famous report the disease has borne Paget's name. Wilks is credited with having published the first case of osteitis deformans; and this case report was included in the five cases described in Paget's classic. All five of the original cases were of the advanced polyostotic or disseminated type. Little has since been added to the clinical description of this form of the disease.

It was not until the past three decades that osteitis deformans was clearly established as an indisputable entity, entirely separate from generalized osteitis fibrosa. Two contributions have been foremost in placing Paget's disease on firm ground. The first was Schmorl's classic description of the microscopic pathology. It was Schmorl who drew attention to the "mosaic" structure of the bone. The second contribution was the discovery by Mandl and others of the relationship between osteitis fibrosa von Recklinghausen and the parathyroids. Such a relationship could not be demonstrated in osteitis deformans.

SKELETAL DISTRIBUTION

As already stated, Paget's first cases were polyostotic, having had involvement of several parts of the skeleton. Subsequent investiga-

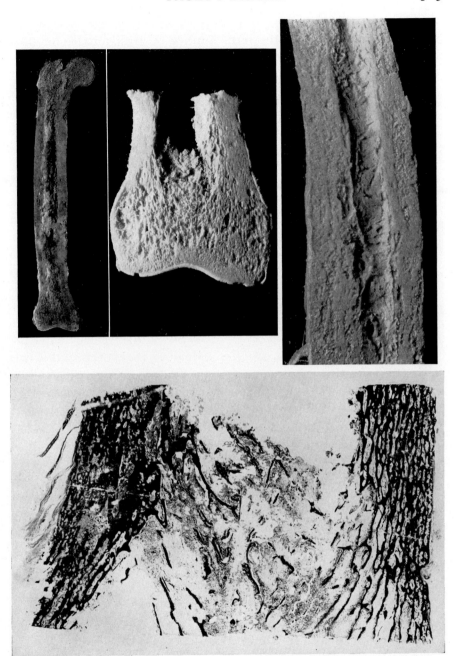

FIGURE 273. Paget's disease of the femur. A. *(Left)* Frontal section of right femur. B. *(Center)* Thin section of the lower femur to show the coarse trabeculation, and thick cortices. Note the elongation of the medullary canal into the metaphysis. C. *(Right)* Femoral diaphysis. D. *(Below)* Histologic section of the distal end of the diaphysis. All periosteal fibrous bone has been replaced by mosaic bone.

tions soon disclosed a monostotic type, in which the disease was localized to one bone as the term implies. A great number of these cases were subclinical, and were discovered in the course of an x-ray examination made for other reasons. The incidence of involvement of the different bones has varied in the many reports in contemporary medical literature. Schmorl, who had the broadest experience from the pathologic standpoint, observed the disease most frequently in the vertebrae and the sacrum. He noted that in the spine the incidence of involvement steadily increases from the first cervical vertebra to the coccyx. The sacrum was found to have the highest incidence of any bone in the body. Lumbar vertebrae were involved twice as often as

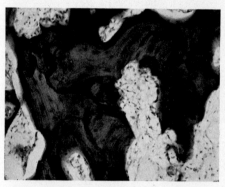

FIGURE 274A. Mosaic structure in Paget's disease. (From region of arrow Figure 278.) High power.

demonstrated in the dorsal vertebrae, and three times as often as in the cervical. Freund and Schmorl demonstrated that areas of the skeleton subjected to the greatest mechanical stress and irritation usually disclosed the highest incidence of involvement. Some unexplained exceptions to this rule are the high incidence of skull involvement and the rarity with which the mandible participates in the disease. Sites of ligamentous and tendinous attachment are often extensively involved. Epiphyses very often present characteristic changes of Paget's disease and, as a result, articular cortices may become distorted and even interrupted in continuity. In a long bone the earliest evidence of the disease is usually observed in a metaphysis from which the pathologic process extends toward the center of the diaphysis. The bones of the lower extremities and pelvis have a much higher incidence of involvement than those of the upper extremities and scapulae.

Distribution of involvement in 139 cases examined by Schmorl:

Sacrum 56%
Lumbar, dorsal, and cervical spine 50%
Right femur 31%
Left femur 15%
Cranium 38%
Sternum 23%
Innominates 21%
Clavicles 13%
Tibiae 8%
Ribs 7%
Humeri 2%

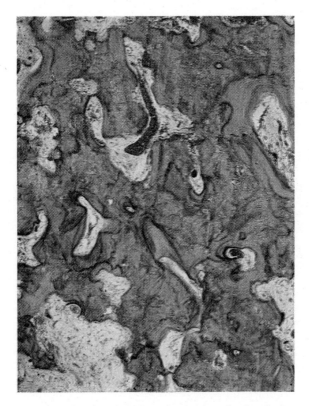

FIGURE 274. *(Continued)* B. See opposite page for description.

The polyostotic form may involve almost every part of the skeleton, but the disease never becomes generalized. This is in contrast to von Recklinghausen's disease which is always generalized, involving even the most remote parts of the skeleton.

LABORATORY FINDINGS

The only laboratory test which is frequently positive and of diagnostic significance is the determination of serum phosphatase activity. In the absence of hepatic disease the serum alkaline phosphatase activity is an index to the extent of new bone formation. Readings of 15 to 100 Bodansky units, and 100 to 200 Jenner Kay units are not uncommon. Gutman and Kasabach found readings of 59 to 103 Bodansky units in the most extensive polyostotic cases, and values ranging from four to eight units when involvement was minimal and monostotic.

ETIOLOGY

Although the etiology of Paget's disease is unknown, it is definitely established that the disease is not due to any known microorganism nor to a parathyroid adenoma. It has been suggested that the disease represents a local

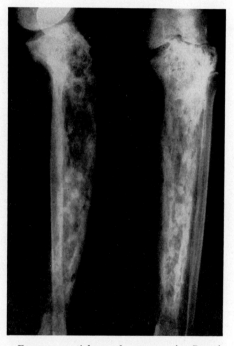

FIGURE 275. Advanced monostotic Paget's disease of the tibia in a 48 year old male.

disturbance of bone metabolism, but this does not tell us much. Explanations based on vitamin deficiencies, heredity, endocrine unbalance, and allergies are untenable.

PATHOLOGY

Mosaic structure—Since Schmorl's description of the mosaic structure of Paget bone, the microscopic differentiation of this disease has been quite simple. Under the microscope the pathogenesis of the bone mosaics is readily visualized as the result of profoundly actively osteoclasia, succeeded by equally active osteoblastic bone apposition (Fig. 274). Bone is absorbed beneath numerous osteoclasts which lie in Howship's lacunae. Sooner or later after the formation of a lacunar line of resorption, the osteoclasts are replaced by osteo-blasts, and osteoid is laid down along the lacunar margin. The osteoid margin then calcifiies to form bone. This process repeats itself over and over at millions of sites to give a complex architecture which is seen as a multitude of multishaped microsegments of bone irregularly morticed together by blue cement apposition lines.

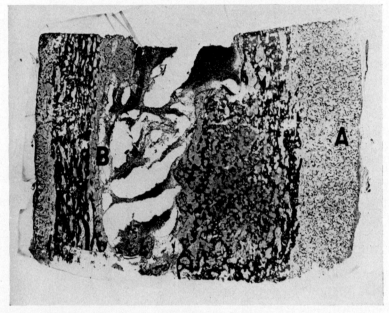

FIGURE 276. Sagital sections of a tibia diaphysis during a predominately osteoblastic stage of Paget's disease. The anterior aspect of the tibia is on the right. Note the thick layer of periosteal fibrous bone, A, and the thin layer of endosteal bone, B. All normal cortical bone has been replaced by coarsely trabeculated mosaics. Periosteal and endosteal fibrous bone generally is rapidly replaced by lamellar bone with a mosaic structure.

Freund has drawn attention to the fact that the cement lines in Paget's disease stain more intensely than normal cement lines due to a greater affinity for hematoxylin. Bone lamellae in the mosaic areas tend to run in all directions. There is no static lamellar alignment, the adjacent microsegments often having lamellae running at right angles to each other. The density of the mosaic structure varies from sclerosis to porosis, but in even the most dense areas there is no tendency toward the formation of haversian systems. Fibrous replacement of mar-row is most extensive during periods of intensive osteoclastic activity. During a phase when osteoblastic activity predominates, there is ex-tensive formation of both fibrous bone and mosaic lamellar bone. Fibrous bone tends to be slowly or rapidly replaced by mosaic lamellar bone.

Stages in the pathogenesis: For descriptive purposes, and to aid in

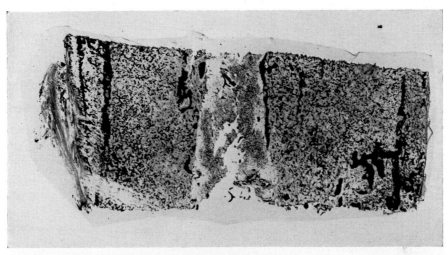

FIGURE 277. Frontal section of a femoral shaft during a predominately osteoclastic phase of osteitis deformans. The bone is diffusely porotic and would have been subject to bending deformities.

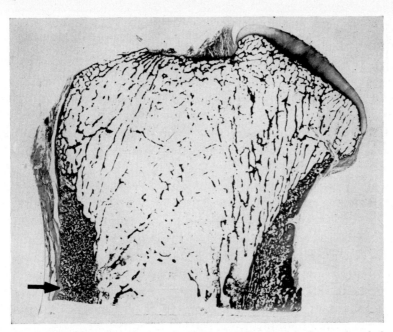

FIGURE 278. Frontal section of an upper humerus. The head is flattened and there is pronounced widening of the cortices and medullary canal. Bone of the shaft cortex is dense and completely transformed to the mosaic structure, indicating an active osteoblastic phase. (Arrow points to region photomicrographed, Figure 274A. and B.)

visualizing the process, the pathogenesis of Paget's disease may be divided into four stages even though these stages are not often well defined, and the same bone may in different fields show different stages of the disease.

FIRST STAGE

The active stage is characterized by a predominance of osteoclastic activity. There is a pronounced degree of hyperemia, and often rapid bone resorption. The cancellous bony trabeculae become thinner and the haversian canals of compact bone become larger to form haversian

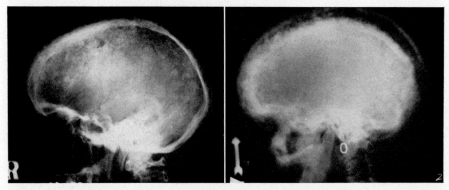

FIGURE 279. Paget's disease of the skull. A. *(Left)* Moderately advanced involvement. Some of the suture lines and vessel markings are still visualized. B. *(Right)* Advanced skull involvement. Suture lines and vessel markings are lost in the profound thickening of the skull. Practically all thickening takes place on the surface of the outer table through periosteal fibrous bone formation.

marrow spaces. Simultaneously, normal marrow elements in involved areas are replaced by young fibrous tissue. New bone then forms on the basis of this fibrous tissue. The system of fine fibrous bone trabeculae is not to be confused with mosaic bone which is, in striking contrast, principally lamellar in type. During this active stage the periosteum may give rise to considerable new bone formation. According to Freund the adjacent para-osseous fibrous tissue, such as the fascia and intermuscular septa, may also give rise to new bone. The result is a widened bone. The long bones may more than double their normal width (Fig. 273). So much of the bone is fibrous in type during this stage that it may be sliced with a sharp knife. However, periosteal fibrous bone in Paget's disease seldom remains in the primitive state but usually is replaced by lamellar bone with a mosaic structure, the transformation extending from the cortex outwards.

In a few instances the endosteum has formed new bone layer upon layer, in the same manner as the periosteum (Fig. 276). Pick has

described cases in which the endosteal bone formation actually pre-
dominated, causing considerable narrowing of the medullary canal.

SECOND STAGE

The second stage is an intermediary stage during which osteoblastic
activity and osteoclasia are about equal.
During this stage, the fibrous bone previously formed in a more active stage is extensively replaced by lamellar bone mosaics.

THIRD STAGE

The third, or healing, stage is marked by
the predominance of osteoblastic bone formation. Mosaic bone is extensively formed,
replacing fibrous bone and any remaining
normal lamellar bone. The mosaic structure
is best studied in this stage. Gradually osteosclerosis replaces osteoporosis, and the
bones become brittle instead of soft.

FOURTH STAGE

Theoretically at least, it is permissable
to speak of a fourth or healed stage. In the
period following cessation of all activity of
the disease, mosaic bone is slowly but steadily replaced by normal lamellar bone with
haversian systems. It is conceivable that

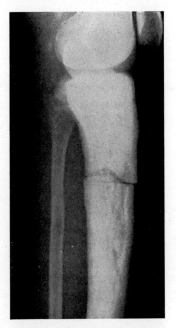

FIGURE 280. Transverse fracture of a tibia in an osteoblastic
phase of Paget's disease. In this
stage the bone is hard and brittle.

with freedom from exacerbations over a period of many years much of
the mosaic structure would disappear.

PSEUDO-CYSTS

True cysts and brown tumors have been described in Paget's disease, but they are rare. Pseudo-cysts are the rule, and are believed to
represent localized areas of marrow necrosis. Microscopically they are
seen to contain necrotic debris which is undergoing resorption by
phagocytes and replacement by regenerative fibrous elements. The
coarse bony trabeculation so frequently seen in Paget's disease may
form patterns which give the false impression of representing cysts.

SKULL CHANGES

Polyostotic Paget's disease usually involves the skull (Fig. 279). The calvarium is most extensively involved and may become greatly thickened by periosteal fibrous bone formation on the outer skull surface. In one of Paget's cases the skull circumference increased from 53.3 cm. to 67 cm. The fibrous bone is gradually replaced by mosaic bone. Both the suture lines and the differentiation of skull tables are lost. In rare instances there is involvement of the facial bones *(leontiasis ossea)*.

COMPLICATIONS

Pathologic Fractures: Pathologic fractures occur during the active stage because of the softness from osteoporosis, and during the healing stage because of the brittleness from osteosclerosis (Figs. 280 & 281). Bending and crumpling is common in the former; and transverse or comminuted fractures, in the latter. Transverse fissures occasionally appear, particularly in the tibia. They either represent fractures or Looser's zones of transformation.

Sarcoma Formation in Paget's Disease: It is estimated that approximately 10 percent of the polyostotic cases develop malignant changes. An interesting characteristic of many of the sarcomas in Paget's disease

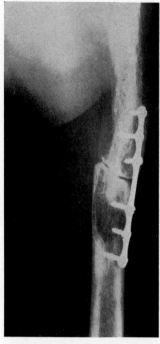

FIGURE 281. Ununited pathological fracture of a femur involved by Paget's disease in its proximal one-half. Note how sharply the disease ends in the mid-femur.

is their multicentric origin. Several widely separated areas of Paget's bone marrow may simultaneously develop sarcomatous changes; formerly the multiple areas of sarcoma were believed to represent metastases from a primary growth.

It has been demonstrated by Freund and Perlman that sarcomatous formations appear where the fibrous marrow is mature, and not immature. Of the two types of sarcomas observed, fibrosarcoma and osteosarcoma, the former is the more common. Coley and Sharp collected 71 cases of osteogenic sarcoma in patients past 50 years of age and found that in 28 percent the sarcoma was associated with Paget's disease. There is no successful treatment for sarcomas complicating Paget's disease; all are fatal in less than five years.

ROENTGENOLOGIC CORRELATION

The roentgenogram is of the utmost importance in the diagnosis of osteitis deformans. In the majority of cases the diagnosis is made first by the roentgenologist.

One of the most conspicuous aspects of osteitis deformans is the abundant periosteal bone formation. Thin lamellations of periosteal bone represent one of the earliest signs of the disease. Pronounced widening of the long bone diaphyses through the formation of thick layers of periosteal bone characterizes the advanced stage. Normal trabecular markings are completely replaced by the coarse, wavy trabeculae that are so typical of Paget's disease. No other entity is capable of such widespread broadening of the shafts of long bones.

Medullary canals may be widened or narrowed, the former type being the more common.

Notwithstanding the fact that more cases are monostotic than polyostotic, the finding of a solitary lesion calls for an x-ray study of the entire skeleton. The monostotic form often involves a single vertebral body. A honeycomb trabecular pattern is a frequent finding, and there may be either sclerosis or porosis. Pathologic compression fractures are not rare.

In the skull, new bone is laid down almost exclusively on the outer table. Osteoporosis is the rule, both in the old bone of the skull and the new fibrous bone. In a late stage all fibrous bone is replaced by mosaics of lamellar bone. Multiple small islands of dense mosaic bone scattered throughout the skull give the bone a woolly appearance.

A localized area of a wild and bizarre overgrowth of bone in osteitis deformans generally represents the worst possible complication of the disease—osteogenic sarcoma.

CLINICAL CORRELATION

Paget's disease usually occurs between the ages of forty and seventy. Schmorl, in a large series of detailed post-mortem examinations, found an incidence of 3 percent in individuals past forty years of age, making the disease a relatively common geriatric entity. However, many of these cases were subclinical during life and were diagnosed only after a study of post-mortem pathologic material. Dickson, Camp and Ghormley reviewed 367 Mayo clinic cases of Paget's disease and found only one patient under 30 years of age; one-third of the patients were in the sixth decade.

Most of the series of cases thus far reported disclose a higher incidence in men than in women; however in a series of 116 cases reported in 1936 by Gutman and Kasaback the sexes were equally affected. The incidence of the disease appears to bear no relationship to nationality or occupation.

Although there is no known hereditary factor, instances of several cases occurring in the same family have been reported.

The monostotic form is much more common than the polyostotic. Many observers believe the monostotic form to be merely an early or arrested stage of the disease. Undoubtedly many cases have existed in a subclinical state for a number of years and even throughout adult life without the disease's ever advancing to clinical manifestations.

In general, osteitis deformans is slowly but steadily progressive. However, remissions are very common and may extend through many years. After a short or long period an exacerbation may occur with extension of the disease to many new parts of the skeleton. The disease *per se* is not fatal, but it may give rise to pathologic fractures and a secondary anemia which indirectly may lead to death. Sarcomas complicating Paget's disease are the principal source of fatalities.

SYMPTOMS

When symptoms occur in osteitis deformans, they are usually in the form of bone pain located over the long bones of the lower extremities. The pain may be dull and boring or sharp and radiating. Occasionally Paget's pain becomes agonizing. Extensive skull involvement may give rise to headaches. The enlarging head requiring a larger size hat each year is a familiar symptom of skull involvement. A pathologic fracture not infrequently ushers in the clinical symptoms that lead to a diagnosis.

DIFFERENTIAL DIAGNOSIS

Clinically it is very important to differentiate Paget's disease from generalized osteitis fibrosa cystica in view of the fact that the latter can be effectively treated. Chronic pyogenic and luetic osteomyelitis and periostitis occasionally require differentiation. Metastatic malignancies have also been confused with osteitis deformans. The periosteal bone formation of Paget's disease with widening of the long bones is a useful point in differential diagnosis. Microscopically the diagnosis seldom is difficult. Occasionally one may see a superficial resemblance to a mosaic structure in the complex blue cement lines of chronic pyogenic and luetic osteomyelitis, von Recklinghausen's disease, and regeneration following aseptic bone necrosis.

REFERENCES

BIRD, C. E.: Sarcoma in Paget's disease: *Arch. Surg., 14*:1187, 1927.

BODANSKY, A. and JAFFE, H. L.: Phosphatase studies. *Arch. Int. Med., 54*:88, 1934.

CAMPBELL, E. and WHITFIELD, R. D.: Osteogenic sarcomata of vertebra secondary to Paget's disease with compression of spinal cord and canda equina." *N. Y. State J. Med., 43*:931, 1943.

COLEY, B. L. and SHARP, G. S.: Paget's disease. A predisposing factor to osteogenic sarcoma. *Arch. Surg., 23*:918, 1931.

DICKSON, D. D., CAMP, J. D., and GHORMLEY, R. K.: Osteitis Deformans. *Radiology, 44*:449, 1945.

FREUND, E.: Osteitis deformans. *Virchows Arch. f. path. Anat., 274*:1, 1929.

GROH, J. A.: Monosteitic Paget's disease as clinical entity. Roentgenographic observations of 9 cases. *Am. J. Roentgenol., 50*:230, 1943.

GUTMAN, A. B., and KASABACH, H.: Paget's disease, analysis of 116 cases. *Am. J. M. Sc., 191*:361, 1936.

JAFFE, H. L.: Paget's disease of bone. *Arch. Path., 15*:83, 1933.

KAY, H. P.: Plasma phosphatase in osteitis deformans and in other diseases of bone. *Brit. J. Exper. Path., 10*:253, 1929.

KIRSHBAUM, J. D.: Fibrosarcoma of the skull in Paget's disease. *Arch. Path., 36*:74, 1943.

KNAGGS, R. L.: On osteitis deformans and its relation to osteitis fibrosa and osteomalacia. *Brit. J. Surg., 13*:206, 1925.

PAGET, SIR J.: On a form of chronic inflammation of the bones. *Proc. Roy. Soc. Med. & Chir. Tr., 60*:39, 1877.

PAGET, SIR J.: Additional cases of osteitis deformans. *Proc. Roy. Soc. Med. & Chir., 9*:147, 1882. *Illust. Med. News, 2*:181, 1889.

PERLMAN, R.: Sarcoma formation in Paget's disease. *J. Bone & Joint Surg., 16*:594, 1934.

PICK, L.: *Verhandl. d. Gesellsch. f. Verdanungs u. Stoffwechseldr., 10*:146, 1931.

PIKE, M. M.: Paget's disease with associated osteogenic sarcoma. *Arch. Surg., 46*:750, 1943.

REIFENSTEIN, E. C. and ALBRIGHT, F.: Paget's disease. *New England J. Med., 231*:343, 1944.

SCHMORL, G.: Uber osteitis deformans Paget. *Virchows Arch. f. path. Anat., 283*:694, 1932.

SUGARBAKER, E. D.: Osteitis deformans. *Am. J. Surg., 48*:414, 1940.

WHITE, E. P. G.: Osteitis deformans in monkeys. *Arch. Int. Med., 30*:790, 1922.

WILLIAMS, H. L. and WATSON, E. M.: Hyperphosphatemia. *J. Lab. & Clin. Med., 26*:1333, 1941.

CHAPTER XI

Melorheostosis

Contents

This rare bone disease was first described in 1922 by Leri and Joanny. Their patient was a woman, aged thirty-nine years, who had had a small deformity of the hand since the age of ten years. Limitation of elbow motion and shoulder pain had slowly developed, but the remainder of the body was negative. Roentgenograms disclosed a peculiar "flowing" type of hyperostosis that previously had never been described in medical literature. In 1925 Lewin and McLeod reported a similar case in a man aged thirty-five who had had symptoms since the age of six. The bone changes were most evident along the course of the ulnar nerve.

Muzii's case was reported in 1926; Putti's case, in 1927. In 1942 Franklin and Matheson reviewed the literature and added the 39th case. Nineteen of the cases were males, twelve were females and in the other eight cases the sex was not stated. The age at the time the diagnosis was made varied from six to forty-nine years. In 20 cases symptoms appeared first in a lower extremity, and in 19, first in an upper extremity. Five of the cases had shortening, up to 4 cm., of an involved limb; and in three cases there was lengthening, the greatest being 5 cm.

Melorheostosis is virtually always a unilateral disease; however, Bury, in 1939, reported the case of a 35 year old female who had bilateral lower extremity involvement, in which the hyperostotic osteosclerotic tract extended from the ilium to the metatarsals on one side and from the ilium to the knee on the other side.

Involvement of the skull and mandible is exceptional, but in the interesting case of Franklin and Matheson the lesions involved the right side of the skull and mandible, and the right upper and lower extremities.

Associated diseases have not appeared relevant unless there is some significance in the associated scleroderma in the Dillehunt and Chuinard case. In their case the scleroderma was in the lower extremity directly over the site of the bone lesions.

Melorheostosis develops incipiently, usually becoming manifest between the ages of five and 20. Pain of moderate severity, dull and boring in character, often worse at night, is characteristic. Pressure over an involved bone, or excessive use of an involved extremity accentuates the pain. Periods of remission of pain are common.

ETIOLOGY

Nothing is known of the etiology. An array of theories have been proposed, but none casts any light on the subject.

ROENTGENOGRAPHIC APPEARANCE

Involvement seldom occurs in more than one extremity, but in the upper extremity the shoulder girdle may be involved on the affected side (Fig. 284), and in lower extremity involvement, the pelvis may be included. Kraft, in reviewing the previously reported cases and in reporting two cases of his own, divided the condition into three types:

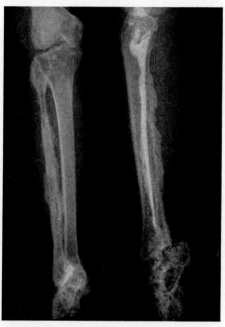

FIGURE 282. Roentgenograms showing the typical lesions of melorheostosis. An elongated, irregular, often wavy, sclerotic periosteal hyperostosis is characteristic. This patient was a 44 year old female who had had multiple deformities of her upper extremities and right leg since childhood. Because of a painful right foot and an equino-valgus deformity, the leg was amputated.

1. Uninterrupted involvement of an entire extremity. A continuous "flowing hyperostosis" from the scapula to the finger tips, or in the lower extremity from the ilium to the toes.

2. Involvement of only the proximal one-half of an extremity.

3. Irregular, interrupted involvement of an entire extremity in which multiple interruptions occur in the "flow."

PATHOLOGIC ANATOMY

The striking alteration of involved bones appears as a narrow, elongated, irregular, sclerotic hyperostosis. The contour of the bony deposits resembles nothing else so much as the pattern made by paraffin flowing down the sides of a burning candle. Leri and Joanny first suggested this resemblance, and it prompted them to name the disease Melorheostosis which means "member flow." This flowing hyperostosis does not often encircle the entire circumference of a bone but occurs more frequently in a linear distribution. In several of the re-

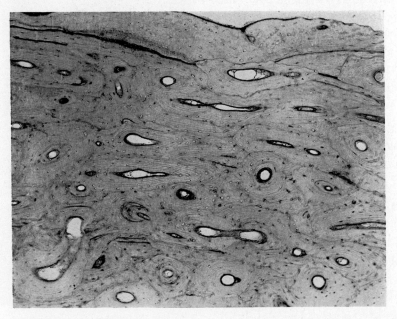

FIGURE 283. Photomicrograph of a section of the fibular periosteal hyperostosis shown in Figure 282. Histologic studies revealed only normal dense compact bone.

ported cases these linear deposits followed the course of a nerve. The involvement is not limited to the formation of dense periosteal bone but in addition alters the cortex by promoting osteosclerosis. Endosteal bone, when it forms, narrows the medullary canal. Deposits of bone and calcium frequently appear in the paraosteal and para-articular soft tissues, the latter being the more common. In several instances para-articular bony deposits enlarge to the point of locking the joint. However, joint involvement does not develop until a late stage of the disease. If a metaphysis becomes involved before the epiphyseal plate fuses, there may be premature fusion with resultant shortening of the extremity. Or there may be epiphyseal plate stimulation with extremity lengthening.

HISTOPATHOLOGY

Biopsies have been few, and there have been no post-mortem studies. Leri's biopsy showed normal dense compact bone. Putti's biopsy showed dense compact bone, in which the haversian canals were constricted or obliterated by perivascular ossification. Few osteoblasts and

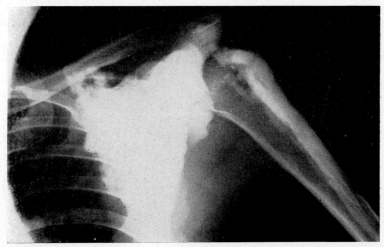

FIGURE 284. Melorheostosis in a 38 year old male with involvement of the bones of the left upper extremity. Involvement of the humerus is limited to the lateral aspect, whereas the scapula is completely enveloped by the dense periosteal hyperostosis.

osteoclasts were in evidence. Histologically there is no inflammation, simply new bone formation.

THEORIES OF ETIOLOGY

The etiology is unknown. Putti explained the condition on the basis of a local ischaemia; Lewin and McLeod, on a neurogenic basis; Zimmer, as a developmental defect; Kraft, as an endocrine imbalance; Moore and de Lorimer, as periosteal telangiectases. All of which means that there is no tenable theory. Perhaps the explanation on the basis of a skeletal developmental defect is the most logical.

DIFFERENTIAL DIAGNOSIS

Melorheostosis must be differentiated from chronic pyogenic osteomyelitis, Paget's disease, leutic osteitis and periostitis, osteopetrosis, and osteoblastic carcinoma metastases.

REFERENCES

Melorheostosis

DILLEHUNT, R. B. and CHUINARD, E. G.: Melorheostosis, Leri. A case report. *J. Bone & Joint Surg., 18*:991, 1936.

FRANKLIN, E. L. and MATHESON, I.: Melorheostosis. Report of a case with review of the literature. *Brit. J. Radiol., 15*:185, 1942.

KRAFT, E.: Melorheostosis Leri: flowing hyperostosis of a single extremity, report of 2 cases. *J. A. M. A., 98*:705, 1932.

LEWIN, P. and MacLEOD, S. B.: Osteosclerosis with distribution suggesting that of ulnar nerve; unclassified bone condition. *J. Bone & Joint Surg., 7*:968, 1925.

LERI, A. and JOANNYS Hyperostose en coulie sur toute la longneur d'un membre ou melorheostose. *Bull. et mém. Soc. méd. d. hop. de Paris, 46*:1145, 1922.

LERI, A. and LIEVERE, J. A.: *Bull. Acad. de méd., Paris, 99*:737, 1928; *Press. méd., 36*:801, 1928.

MOORE, J. J. and DeLORIMER, A. A.: Melorheostosis, Leri. Review of the literature and report of case. *Am. J. Roentgenol., 11*:161, 1933.

MUZII, M.: Iconograpia rara di malattie delle ossa. *Radiol. med., 13*:435, 1926.

PUTTI, V.: L'osteosi eburneizzante monomelica. *Chir. d'org. di movimento, 11*:335, 1927.

CHAPTER XII

Hypertrophic Osteoarthropathy

Contents

Bamberger in 1889 and Marie in 1890 described a syndrome consisting of clubbed fingers, ossifying periostitis, and mild chronic arthritis. This syndrome is associated in most instances with chronic suppurative pulmonary lesions, such as chronic bronchiectasis, and chronic empyema. A few cases have been reported in which pulmonary tuberculosis and heart disease have been associated with the bone and joint changes. A case was reported by Beclere in which a left subclavian aneurysm caused edema of the left upper extremity and osteoarthropathic changes localized to that extremity. In this instance the changes must have been related to vascular congestion. In those cases in which there is an associated suppurative pulmonary lesion, the osteoarthropathy is believed by some investigators to represent chronic inflammation created by hematogenous toxins originating in the pulmonary focus. More than likely there are instances in which both the vascular congestion and the toxins play a role in the etiology. It has been claimed, in those rare cases attributed to malignancies (sarcoma and carcinoma), that the tumor produced a toxin which caused the osteoarthropathy; this theory has a weak foundation.

EXPERIMENTAL PRODUCTION

Mendlowitz and Leslie, in 1941, produced hypertrophic osteoarthropathy in dogs by anastomosing the pulmonary artery to the left auricle. Circulatory shunts of 13 to 46 percent of the ventricular output were produced. An increased systemic cardiac output with an accelerated peripheral blood flow was considered to be the most significant alteration. Typical periosteal bone formations of hypertrophic osteoarthropathy gradually developed. Mendlowitz and Leslie concluded that any theory devised to explain hypertrophic osteoarthropathy should not disregard the factor of increased peripheral blood flow.

The brothers Compere, and Adams attempted to produce the disease experimentally through the creation of lung abscesses in dogs. The experiments failed to produce skeletal changes, but led these investigators to believe that a circulatory disturbance and an upset acid-base equilibrium are more important than toxic factors in causing hypertrophic osteoarthropathy.

BONE MANIFESTATIONS

The bone changes are variable, involving a small localized portion of the skeleton to virtually every bone in the body; the most frequently involved bones are the humerus, tibia, metatarsals, and metacarpals. The major manifestation is an ossifying periostitis in which the diaphyses of involved bones become covered with a thin or thick layer of fragile fibrous bone having a smooth or slightly undulated symmetrical outline (Fig. 285). If the disease is protracted and the lung lesion unchanged, the periosteal bone gradually increases in density eventually becoming indistinguishably assimilated to the cortex. Involved diaphyses of long bones may achieve the same width as the epiphyses, a phenomenon giving the bones a straight-sided outline. Instances are reported where, following the healing of the lung lesion, the periosteal bone absorbed. Exacerbations of the underlying cause of the periosteal bone often lead to lamellations in the epicortical bone formations.

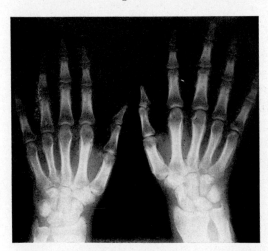

FIGURE 285. Ossifying periostitis of hypertrophic osteoarthropathy. (Courtesy, *U. S. Army Institute of Pathology*, Acc. No. 121454.)

Osteoporosis of the involved bones is frequent.

Fried described cases in which periosteal bone partially enveloping vertebral bodies resembled that seen in acromegaly. Fried emphasized, as did Marie, that hypertrophic osteoarthropathy must sometimes be differentiated from acromegaly.

Histologically the periosteal bone is not remarkable. It results from cambium proliferation and is non-specific, and non-pathognomonic in character.

JOINT MANIFESTATIONS

The joint changes are less well defined than the bone changes. Involved joints that have been examined histologically revealed chronic inflammatory changes in both fibrous and synovial layers of the capsule. Round cell infiltration is in evidence but there is little destruction. The inflammatory picture may be both fleeting and recurring. Cartilage necrosis and erosion have been reported but are exceptional. Joint manifestations are not very disabling.

CLUBBED FINGERS

This, the most consistent and obvious clinical manifestation of pulmonary osteoarthropathy, was first described by Hippocrates. The enlargement of the finger tips may be slight to pronounced. In the more pronounced cases the nail becomes widened, brittle, and often splits. The dome shaped contour of the nails is due to curving over the end of the finger, a contour that has been compared to a parrot's beak.

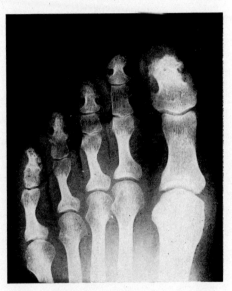

FIGURE 286. Hypertrophic osteoarthropathy manifest in the feet by prominent distal phalangeal tufts and clubbing of toes. This patient, a 20 year old male, had a congenital heart lesion manifest since birth by pulmonary congestion and cyanosis.

Clubbing of the fingers represents hyperplasia of the soft tissue portion of the finger. In most cases the terminal phalanx is not the site of periosteal bone formation. The fact that the tips of fingers and toes are the most dependent portions of the body is offered as an explanation of the vascular congestion and connective tissue hyperplasia localized at these sites. Weens and Brown reported two cases in which the terminal phalanges of the clubbed fingers were atrophic. Lock, on the other hand, noted enlargement and tufting of the terminal phalanges in five consecutive cases.

REFERENCES

Hypertrophic Osteoarthropathy

Bamberger, E.: Bronchiektosie und Veränderung einzelner Röhrenknochen. *Wien klin. Wchnschr.*, *2*:226, 1889.

Bamberger, E.: Uber Knochenveränderung bei Chronischen Lungen und Herzkrankheiten. *Ztschr. klin. Med.*, *18*:193, 1891.

Compere, E. L., Adams, W. C., and Compere, C. L.: Possible etiologic factors in the production of pulmonary osteoarthropathy. *Proc. Soc. Exper. Biol. & Med.*, *28*:1083, 1931.

Crump, C.: Histologie der allgerneinen Osteophytose (Osteoarthropathie hypertrophante pneumique). *Virchows Arch. path. Anat.*, *271*:467, 1929.

Freund, E.: Idiopathic familial generalized osteophytosis. *Am. J. Roentgenol.* *39*:216, 1938.

Fried, B. M.: Chronic pulmonary osteoarthropathy. *Arch. Int. Med.*, *72*:565, 1943.

Hasbrouck, E. M.: Case of hypertrophic pulmonary osteoarthropathy. *New York State J. Med.*, *67*:665, 1896.

Locke, E. A.: Secondary hypertrophic osteoarthropathy and its relation to simple club fingers. *Arch. Int. Med.*, *15*:659, 1915.

Marie, P.: De l'osteo-arthropathie hypertrophiante pneumique. *Rev. de méd. Paris*, *10*:1, 1890.

Mendlowitz, M.: Clubbing and hypertrophic osteoarthropathy. *Medicine*, *21*:269, 1942.

Mendlowitz, M. and Leslie, A.: Pulmonary artery to left auricle anastomosis with hypertrophic osteoarthropathy. *Am. J. Path.*, *17*:458, 1941.

Shaw, H. B. and Cooper, R. H.: Pulmonary hypertrophic osteoarthropathy occurring in a case of congenital heart disease. *Lancet*, *1*:880, 1907.

Thorburn, W.: Three cases of hypertrophic pulmonary osteoarthropathy. *Brit. M. J.*, *1*:1155, 1893.

Weber, F. P.: Histology of new bone formation in case of pulmonary hypertrophic osteoarthropathy. *Proc. Roy. Soc. Med.*, *2*:187, 1908-09.

Weens, H. S. and Brown, C. E.: Atrophy of terminal phalanges in clubbing and hypertrophic osteoarthropathy. *Radiology*, *45*:27, 1945.

CHAPTER XIII

Skeletal Manifestations of Endocrine Disorders

Contents

The more important endocrine glands, capable in a pathologic state of altering the skeleton, include the pituitary, thyroid, parathyroids, adrenals, and the gonads. During the period of growth the hormones exert their influence principally upon enchondral ossification; after full growth the influence is on all elements: bone, periosteum, marrow, and cartilage.

PITUITARY GLAND

From many standpoints the anterior lobe of the pituitary gland is the most important structure in the endocrine system. At least six distinctly different skeletal system disturbances have their origin in lesions of the anterior lobe:

1. **Gigantism:** Hyperplasia or adenoma of the eosinophil cells, causing hypersecretion during the period of skeletal growth.

2. **Acromegaly:** Hypersecretion of eosinophil cells during adulthood.

3. **Basophilism** *(Cushing)*: Hyalinization (degranulation) of the ba-

sophil cells of the anterior lobe. Hypersecretion "S" harmone of the adrenal cortex.

4. **Pituitary dwarfism:** Hyposecretion of the eosinophil cells and frequently of other componet cells of the anterior lobe during infancy and childhood.

5. **Fröhlicks syndrome,** Simmonds Syndrome, and probably the Laurence-Moon-Biedl Syndrome, are caused by anterior lobe lesions.

THYROID GLAND

The thyroid gland, is responsible for two skeletal disturbances:

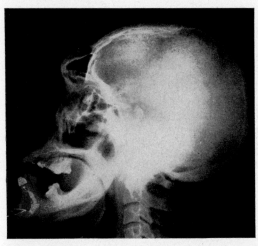

FIGURE 287. Acromegalic skull of a male age 40, showing pronounced prognathism, hyperpneumatization, and a deepened eroded sella turcica. An old fracture of the mandible accounts for the wire loop.

1. **Cretinism:** Hyposecretion in infancy and childhood produces cretinism with its associated growth retardation.

2. **Skeletal porosis:** Hypersecretion (exophthalmic goiter) can cause profound skeletal porosis.

GONADS

Hypergonadism produces premature closure of epiphyses and a resulting shortened stature.

Hypogonadism delays closure of epiphyses and in males causes a feminine body configuration. In adults hypogonadism plays an important part in senile and post-menopausal osteoporosis.

GIGANTISM (PITUITARY)

The preadolescent eosinophilic adenoma or hyperplasia, by secreting excessive quantities of growth promoting hormone, accelerates skeletal growth, the bones ultimately assuming giant proportions. Bones developing both by enchondral and membranous ossification show the same stimulated growth. At the enchondral lines there is hyperemia, pronounced osteoblastic activity, and in some cases it is said that the orderly column arrangement of normal enchondral ossification is disturbed. Periosteal bone formation is also accelerated and leads to an increase in thickness of the bones, the new bone frequently possessing irregular contours. Feet and hands may become immense, the skull, thickened; and the lower jaw, enlarged. The muscles do not often keep pace with the skeletal growth; many such giants are neither very strong nor very intelligent. When growth finally ceases, acromegalic signs may develop if the hypersecretion of the eosinophil cells continues.

ACROMEGALY

Pierre Marie in 1886 recorded a classical description of acromegaly and was the first to identify the pituitary origin of the disease. He named the disease acromegaly from the Greek words *akros*, meaning extremities and other prominent parts of the body, and *megale*, meaning large. According to Marie, Brigidi in 1877 was the first to describe the skeletal changes associated with acromegaly. Other descriptions of the bone and joint changes have been reported by von Recklinghausen, Virchow, Erdheim, Keith, Hunter, Cushing and Davidoff, and Waine, Bennett, and Bauer.

The advanced clinical picture of acromegaly is familiar and well defined. In advanced stages the individual presents a picture bordering on the grotesque, with his lantern jaw, massive hands and feet, barrel chest, large coarse facial features, and dorsal kyphosis.

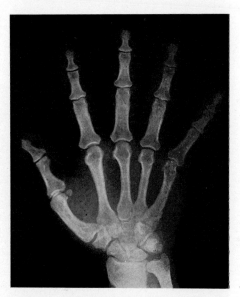

FIGURE 288. Acromegalic hand of the patient whose skull is shown in Figure 287. Hands were large and spade-like with tufting of the terminal phalanges.

There may be protracted headaches (bitemporal), and because of pressure of the tumor on the optic nerves, tracts, or chiasma, there may be impairment of vision and narrowing of visual fields.

Knaggs believes that in gigantism and acromegaly the increased secretion of growth-stimulating hormone makes the osteoblasts more sensitive and more responsive to mechanical stresses. The greatly enlarged lower jaw is thought to result from bone formation stimulated by muscles of mastication. There is hyperplasia of bone at almost all muscle and ligament attachments, giving the bones a pronounced surface irregularity.

VERTEBRAE

Vertebral changes are a prominent part of acromegaly and have been described in detail by Erdheim. Dorsal and lower cervical vertebral bodies become enlarged anteriorly and laterally through a combination of periosteal bone apposition and reactivated enchondral ossification (Fig. 289). The newly formed bone remains sharply demarcated both grossly and roentgenographically. Lateral and anterior lipping develops and is similar to, but more uniform than, the lipping in osteo-arthritis.

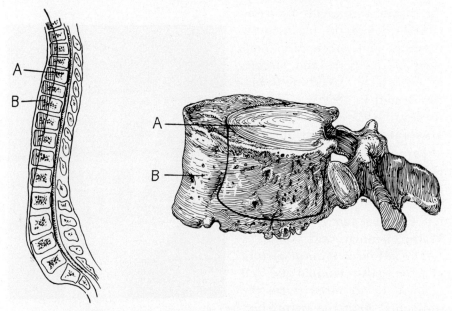

FIGURE 289. Vertebrae in acromegaly. Dorsal and lower cervical vertebral bodies, *A*, become enlarged anteriorly and laterally, *B*. (After Erdheim.)

In one of Waine, Bennett, and Bauer's cases the lipping produced a fusion of the 6th and 7th dorsal vertebral bodies. Marginal lipping is created principally by reactivated enchondral ossification, the remainder of the vertebral body enlargement arising from periosteal bone formation. A serrated, saw-tooth border is characteristic of the marginal lipping of acromegalic vertebrae.

As the vertebrae enlarge so also do the intervertebral discs, and this is accomplished by activity of the anterior and lateral perichondrium of the annulus fibrosis. A fibrous and fibrocartilaginous expansion of the discs keeps pace with the enlarging vertebral bodies. Narrowing of intervertebral discs in late stages is quite common.

In acromegaly the vertebral changes are not dependent upon degenerative changes in the discs as are the changes in osteo-arthritis. Acromegaly in young adults and the middle-aged often shows no degeneration whatever in the intervertebral discs. In the aged it is only natural that the two conditions would be found together.

Roentgenograms of the vertebral bodies generally show the dorsal to be wider than the lumbar vertebrae. At first glance the dorsal bodies appear flattened but this is an illusion. Actually there is no flattening, but simply an increase in the antero-posterior and lateral diameters.

SKULL AND MANDIBLE

Skull changes are characterized by greatly expanded air sinuses, accentuation of surface markings, and enlargement of the sella turcica (Fig. 287). The sella may encroach on the underlying sphenoidal sinus; cases have been reported in which the entire sinus was filled by an adenoma-expanded sella. Some degree of erosion and thinning of the clinoid processes is the rule.

Elongation of the mandible (prognathism) in acromegaly represents a diffuse enlargement (Fig. 287). The teeth tend to become separated from each other and occlusion anteriorly is lost.

PHALANGES

Tufting of the terminal phalanges of the fingers and toes is a consistent finding in acromegaly (Fig. 288). Cushing considered it pathognomomic, and described the tufting as "arrow head terminal phalanges." Similar tufting has been observed in a number of cases of hypertrophic osteoarthropathy.

RIBS

The bovine or barrel chest in acromegaly is due to reactivated growth at the costochondral junction of the ribs. Erdheim, and Waine, Bennett and Bauer, found fusiform enlargement of the costochondral junctions (acromegalic rosary) which histologically was due to a combination of perichondrial proliferation on the cartilage side of the junction and rekindled enchondral ossification on the bone side. The diffuse broadening and thickening of the ribs is the result of periosteal bone apposition.

JOINTS

Erdheim made the first detailed study of the joint changes in acromegaly. Recently (1945) Waine, Bennett and Bauer reported that they had observed changes in acromegalic joints, similar to those described by Erdheim.

In osteo-arthritis the initial change is impairment and loss of the binding substance in the superficial layers of the articular cartilage, with
the result that fibrillation of the collagenous bundles takes place, and
is followed by erosion. In acromegaly the initial lesion in the articular
cartilage was found to be hyperplasia and hypertrophy of the zone of
columns. In place of a decrease in matricial substance, there was an
initial increase. In both entities there is reactivated enchondral ossifi-

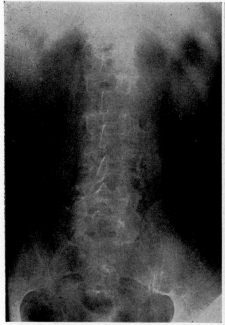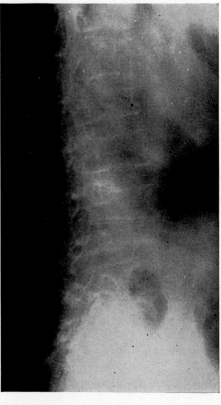

FIGURE 290. Pituitary basophilism in 41
year old male with basophilic adenoma of
pituitary. Profound generalized skeletal deossification is characteristic. A. *(Left)* Antero-posterior roentgenogram of the lumbar
spine. B. *(Right)* Lateral view.

cation leading to the formation of marginal osteophytes. Eventually
the involved areas of articular cartilage in acromegaly become fibrillated
and eroded, giving a picture identical with advanced osteo-arthritis.
Thus the joint pathology in acromegaly differs from that in osteo-arthritis only in the early stages.

BASOPHILISM

(Cushing's Syndrome)

In 1932 Cushing described a syndrome characterized by pronounced skeletal deossification, obesity of the trunk, neck and face, hypertension, hirsutism, glycosuria, and purple abdominal striae. In each instance in the 16 cases studied Cushing found either hyperplasia or an adenoma of the basophil cells of the anterior lobe of the pituitary gland. Cushing contended that the syndrome was a response to an excessive secretion of the basophil cells. Eleven of the sixteen cases studied were females.

SKELETAL CHANGES

The skeletal deossification often becomes profound (Fig. 290). In a case reported by Zondek, some of the bones, particularly the ribs and

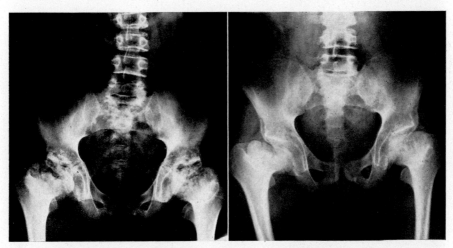

FIGURE 291. Disturbed epiphyseal ossification associated with combined hypothyroidism and hypopituitarism. A. *(Left)* Roentgenogram of pelvis of a male age 21. B. *(Right)* Roentgenogram of pelvis when patient was age 23. Ossification of the flattened femoral heads is complete.

vertebrae, had become so soft that they could be cut with a knife. The process is one of simple osteoporosis and is not associated with a significant fibrous osteitis. The frequently associated spondylarthralgia and dorsal kyphosis appear to be related to the osteoporosis and pathologic vertebral body compression. Changes in the sella turcica are rare.

PROGNOSIS

The prognosis is grave since the majority of patients succumb within five years; however, several have survived more than 20 years.

ETIOLOGY

The basophil cell origin of the syndrome has been contested by Kraus and Susman. Kraus considered the basophil cell findings to be incidental and not causative; he believed that the associated adrenal and gonodal lesions were more significant. Susman examined 260 hypophyses at post-mortems and found 21 instances in which there was an increase in basophil cells unassociated with the Cushing syndrome. Susman concluded that there was no histological basis for believing that the syndrome is caused by hypersecretion of the basophil cells.

Crooke reported a series of 12 cases of basophilism. In six of the cases there was a basophil adenoma, in three cases an adrenal tumor and in three cases a thymus tumor. In all 12 instances the basophil cells disclosed hyalinization, also described as degranulation. The regressive basophil changes are now believed to be the fundamental alteration in the Cushing syndrome. The primary etiologic factor may be a benign or malignant tumor of the adrenal cortex, thymus or ovary. Heinbecker has shown evidence that the primary cause may also reside in atrophy of the paraventricular and other nuclei of the hypothalmus.

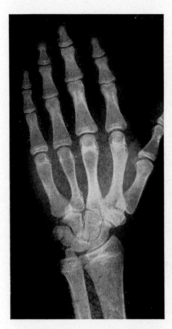

FIGURE 291 Continued. C. Roentgenogram of the right hand when patient was age 21, demonstrating the delayed closure of epiphyseal plates.

Most of the symptomatology of basophilism is explainable on the basis of the pattern of the endocrine unbalance. Destruction of the basophil cells leads to hypothyroidism and hypogonadism.

Albright and his co-workers contend that the osteoporosis in Cushing's syndrome is due principally to an excessive secretion by the adrenal cortex of sugar hormones ("S" hormones). These hormones convert proteins into sugars (glycogenesis) and inhibit anabolism of protoplasm, including bone matrix. With the catabolic process undiminished and anabolism suppressed, all body tissues including the skeleton undergo progressive atrophy. The hypogonadism of Cushing's syndrome also appears to play an important part in the disease by the loss of the stimulus to osteoblastic activity associated with gonadal internal secretions. Albright noted beneficial effects from the use of estrogens and androgens to improve the calcium balance and stimulate osteogenesis. During this form of therapy there was a decrease in calcium and phosphorus excretions.

Histologically, the bone changes are those of osteoporotic deossification; no osteoid seams are present as seen in calcium and vitamin D deficiencies. The paucity of osteoblasts and osteoblastic bone apposition is striking.

ANTERIOR LOBE HYPOPITUITARISM

Several distinctly different syndromes have their origin in hypofunction of the anterior lobe of the pituitary gland. Lesions responsible for these syndromes have a wide variety of underlying origins which include tumors, infections, emboli, and hematomata. Replacement of the anterior lobe by dense fibrous scar tissue has been a frequent finding.

PITUITARY INFANTILISM

When the defect of the anterior lobe develops in infancy the so-called Loraine type of dwarf frequently follows (Fig. 293). Bodily features remain childlike, but well-proportioned. Mentality is normal. In addition to hyposecretion of growth-promoting hormone, there is diminution of the gonadotrophic factor to the extent that secondary sex characteristics do not evolve during puberty. Epiphyses ossify late, and epiphyseal plates close late.

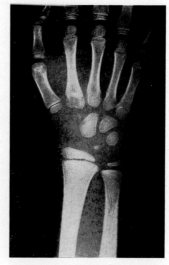

FIGURE 292. Hypothyroidism. Hand of patient age 10 years demonstrating the delay in carpal ossification.

FRÖHLICH SYNDROME (ADIPOSOGENITAL DYSTROPHY)

Fröhlich described a syndrome consisting of preadolescent obesity, retarded growth, and retarded sexual development. The skeleton is underdeveloped, the epiphyses having delayed ossification; this aspect of the syndrome is emphasized when there is an associated hypothyroidism. Obesity is the girdle type and gives the male a female configuration. Terminal phalanges are tapered, and there is dorsal padding of the proximal one-half of the fingers. Fröhlich attributed most cases to anterior lobe tumors.

SIMMONDS SYNDROME (PITUITARY CACHEXIA AND SENILITY)

Simmonds described a rare syndrome, in which destruction of the anterior lobe of the pituitary led to emaciation and premature senility, and in children, it also produced dwarfism (Progeria). Destruction of the anterior lobe is virtually total leading to inadequate secretions of all anterior lobe factors (growth, gonadotrophic, adrenotrophic, and thyrotrophic). Typical cases are manifest by a startling clinical appearance. The childhood form of the disease is associated with skeletal underdevelopment, and in both childhood and adult forms the skeleton undergoes premature senescent changes. The prognosis is poor.

LAURENCE-MOON-BIEDL SYNDROME

In 1886 Laurence and Moon, and in 1922 Biedl, described a very rare syndrome presumably due to a lesion of the anterior lobe of the pituitary.

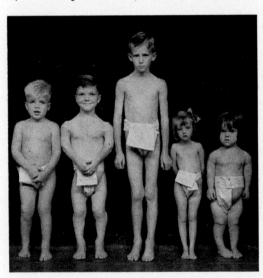

The disease is characterized by adiposogenital dystrophy, polydactylism, retarded skeletal development, pigmented retinitis and mental deficiency. It has a familial character, Laurence and Moon's patients being four brothers and sisters in a family of eight born of normal appearing parents. Biedl's two patients were a brother and a sister.

FIGURE 293. Dwarfism. From left to right: cretin dwarf, achondroplastic dwarf, normal boy for comparison, pituitary dwarf of the Loraine type, and a second achondroplastic.

HYPERTHYROIDISM

Hyperthyroidism can cause the calcium balance to become positive and ultimately lead to pronounced generalized skeletal porosis. Von Recklinghausen in 1891 reported the autopsy findings of a 23 year old female that had died of Basedow's disease (exopthalmic goiter). Large numbers of osteoclasts and generalized osteoporosis were noted and he stated that "all the bones saw like rotten wood, the sternum and calvaria being readily cut with a knife." The osteomalacic skeleton was viewed as secondary to the hyperthyroidism.

Aub and associates reported in 1926 and 1929 that calcium excretion in hyperthyroidism was in direct proportion to the elevation of the basal metabolic rate. A positive calcium balance ceased to exist when the basal metabolic rate returned to normal. A negative balance was observed in myxedema. Normal individuals, administered sufficient thyroxin to elevate their B.M.R., developed a positive calcium balance.

Hunter and others have noted that neither clinically nor experimentally has the hyperthyroid state influenced serum calcium and phosphorus. Slight to moderate elevation of the serum alkaline phosphatase is the rule.

Skeletal deossification may extend over a period of many months or years. Aub and colleagues, in a series of radiograms taken by a uniform technique during a protracted period of hyperthyroidism, recorded the gradually diminishing density of the hand bones.

Plummer and Dunlap studied three cases of generalized skeletal deossification in hyperthyroidism and noted that the most advanced porosis was in the calvarium and ribs. In one of the cases the ribs were so friable that multiple fractures had occurred. These investigators considered the generalized deossification a usual rather than unusual finding. Hunter, on the other hand, detected osseous atrophy in less than half of his cases.

HYPOTHYROIDISM

In infancy and childhood hypothyroidism begets cretinism and in adults, myxedema. Skeletal changes are limited to pre-adolescent thyroid hypofunction.

Cretinism produces dwarfism (Fig. 293). Ossific nuclei appear late in the epiphyses and grow slowly; epiphyseal plates often remain open far into adult life. In most instances the process of enchondral ossification is normal, except for the retardation, and the bones are normal in structure. In a few instances, particularly when other endocrine factors enter the picture, the epiphyses ossify in a bizarre fashion leading to deformations which include irregularities of joint contour.

HYPERGONADISM

Pre-adolescent hypergonadism leads to premature closure of epiphyses. A short, stocky stature results and is characterized by a head and torso that is longer, often by several inches, than the lower extremities. Both the upper and lower extremities appear relatively shortened. Enchondral ossification and bone structure are normal.

HYPOGONADISM

In pre-adolescent hypogonadism (eunuchoidism) the torso-head measurement generally is shorter than the lower extremities, and the span of the upper extremities tends to be greater than the height. In males there are feminine body contours. Secondary sex characteristics are underdeveloped or absent in both sexes.

Hurxal and Hare have summarized the skeletal changes as follows:

1. A tendency to longer bone growth.
2. Delayed epiphyseal closure.
3. Subcalcification.
4. Thinning of cortices.
5. Thin walled, normal sized trabeculation.
6. Roughening of the metaphyseal margin of growing bone.

Post-menopausal osteoporosis is a hypogonadal symptom. The most important single factor in the production of this condition is the loss of the endocrine secretion (estrogen) of the ovaries. Estrogen is, in the female, essential to normal osteogenesis. Osteoblastic activity (osseous anabolism) diminishes in the absence of estrogen, and this factor in the presence of normal osteoclasia (osseous catabolism) creates a negative calcium balance which eventually is manifest as a generalized osteoporosis.

Testes and ovaries have an endocrine function in addition to their reproductive function. The sex hormone produced by the ovaries, the estrogens (theelin, estradial stilbesterol etc.), are created by the preovulation cells of the ovarian follicles. In the male, the sex hormone, the androgens (testosterone compounds), are produced by cells between the seminiferous tubules.

Albright administered estrogens (and androgens) to patients with post-menopausal osteoporosis. Pain (principally spinal) was relieved, the excretions of calcium and phosphorus were diminished, and there was "fairly convincing" evidence by roentgenogram that the bones increased in density. The spine and pelvis regularly show the most advanced porosis.

Senile osteoporosis is undoubtedly caused, in part at least, by the loss of gonadal function. Testosterone and estradiol were used by Reifenstein and Albright for the therapy of a male age seventy-two who has senile osteoporosis. During the therapy there was a dimunition of the calcium and phosphorus excretions that was directly attributable to the steroid hormones administered.

PARATHYROID GLANDS

The generalized fibrous osteitis of hyperparathyroidism was described in Chapter IX.

REFERENCES

ALBRIGHT, F., SMITH, P. H., and RICHARDSON, A. M.: Post-menopausal osteoporosis; its clinical features. *J. A. M. A., 116*:2465, 1941.
ALBRIGHT, F.: Cushing's Syndrome. *The Harvard Lecture Series. 38*:123, 1942-43.
AUB, J. C., HEATH, C. W., and BAUER, W.: Effect of thyroid on calcium metabolism.

Proc. Soc. Exper. Biol. & Med., *23*:699, 1926.

AUB, J. C., BAUER, W., HEATH, C., and ROPES, M.: Studies of calcium and phosphorus metabolism. Effects of thyroid hormone and thyroid disease. *J. Clin. Investigation*, 7:97, 1929.

BIEDL, A.: *Deutsche. Med. Wchnschr.*, *48*:1630, 1922.

BRIGIDI, V. (quoted by Marie): N.iconog. Sal petière. *1*:247, 1888.

CHESTER, W. and CHESTER, E. M.: Vertebral column in acromegaly. *Am. J. Roentgenol. 44*:552, 1940.

CUSHING, H.: The basophil adenomas of the pituitary body and their clinical manifestations (Pituitary basophilism). *Bull. Johns Hopkins Hosp.*, *50*:3, 137, 1932; *J. A. M. A.*, *99*:4, 1932.

CUSHING, H. and DAVIDOFF, L. M.: The pathological findings in four autopsied cases of acromegaly with a discussion of their significance. *Monographs of the Rockefeller Inst. Med. Res.*, No. 22, New York, 1927.

ERDHEIM, J.: Die pathologisch-anatomischen grundlagen der hypophysären Skelettveränderungen. *Fortsch. a. d. Geb. d. Röntgenstrahlen*, *52*:234, 1935.

ERDHEIM, J.: Ueber Wirbelsäulenveränderungen bei Akromegalie. *Virchows Arch. f. path. Anat.*, *281*:197, 1931.

GOLDZIEHER, W. A.: *The Endocrine Glands*. D. Appleton-Century Co., New York, 1939.

HUNTER, W.: A case of acromegaly. Hypertrophy of the pituitary body and thyroid; changes in the bone marrow. *Tr. Path. Soc. London*, *49*:246, 1897.

HUNTER, D.: Calcium and phosphorus metabolism. *Lancet*, *1*:995, 1930.

HURXTHAL, L. M. and HUGH, H. F.: The bone changes in primary hypogonadism. *Radiology*, *32*:521, 1939.

KEITH, A.: An inquiry into the nature of the skeletal changes in acromegaly. *Lancet*, *1*:993, 1911.

KRAUS, E. J.: Morbus Cushing and Basophiles Adenom. *Klin. Wchnschr. 16*:533, 1937; and *13*:487, 1934.

LAURENCE, J. Z. and MOON, R. C.: *Brit. Ophth. Rev.*, 2:32, 1866.

MARIE, P.: Surdeux cas d'acromégalie. *Rev. d. méd., Paris*, *6*:297, 1886.

MARIE, P. and MARINESCO, G.: Sur l'anatomie pathologique de l'acromégalie. *Arch. de Méd. expér et d'anat. path.*, *3*:539, 1891.

PLUMMER, W. A. and DUNLAP, H. F.: Cases showing osteoporosis due to decalcification in exophtholmic goiter. *Proc. Staff Meet., Mayo Clin.*, *3*:119, 1928.

VON RECKLINGHAUSEN, F.: *Die fibröse oder deformirende ostitis, die osteomalacie und die osteoplastische carcinose in ihren gegenseitigen Beziehungen.* Festschrift Rudolf Virchow. George Reimer, Berlin, 1891.

VON RECKLINGHAUSEN, F.: Ueber die acromegalie. *Arch. Path. Anat.*, *119*:36, 1890.

REIFENSTEIN, E. C., JR. and ALBRIGHT, F.: The metabolic effects of the steroid hormones in osteoporosis. *J. Clin. Investigation*, 26:24, 1947.

SUSMAN, W.: Adenoma of the pituitary with special reference to pituitary basophilism of Cushing. *Brit. J. Surg.*, 22:539, 1934-35.

VIRCHOW, K.: Ein Fall und ein Skelet von Akromegalie. *Klin. Wchnschr.*, 26:81, 1889.

WAINE, H., BENNETT, G. A., and BAUER, W.: Acromegaly associated with joint disease. *Am. J. M. Sc.*, *209*:671, 1945.

WERNER, A. A.: *Endocrinology. Clinical Application and Treatment,* 2nd. ed. Lea and Febiger, Philadelphia, 1942.

ZONDEK, H.: *The Diseases of the Endocrine Glands,* 4th ed. Williams and Wilkins Co., Baltimore, 1944.

CHAPTER XIV

Congenitally Defective Skeletal Ossification

Contents

Congenital defects in ossification of the skeleton are said to stem from defective bone cells (osteoblasts and osteoclasts), defective en-

Pattern of Lesions

Wide variation exists in the pattern of the cartilaginous masses. They may be rounded or oval, resembling solitary chondromata, or they may be elongated and appear as streaks or striae in the roentgenogram. In the metaphyses an expansion near the epiphyseal plate, by the cartilage accumulation, often gives an appearance referred to as trumpeting. Widespread elongated expansion of the metaphyses giving a club shaped outline has been observed but is less common in dyschondroplasia than in hereditary multiple exostoses.

There are occasions when a peripheral lesion taken alone might easily be mistaken for an exostosis; when the picture is studied in its entirety, confusion is unlikely.

Lesions in the ilium often present an interesting fan-shaped pattern created by multiple stria of cartilage which are more widely separated at the iliac crest and come to a point toward the acetabulum.

Variation in calcification of the cartilage leads to the various types of stippling and streaks seen in roentgenograms. When no cal-

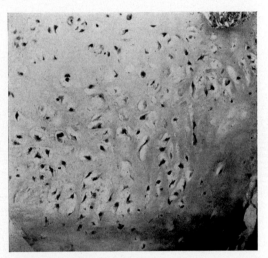

FIGURE 295. Ollier's Disease. Photomicrograph of a field of dysplastic cartilage.

cium exists in a circumscribed mass of cartilage, the appearance in the roentgenogram may be that of a cyst. The error of calling these radiolucent areas "cysts" is not made when the pathology of dyschondroplasia is understood. Sanderson and Smith reported an interesting case of Ollier's disease that had been erroneously diagnosed osteitis fibrosa.

CLINICAL CORRELATION

Dyschondroplasia generally begins in infancy. Most cases are detected in early childhood but in a few instances the disability is minimal and the diagnosis cannot be made until later years.

Disability ordinarily has its origin in the disturbance of length growth in an extremity. Occasionally an epicortical mass leads to disability, particularly when the fingers are involved. Shortening of many centimeters has been observed in extremities. In the lower extremity epiphyseal arrests have been utilized to affect equalization of leg length. When Phemister orginated the important operation of epiphyseal arrest, his first case was that of a girl with Ollier's disease. The end-result was excellent.

HEREDITARY MULTIPLE EXOSTOSES

Synonyms

Multiple exostoses, hereditary multiple cartilaginous exostoses, hereditary deforming chondrodysplasia (Ehrenfried), diaphyseal aclasis (Keith), metaphyseal aclasis (Greig).

Pathologic Anatomy

The two lesions that characterize this entity are multiple exostoses and irregularly expanded metaphyses. Exostoses are always multiple and vary from pointed spike-like processes to broad mushroom shaped tumors. While most exostoses are found to project from metaphyses of the long bones, they generally have their origin at epiphyseal plates.

Exostoses

Exostoses are composed of normal compact and cancellous bone, capped by a zone of hyaline cartilage which forms the enchondral line responsible for the underlying bone. Cortex of the host bone is continuous with the cortical periphery of the exostosis. Larger exostoses have a medullary canal that communicates with the marrow canal of the host bone. As with a solitary osteochondroma, the bone of an exostosis is most dense at the junction with the host bone.

Expansion of Metaphyses

Expansion of metaphyses does not take place in all cases, may involve few or many metaphyses, and is most frequently observed in the tibia, femur, and humerus. An involved metaphysis, in place of tapering at its junction with the diaphysis, is roughly cylindrical shaped. Spike-like exostoses and numerous, excrescences frequently project in an irregular pattern from the metaphysis.

Pathogenesis-Exostoses

Through some mechanism, not yet clearly understood, small fragments of hyaline cartilage, at or adjacent to an epiphyseal plate, grow, develop an enchondral line, and through the process of enchondral ossification form an exostosis. Wide variation exists both in the time during the growing period when the exostoses appear, and in the size attained.

Histologically the enchondral line in and beneath the cartilaginous cap is similar to the normal enchondral line of an epiphyseal plate. A zone of columns generally is discernable, as is a zone of provisory calcification. Growth takes place in the exostosis during the growing period of the host bone. Growth is indicated microscopically by the presence of intratrabecular islands of calcified cartilage. The farther from the enchondral line that such islands can be identified, the more rapid the rate of growth. At the end of the growing period of an exostosis, a lamellar plate of bone forms beneath the cartilage cap and most or all of the overlying cartilage disappears.

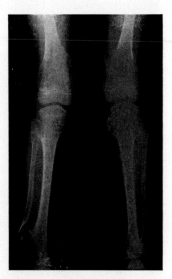

FIGURE 296. Hereditary multiple exostoses of the tibia, fibula, and femur.

Reactivated growth in an exostosis during adult life should arouse suspicion of superimposed malignant changes. Such changes, which occur only rarely, take place in the remains of the cartilaginous cap, giving rise to a chondrosarcoma. Ordinarily, growth of the tumor is slow and pulmonary metastasis, late. The percentage of cases in which chondrosarcoma develops has not been definitely established but the available evidence indicates that it is less than ten percent. A chondrosarcoma developed in three of Jaffe's 28 cases. In Fennel's patient a chondrosarcoma developed in an exostosis of the lower femur that grew rapidly following violent trauma associated with a high fall. The patient was well after a 13 year follow-up of a local excision of the tumor.

Metaphyseal Expansion

The pathogenesis of the irregular widening of the metaphyses is not nearly so well understood as the genesis of exostoses. Keith's theory is the most tenable. He explained the changes on the basis of unrestrained proliferation of the periphery of epiphyseal plates. A defective periosteal ring was given as the basis for the unrestrained cartilage proliferation. Replacement of the peripheral cartilage deposits by bone gives rise to the metaphyseal expansion. As length growth takes place in the bone the expanded area of metaphysis elongates, giving an index to the time of onset of the supposed defect in the epiphyseal plate.

Etiologic Theories

1. Virchow contended that exostoses and excrescences represented independently growing fragments of epiphyseal plate pinched off at the periphery during growth. This theory, long accepted, is now considered untenable by most oncologists.

2. Cartilage islands have been identified subperiosteally in cases of multiple exostoses. Such islands of cartilage have been viewed as the underlying cause of the bone changes that characterize this entity.

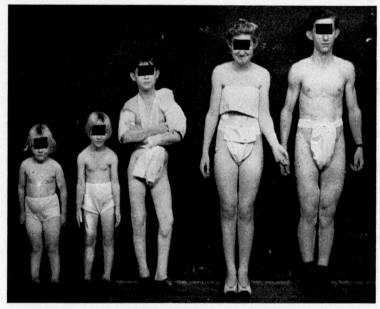

FIGURE 297. Hereditary multiple exostoses. A. Five children of one family all of whom developed multiple exostoses.

There is considerable evidence that subperiosteal foci of cartilage do give rise in some instances to individual exostoses. The origin of the cartilage islands is unknown, but may represent cell rests or direct metaplasia.

3. Keith's theory of a defective periosteal ring around the epiphyseal plate has already been mentioned. The remodelling of the metaphysis is believed to be disturbed by the changes associated with hereditary multiple exostoses. There has been a tendency to explain all of the bone changes by one theory. Jaffe, on the other hand, believes that the lesions are best explained by combining the theory of subperiosteal cartilage islands with the Keith theory of a defective periosteal sleeve.

Hereditary Factor

Stocks and Barrington reviewed 1,124 cases of multiple exostoses and found that there was a hereditary factor in 64 percent. Transmission by the father occurred in 73 percent and by the mother in 27 percent. In general, when a parent had extensive lesions, the children inheriting the disease also developed lesions. Typical lesions have been traced through as many as five generations. The hereditary factor is tremendously important, both in the etiology and in differential diagnosis. Heredity, however, does not play a significant part in either solitary exostoses or dyschondroplasia.

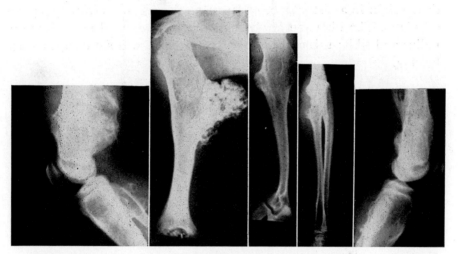

FIGURE 297 Continued. B. Roentgenograms of several extremities of the children in Figure 297A.

ROENTGENOGRAPHIC CORRELATION

Roentgenograms should be taken of the spine, pelvis, and all extremities whenever multiple exostoses are identified or suspected. In many instances the lesions can be detected in the roentgenograms when clinical evidence is lacking.

During growth, the cap of an exostosis is poorly defined; whereas, at the completion of growth a thin, well-outlined cortex demarcates the entire lesion. The bone beneath the cartilage cap resembles articular cortex in that it is composed in maturity of a continuous plate of lamellar bone. Reactivation of growth in an exostosis during adult life on the basis of a chondrosarcoma soon destroys the definition of the crown of the lesion.

In their lateral roentgenograms, exostoses are well visualized and dimensions clearly reflected. In their antero-posterior views, the exostoses often appear as round radiolucent lesions resembling (only in this one view) an enchondroma or bone cyst. The relative osteoporosis at the site of the lesion, in this view, deserves explanation. Since the cap of the exostosis is cartilage and the bone beneath the cap is porotic, there is no bone of density comparable to that of the metaphysis (or diaphysis) from which the exostosis projects.

Exostoses of long bones tend to deviate toward the center of the diaphysis of the host bone. This is the result of compression by overlying soft tissues during growth of the host bone and the exostoses.

Deformities are frequent in hereditary multiple exostoses and have their origin in a disturbance of enchondral ossification in the epiphyseal plates. The ulna and fibula generally are shortened more than the radius and tibia; this condition creates radial and tibial compensatory bowing.

CLINICAL CORRELATION

Exostoses are painless unless they impinge upon a sensitive structure. Occasionally a muscle or a fascial surface, by gliding over an exostosis during joint motions, creates an adventitious bursa. Such a bursa may become inflamed and painful.

Diagnosis

Most cases have been diagnosed in childhood, although in a few instances the lesions have not been detected until adulthood. No clinical evidence of the lesions exists at birth. Males predominate; in the cases reported, the incidence of males has been more than two times that of females. While long bones are the dominant sites, characteristic lesions may be found in the pelvis, vertebrae, ribs, scapulae, phalanges, and those bones of the skull formed by enchondral ossification. Lesions tend to be bilateral, symmetrical, and to grow most extensively at the sites of the most rapid metaphyseo-epiphyseal growth.

Exostoses are excised only if they become symptomatic, impinge on a vital structure, cause serious cosmetic distortion, or begin to grow during adult life. To prevent recurrences following excision of an exostosis, it is important to remove both the cap and the periosteum covering the exostosis.

LIPOCHONDRODYSTROPHY
SYNONYMS

Gargoylism, Hurler-Pfaundler syndrome, and dysostosis multiplex (Engle).

Lipochondrodystrophy is a rare disease of congenital origin characterized by defective lipoid metabolism, multiple skeletal system deformities, and corneal clouding.

SKELETAL SYSTEM

The skull is enlarged in circumference but not in thickness. Prominent frontal bones, a depressed nasal bridge, and widely spaced orbits give the face a gargoyle-like appearance. Retarded mentality, defective teeth and thick tongue frequently contribute to the facies of this syndrome.

A dorso-lumbar kyphosis or gibbus is a consistent feature and is the result of anterior wedging of the vertebral bodies at this junction (Fig. 298). All joints show somewhat limited mobility and the short thick hands frequently have flexion contractures of the fingers. The long bones have thickened diaphyses and in some instances, fragmented epiphyses.

Other Characteristics: Both the liver and the spleen are generally enlarged and lipoid laden cells

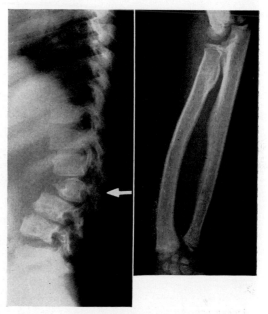

FIGURE 298. Lipochondrodystrophy. Roentgenograms of the spine and an upper extremity of a male age 16. (Children's Hospital, Los Angeles.)

have been noted in the lymph nodes, pituitary gland (anterior lobe), the brain, and the corneas. Diffuse clouding of the cornea is a prominent feature and is present in no other of the cranial dysostoses. Many of the reported cases have also developed inguinal or umbilical hernias.

Etiology: The etiology is unknown. A defective germ plasm is surmised.

ACHONDROPLASIA

(Chondrodystrophia foetalis)

This, the most profound of the disturbances of enchondral ossification, is characterized by the dwarfism accruing from poorly proliferating enchondral lines. Nothing is known of the etiology. There has been a definite hereditary factor in numerous reported cases, the disease being transmitted either by the father or the mother. Sexes and races are equally divided.

The disease is characterized by retarded enchondral ossification, not a complete loss of growth as the term achondroplasia implies. Parrot in 1878 coined the name achondroplasia and it is still in general use. Kaufmann's term, chondrodystrophia foetalis has not been widely adopted.

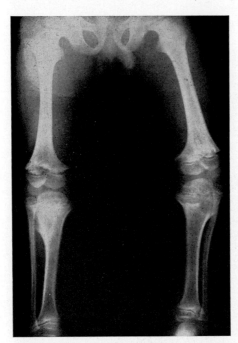

FIGURE 299. Achondroplasia. The lower extremities of the achondroplastic boy shown in Figure 293.

PATHOLOGIC ANATOMY

The description of the pathologic changes will be divided on an anatomical basis into: (a) Epiphyseal plates, (b) Periosteum, and, (c) Skull.

Epiphyseal Plates

A discussion of the histopathology and pathogenesis of achondroplasia centers principally around the epiphyseal plates. All growth centers are affected in one degree or another, varying from near-complete aplasia to merely a substantial retardation of normal enchondral ossification. In the former, profound dwarfism is the outcome; in the latter, a shortened stature.

In a typical case, the epiphyseal plates present outstanding histologic evidence of their disturbance. Whereas a normal epiphyseal plate is flat or slightly dome shaped, with an even contour, the achondroplastic epiphyseal plate is crenated and even jagged in outline. Microscopically the plates reveal none of the orderliness of the normal plate. In place of a zone of columns there is only an irregular, purposeless distribution of the chondrocytes. The zone of calcified cartilage likewise presents an irregular and often incomplete line at the metaphyseal junction. In place of a row of projecting bars of calcified cartilage matrix there are scattered small excrescences or pinched off islands. Intratrabecular islands of calcified cartilage, the index of the rate of growth, do not appear beyond a point closely adjacent to the epiphyseal plate. In less severe cases there may be scattered areas in which a zone of columns can be detected, as well as a semblance of order in the zone of provisory calcification.

The key to the epiphyseal plate disturbance appears rather definitely to reside in the zone of mother cells, also known as the zone of proliferation, where the chondrocytes required for a continuous cartilage replacement process (enchondral ossification) are created. Nothing in the histological study suggests an explanation for the failure of chondrocytic proliferation. Even those chondrocytes that are delivered to the zone of calcified cartilage are abnormal, and are unprepared to receive the cells from the metaphyseal marrow spaces in the process of building new bony trabeculae.

When growth ceases, the epiphyseal plate may disappear or it may remain in place in a totally inactive state far into adult life. No explanation for this variation can be offered. On the metaphyseal side of the epiphyseal plates, there may be pronounced vascularity and an associated osteoporosis; or there may be few blood vessels and osteosclerosis.

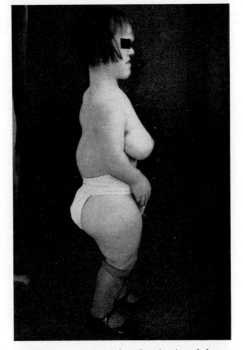

FIGURE 300. An achondroplastic adult.

Periosteum

The periosteum is normal in achondroplasia, as are the osteoblasts and osteoclasts. Whatever length of shaft the epiphyseal plates succeed in building, the periosteal bone apposition can be depended upon to construct a heavy diaphysis. Cortical walls tend to be thick and broad, although instances of osteoporosis have been reported. Likewise, the mechanism through which metaphyses are reconstructed to diaphyses during growth is quite normal. Histologic studies disclose nothing abnormal in either the periosteum or the diaphyses.

Skull

Important changes take place in the achondroplastic skull, changes that are sharply reflected by the gross appearance and at times by clinical symptoms. Narrowing and shortening of the base of the skull, so characteristic of achondroplastics, is caused by ossification and fusion

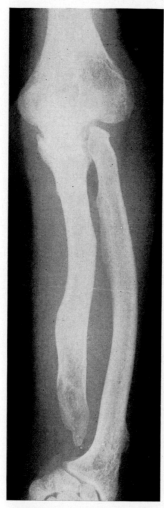

of the sphenoid and occipital bones (Fig. 300). This process normally occurs in early adult life, but in achondroplasia it often occurs during intrauterine life or in infancy. Premature ossification and fusion take place in all four of the bones that make up the foramen magnum. It has been claimed that in many of the achondroplastics that die before birth or during infancy a compression of the medulla oblongata by a stenosed foramen magnum may have been contributory.

Virtually all achondroplastics have a slight degree of hydrocephalus, and this is a factor in the actual and relative enlargement of the head.

Roentgenologic Correlation

The shortened diaphyses and large epiphyses of long bones have a striking roentgenographic appearance (Fig. 299). Epiphyses are considerably expanded and flared beyond normal dimensions. Centers of ossification may appear many years prematurely or be long delayed. In the same manner the epiphyseal plates may remain open to middle age, or close in early childhood.

Vertebrae develop bizarre patterns of ossification and very often become wedge-shaped anteriorly in the dorsal and upper lumbar areas. Wedged vertebrae account

FIGURE 301. Roentgenogram of a forearm of an achondroplastic adult.

for the characteristic dorsal and dorso-lumbar kyphosis. A dorso-lumbar gibbus is not unusual. Ribs tend to be broad and to flare anteriorly. Acetabulae often ossify improperly leading to shallowness. Bowing of the long bodies is common.

Clinical Correlation

The achondroplastic dwarf is a most striking figure. Having normal intelligence and a genial nature he usually gets along well in the world. Several important figures in history and mythology have been achondroplastics. In centuries past they were particularly adept at serving as court jesters.

Their abbreviated stature is made all the more conspicuous by a

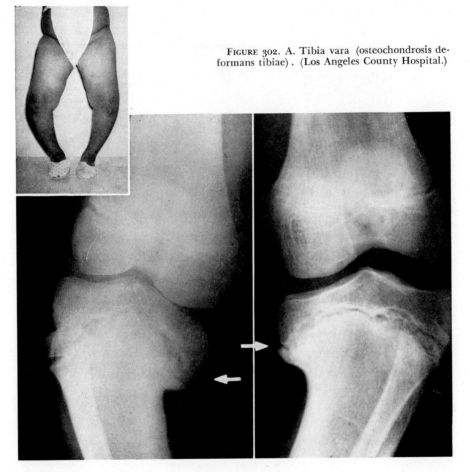

FIGURE 302. A. Tibia vara (osteochondrosis deformans tibiae). (Los Angeles County Hospital.)

large head with frontal bossing, pug nose, prognathism, and stubby fingers, arms and legs. Although normal in appearance at birth, the characteristic changes become evident within a few months.

OSTEOCHONDROSIS DEFORMANS TIBIAE
(Tibia vara)

Osteochondrosis deformans tibiae, a name suggested by Blount, is an osteochondrosis of the medial aspect of the proximal tibial epiphysis. This localized disturbance of enchondral ossification leads to tibial bowing referred to as tibia vara (Fig. 302).

Two forms of the disease are described, an infantile form and an adolescent form. Only the infantile or congenital form can be viewed as a congenital defect in enchondral ossification.

In 1937, Blount reported 13 new cases and reviewed the 15 cases in the literature. He stated that, "The appearance is strikingly that of a

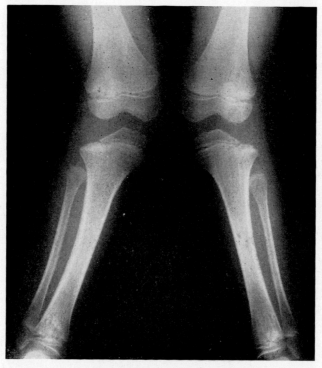

FIGURE 302. *(Continued)* B. Tibia valga. (Los Angeles Children's Hospital.)

localized chondrodysplasia." Histological studies of material from the site of the lesion showed an irregular alignment of chondrocytes in the epiphyseal plate and no zone of orderly columns. Islands of cartilage were found in the metaphysis.

Growth of the medial aspect of the upper tibia is retarded, leading gradually to a medial deviation of the tibial diaphysis. Clinically the disturbance is reflected by bowing of one or both legs, similar to the bow of rickets. Osteochondrosis deformans tibiae must, of course, be differentiated from rickets. An osteotomy of the tibia frequently is necessary to correct the malignment, but will be followed by recurrence of the deformity if done prior to cessation of growth in the epiphyseal plate.

Twenty of the 28 cases reviewed by Blount were the infantile form; 18 were females, two were males and in one the sex was not stated.

MADELUNG'S DEFORMITY

Madelung's deformity represents a dyschondroplasia of the medial aspect of the distal radial epiphysis (Fig. 303). This localized defect in enchondral ossification usually begins early in childhood and appears to be similar to osteochondrosis deformans tibiae except for the difference in location.

Premature fusion takes place in the medial half of the distal radial epiphyseal plate. The ulnar deviation of the hand and the prominence of the distal end of the ulna have their origin in the retarded growth in the medial aspect of the distal radial epiphyseal plate. Dannenberg, Anton, and Spiegel urge that the name Madelung's deformity be replaced by the term dyschondroplasia of the distal radial epiphysis.

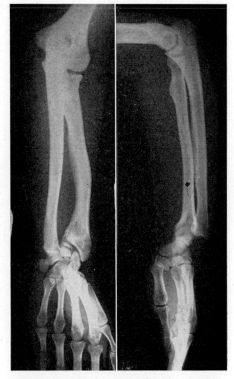

FIGURE 303. Madelung's deformity (dyschondroplasia of the medial aspect of the distal radial epiphysis).

MORQUIO'S DISEASE
(Chondro-osteodystrophy)

In 1929 Morquio described a familial form of generalized chondo-osteodystrophy. This rare entity is characterized by a bizarre congenital disorder of skeletal ossification. Certain parts of the skeletal system became more involved than others, the spine being a center of maximum involvement. A subnormal intellect has been a frequent finding.

HEREDITARY FACTOR

Morquio reported four cases, and all were from the same family, a family of five. Jacobsen discovered 20 cases in five generations of the same family. The frequent familial distribution of the cases is a prominent feature of the disease.

Skeletal Changes

Little evidence of the disorder exists until the child begins to walk, at which time a dorso-lumbar kyphosis or gibbus develops (Fig. 304). The kyphosis, which frequently is severe, is the response to defective vertebral body ossification manifest by anterior wedging, a biconvex shape, and an anterior exostosis-like prominence. Maximum anterior wedging generally centers in the vicinity of the dorso-lumbar junction. A short neck supports a misshapen head and both rest on a pigeon breast. Fragmentation and distorted retarded ossification lead to short extremities and enlarged joints. Generalized ligamentous relaxation is in part responsible for the genu valgum, pes planus, and coxa vara. Generalized deossification has been described, as has failure of many epiphyses to ossify.

Russo reported the case of a 26 year old negro girl who was 36″ tall, weighed 58 pounds, and was seven months pregnant. A stillborn, showing no signs of Morquio's disease, was delivered by Cesarean section. All of the vertebral bodies of Russo's patient were flat and tongue shaped.

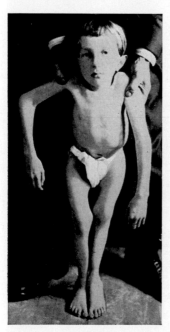

FIGURE 304A. Morquio's disease of a child.

Pathology

Little is known of the pathology; there have been no autopsy reports and very few biopsies. Shelling examined biopsies from three different sites in the lower end of the femur. The biopsy from the shaft disclosed normal bone, but the epiphyseal sections showed an irregular, defective line of enchondral ossification. Metaphyseal bony trabeculae were porotic and many contained cartilaginous islands.

Clinical Correlation

Morquio's disease is rare but probably not so rare as the few cases in the literature (approximately 50) indicate. The deformities are not associated with pain or muscle spasm and this helps differentiate the spine lesions from tuberculous spondylitis. A few cases have been misdiagnosed as rickets.

DYSOSTOSIS CLEIDOCRANIALIS

In 1897 Marie and Sainton described a rare syndrome, characterized by incomplete ossification of the clavicles and part of the membrane bones of the skull; they named it dysostosis cleidocranialis.

The defect in clavicular ossification varies from a narrow transverse zone in the middle one-third which resembles a pseudoarthrosis (Fig.

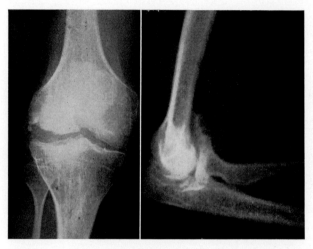

FIGURE 304B. Morquio's disease of an adult. Roentgenograms of the knee and elbow.

305), to a total failure of ossification. The non-ossified portion of the clavicle is a fibrous cord.

Although the sites at which ossification fails to take place are principally in membranous bone, there have been cases in which sites of enchondral ossification have been defective. The ends of the clavicles form by enchondral ossification, so in those instances when the failure of ossification is complete the enchondral zones obviously are affected. Other anomalies, such as finger defects, have been noted. Incomplete ossification of the vault of the skull leads to broadening of the head. Delayed closure of the fontanelles is the rule.

Sites of defective ossification are readily visualized roentgenographically. Clinically, there is the striking feature in many instances of the patient's being able to bring his shoulders together in front of his chest. The reported cases indicate that there has often been an hereditary factor, the condition being transmitted by either the father or mother to either sons or daughters (Fitchet). Sexes are equally divided.

OSTEOPOIKILOSIS

(Osteopathia condensans disseminata)

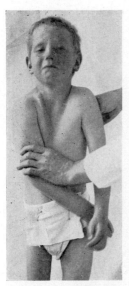

Osteopoikilosis was first described in 1915 by Albers-Schönberg, the same investigator that in 1904 described osteopetrosis. It is a pathologic and radiologic entity characterized by multiple round or oval islands of compact or dense cancellous bone, measuring one-sixteenth to one-fourth inch in diameter and located principally in the pelvis and extremity bones (Fig. 306). Most of these dense bony islands are concentrated near the ends of the bones. Their histological character was described by Schmorl who found them to represent small foci of normal bone set apart and identified by their having greater density than adjacent areas of the host bone. No such bony islands have been seen in the vertebrae or the skull.

Voorhoeve has described osseous condensations in the form of short striae or rods which run in the longitudinal axis near the ends of long bones, and in the pelvis.

FIGURE 305. Dysostosis cleidocranialis. A. Photo of patient.

Osteopoikilosis, rounded or striated, is not associated with symptoms and has no clinical significance.

OSTEOGENESIS IMPERFECTA

(Fragilitas ossium, Brittle bones, Idiopathic Osteopsathyrosis)

Osteogenesis imperfecta was identified as a separate entity by Vrolik in 1849. Previous to that time it was often described with the chondrodystrophies. The etiology is unknown, but there is a strong hereditary factor. Fifteen percent or more of the cases have a family history of the condition. Many cases have occurred in the same family and cases have continued to appear for three and four generations.

Bickel, Ghormley and Camp reviewed 40 Mayo Clinic cases and found 27.5 percent to be hereditary, the other 72.5 percent having no known family history of the syndrome. Blue sclerotics were consistently associated with the hereditary type but not with the non-hereditary type. The underlying cause of the blue coloration of the sclerae is not known; histologically the blue sclerae appear normal.

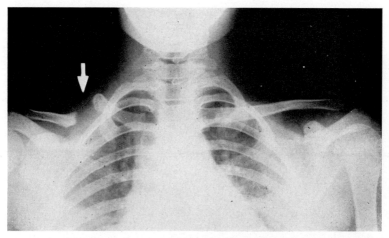

FIGURE 305. *(Continued)* B. Roentgenogram to demonstrate the defect in the right clavicle (arrow).

As the name implies, osteogenesis imperfecta is characterized by defective skeletal ossification. Knaggs has explained the failure of ossification on the basis of defective evolution of the osteoblasts. This explanation has a sound foundation in the histological findings.

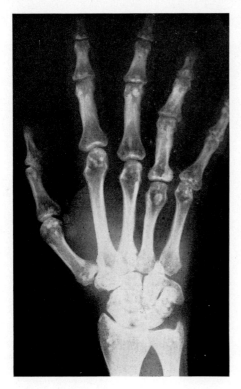

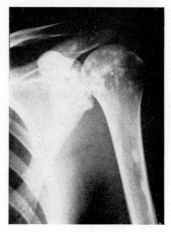

FIGURE 306. Osteopoikilosis. A. *(Left)* Wrist and hand. B. *(Right)* Humerus and scapula.

The term osteogenesis imperfecta is now made to include all types of the disease. Such terms as osteopsathyrosis and fragilitas ossium are no longer widely used.

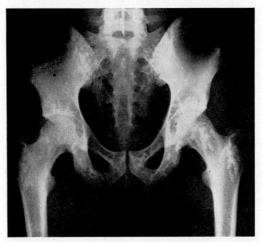

FIGURE 306 Continued. C. Pelvis and femora.

CLINICAL TYPES

Osteogenesis imperfecta has been observed in all age groups but is much more common in infancy and childhood. Four clinical types are recognized: (1) foetal, (2) infantile, (3) childhood and adolescence, and (4) adult.

Foetal Type

If not stillborn they rarely survive more than a few hours. This is the most extreme type that exists and is characterized by great numbers of fractures and deformities. At birth the skull is usually collapsed for it possesses little ossification. Knaggs described such a skull as a "membranous bag." The passage of the foetus through the parturient canal is sufficient trauma to crush the fragile skeleton.

Infantile Type

This type represents a less extreme degree of skeletal deficiency. These cases usually live for several months. During this time they sustain innumerable fractures from even the mildest trauma.

Childhood and Adolescent Type

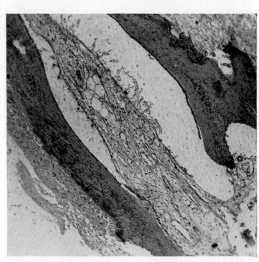

FIGURE 307. Osteogenesis imperfecta. Photomicrograph of trabeculae in a specimen removed during an osteotomy.

This type is frequently referred to as osteogenesis imperfecta tarda (Fig. 308). Ossification of the skeleton at birth is far more substantial than in the foetal and infantile types; in fact, some of these patients pass through an uneventful infancy and early childhood, before beginning their career of fractures. Even though there may be few or no fractures in infancy there is delayed closure of the anterior fontanelle. If adolescence is survived, and it frequently is, these patients sustain few fractures as adult life advances.

Adult Type

Although rare, cases have been described as occurring even in the aged, and there have been instances where the patient appeared to recover from the condition in infancy only to develop skeletal fragility again in adult life.

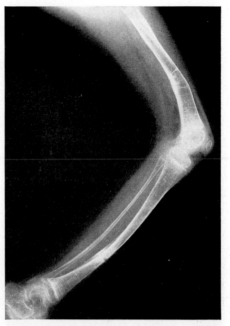

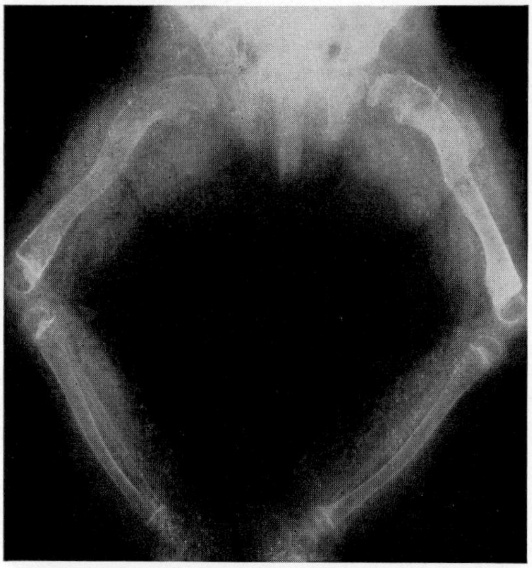

FIGURE 308. Osteogenesis imperfecta. Multiple transverse arrest lines are mementos of the many fractures incurred through infancy and childhood.

FIGURE 309. Osteogenesis imperfecta. Lower extremities after healing of multiple fractures. (Childrens Hospital, Los Angeles.)

PATHOLOGY

As previously stated, the skeletal fragility that characterizes this condition appears to be the result of a defect in the development of osteoblasts. The defect appears early in embryonic life and probably occurs in the mesoblast itself.

Enchondral ossification proceeds normally except during the last stage. The zone of provisional calcification forms in a normal orderly manner. Chondrocytes are released into the metaphyseal marrow, and the calcified matrical bars project into the metaphysis. It is from this point on that the process becomes pathologic. The projecting bars of calcified cartilage await the arrival of a row of osteoblasts to begin the formation of an osteoid trabeculum; few osteoblasts arrive. In less severe cases a fair number of osteoblasts align themselves on the surface of the calcified cartilage, but they appear to be relatively impotent as far as bone formation is concerned. Some of the calcified cartilage is said to form bone trabeculae by direct metaplasia.

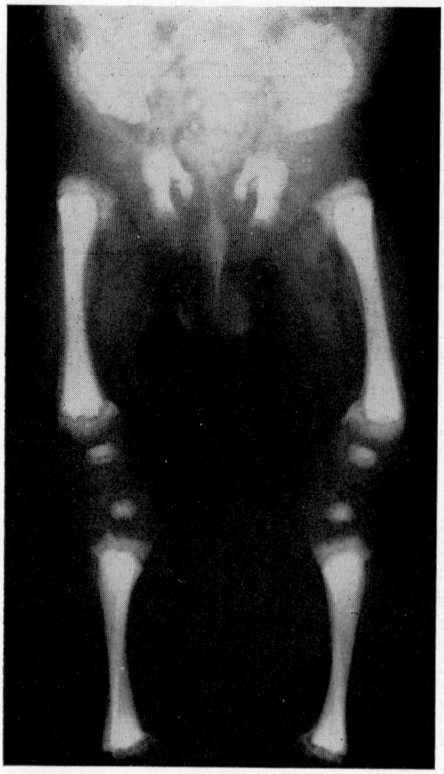

FIGURE 311. Osteopetrosis in a new-born.

Periosteal bone formation is also impaired, and this too is caused by the paucity of osteoblasts. The fibrous layer of the periosteum is somewhat thickened, but the cambium layer is thin and is less cellular than normal. Klotz describes having seen cartilage cells subperiosteally. It is his opinion that their presence represented a reversion of the periosteum to its foetal role as a perichondrium.

In the skull, ossification is widely variable. It may be impaired only to the extent of a delayed anterior fontanelle closure, or so extremely that there are only scattered small foci of ossification. Thus we see that, regardless of the type of ossification, it is defective.

Fractures

Most of the fractures are of the crumpling type and do not often perforate the periosteum. Compression fractures are also common. In contrast to the fractures in scurvy, which are usually metaphyseal, osteogenesis imperfecta fractures are most often diaphyseal. Non-union occurs but is not the rule. Callus, often abundant, may be meager in severe cases. Fractures generally lead to extremity shortening, and angulation deformities are very common. Looser's zones of transformation no doubt account for part of the fractures and bending deformities.

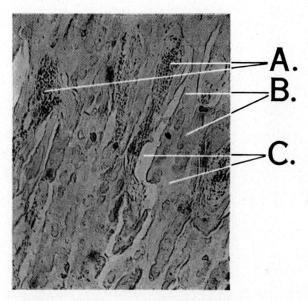

FIGURE 310. Osteopetrosis (marble bones). Photomicrograph demonstrating the persisting elongated bars of calcified cartilage matrix (C). Bone (B) borders the cartilage matrix. The narrowed marrow spaces (A) contain hematogenous marrow.

OSTEOPETROSIS

(Alber-Schönberg's Disease, Marble bones, Congenital Osteosclerosis)

Osteopetrosis, a rare disease manifest in the skeleton, was first described by Albers-Schönberg in 1904. The widely used term, osteopetrosis, was suggested by Karshner in 1926. There has been a hereditary factor in many of the reported cases; Pirie reported four cases from the same family—a mother and her three children. Involved bones present a striking x-ray appearance principally because of the profound increase in density from increased calcium content.

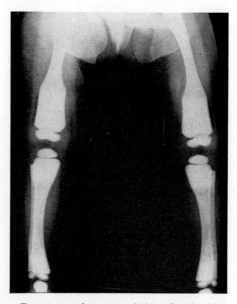

Although the etiology of osteopetrosis is unknown, the condition appears to represent a defect in bone formation, presumably congenital.

Clinically the disease is characterized by a number of symptoms, almost all of which are attributable to the skeletal alterations. Optic atrophy, nystagmus, and blindness develop when the optic foramen becomes narrowed during the skull changes. Hydrocephalus has occurred in several instances. Pressure on the pituitary gland may give rise to thyropituitary symptoms. Secondary anemia

FIGURE 312. Osteopetrosis in a female child age two. This patient became blind during early infancy, and expired following an increasing secondary anemia at age four.

often results from medullary canal stenosis or obliteration. Enlargement of the spleen and liver and impaired dentition have been reported. Pathologic fractures are frequent, and often represent the symptom that leads to a diagnosis of the disease. Fractures heal and the callus that forms generally possess the same increased density and character as the bone fractured.

The skeletal changes may involve part of the bones or the entire skeleton. Bones formed on the basis of membranous ossification are involved as frequently as bones formed by enchondral ossification. The process may begin during foetal life or at any time during the growing period; occasionally a case is first diagnosed in adult life, but presumably the disease has existed since the growing period.

PATHOGENESIS

It has been repeatedly noted that the process begins in the metaphysis at the enchondral line. Enchondral ossification proceeds normally to the point of osteoid apposition on the projecting bars of calcified cartilage matrix. Because of the paucity of osteoblasts, only a thin

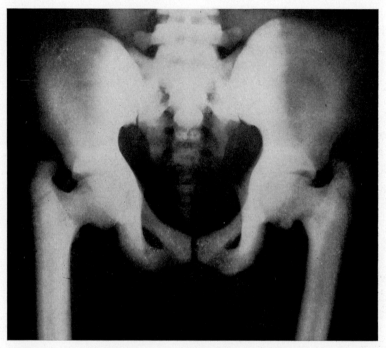

FIGURE 313. Osteopetrosis in a 24 year old male. No symptoms; the disease was detected on a routine pre-employment chest film. (Courtesy, Douglas Aircraft Co.)

layer of osteoid is applied. The zone of provisional calcification continues to proliferate thus producing long, heavy bars of calcified cartilage matrix. Instead of the calcified ground substance absorbing as it normally should, it persists, and it is the persisting concentration of calcified matrical substance that is responsible for the striking clinical, roentgenological, and pathological characteristics of osteopetrosis. As would be expected, the bone cuts like chalk and breaks transversely like chalk; this led Pirie to suggest that the name chalk bones replace the inaccurate term, marble bones. The osteoid which is applied to the surface of the long calcified bars of cartilage matrix may calcify, but it rarely attains the laminated orderly internal architecture of normal mature bone (Fig. 310).

Another important characteristic of this remarkable entity is the narrowing of the medullary canal in involved portions of tubular bones. Since enchondral ossification is interrupted in its last step, the stimulus or capacity of the bone to proceed with the formation of a medullary canal and cortex, is lacking. If the process begins in foetal life, the entire skeleton may be involved. The hematopoetic system in such cases is profoundly disturbed because of medullary canal obliteration. Death has occurred in several of the reported cases from the associated secondary anemia. If osteopetrosis begins in infancy or childhood, the prognosis is not so bad, since the diaphyses formed at the time the disease actively begins are never extensively involved. The portion of the bone that forms by growth after the disease becomes established bears the major portion of the alteration. This is logical in view of the origin of the changes at the enchondral line. The same characteristic apparently applies equally to the membranous bones. However, in the several post-mortem examinations that have been made it was noted that parts of the skeleton which appeared normal grossly and roentgenographically showed, in a small degree, the microscopic changes characteristic of the grossly involved portions. To be more specific, the entire skeleton

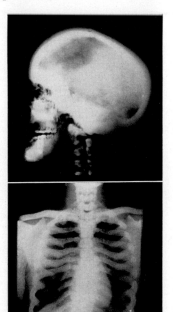

FIGURE 314. Osteopetrosis in a 20 year old male.

showed at least some evidence of persisting intratrabecular islands of calcified cartilage. This presumably means that all cases begin during intra-uterine life, but some become fully developed early, and others later.

Enchondral ossification within epiphyses proper and in the short bones does not form long projecting bars of calcified matrical substance. Instead, the calcified matrix forms a hemo-genous mass through which great numbers of small irregular marrow canals may be seen communicating and interconnecting. These marrow spaces are bordered by osteoid which later calcifies to form bone. The picture is that of an ever-widening zone of provisional calcification. Growth in osteopetrosis is achieved virtually by widening of the zone of calcified cartilage.

Clubbing occurs at the ends of long bones, the upper tibia and lower femur in particular (Fig. 312). This characteristic alteration, which develops at sites of most rapid growth, is explained on this basis: with interruption of normal bone formation, the remodelling and narrowing of the diaphyseal-metaphyseal junction cannot take place. In normal long bones during normal growth, the broad metaphyseal regions gradually narrow with formation of thickened cortices and a medullary canal where the metaphysis joins the diaphysis. In osteopetrosis the persistence of the metaphyseal width as growth continues eventually gives the bone ends a club, or pestle, shape, the area actually representing an elongated metaphysis. In an involved area one may observe, roentgenographically, a few or many narrow transverse lines of decreased density. These transverse lines appear to represent periods of variation in activity of the etiological factor, whatever that factor may be.

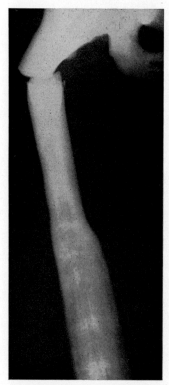

FIGURE 315. Osteopetrosis in an 18 year old girl who had had eight fractures. A fracture in the lower 1/3 of the femur is healed; the upper 1/3 fracture is recent.

Periosteal bone formation in osteopetrosis may be stimulated once the disease is actively established. The shafts widen principally from calcified cartilage deposited by a periosteum reverting to its embyronal state as a perichondrium.

Skull

Skull changes are conspicuous (Fig. 314) and frequently are the source of alarming clinical symptoms. Foramina giving passage to cranial nerves may stenose and cause pressure on the nerves. Blindness has occurred in several cases from pressure on the optic nerve as it passed through the optic foramen. Pressure on the pituitary gland from hypertrophy of the sella turcia has produced hypopituitary symptoms.

ETIOLOGIC THEORIES

Pirie, after observing five cases, believed the disease represented a chronic infection. There is little proof to support this theory. Other investigators have suggested that there is a disturbance of calcium metabolism similar to that existing in osteomalacia and rickets. Several German observers reported hypercalcemia, but this has not been observed by American investigators. Perhaps the most logical explanation is simply to consider the condition a genital defect in evolution of chondroclasts and osteoblasts. New bone does not form properly and adequately, and the calcified matricial substance is not properly absorbed.

PLATYSPONDYLIA

A generalized flattening of the vertebral bodies, a condition of congenital origin, is referred to as generalized platyspondylia. While it may be associated with other congenital abnormalities it often occurs alone. A shortened trunk in these cases is a manifestation of actual narrowing of the superior inferior diameter of the vertebral bodies. A hereditary factor is common.

There has been disagreement as to whether platyspondylia represents a type of chondro-osseous dysplasia or a congenital anomaly. Nové-Josserand and Pouzet reported a case of platyspondylia associated with bilateral congenital coxa vara. They believe that this is evidence that the disorder represents a congenital anomaly.

ATELEIOTIC DWARFS

Ateliotic dwarfs are people in minature. Their proportions are normal, they have no known endocrine disturbance, have a normal sella turcica, and normal intelligence. There is an important hereditary factor. Families of these midgets are known to exist, and some of the children are normal. Brailsford had the opportunity of taking roentgenograms of several ateliotic dwarfs and found that the epiphyses unite much later than normally. In one instance lines of epiphyseal plates were still well defined at the age of 38. A fine stippling was seen in x-rays of the phalanges in place of the normal trabecular pattern. No histological studies could be found in the literature, but the condition appears to represent a generalized congenital retardation of both enchondral and intramembranous ossification.

ARACKNODACTLY
(Spider hands and feet)

Aracknodactly is characterized by long slender bones, particularly the metacarpals, metatarsals and phalanges. The very long tapered fingers prompted the name "spider hands." A generalized muscle weakness and ligamentous relaxation lead to hypermobility of all joints, and frequently to dislocations. The aracknodactylic individual has a pinched appearance from a paucity of subcutaneous fat.

A familial and hereditary factor is present in 30 percent of the cases (Baer); 60 percent of the cases are in females. A congenital heart disease is a frequent associated finding. Phalanges may be porotic. Aracknodactly represents a congenital defect in skeletal development but nothing is known of the etiology.

ACROCEPHALOSYNDACTYLISM
(Apert Syndrome)

Apert in 1906 gave a classical description of the entity he termed acrocephalosydactylism. It is a rare entity characterized by a long head pointed at the top, and by partial or complete syndactylism. A comprehensive report of this subject was made by Park and Powers in 1930.

REFERENCES

BAER, R. W.: Aracknodactly in *Brennemann's Practice of Pediatrics*. Vol. IV, Chap. 26. W. F. Prior, Inc., 1945.

BRAILSFORD, J. F.: *Radiology of Bones and Joints*. Wm. Wood and Co., Baltimore, 1935.

NOVE-JOSSERAND, G. and POUZET: Forme spéciale de coxa-vara congénitale avec platyspondylie. *Lyon Chir., 31:*469, 1934.

PARK, E. A. and POWERS, G. F.: Acrocephalosyndactylism. *Am. J. Dis. Child., 20:*235, 1920.

HEREDITARY MULTIPLE EXOSTOSES

BENNETT, G. E. and BERNHEIMER, G. A.: Malignant degeneration in a case of multiple benign exostoses. *Surgery, 10:*781, 1941.

FENNEL, E. A.: Osteogenic sarcoma from exostosis. *Am. J. Surg., 39:*121, 1938.

JAFFE, H. L.: Hereditary multiple exostoses. *Arch. Path., 36:*335, 1943.

KEITH, A.: Studies on the anatomical changes which accompany certain growth-disorders of the human body. *J. Anat., 54:*101, 1920.

MILLER, E.: Uber hereditare multiple cartilagmare exostosen und ecchondrosen. *Beitr. z. Path. Anat. u. z. allg. Path., 57:*232, 1913-14.

STOCKS, P. and BARRINGTON, A.: Hereditary disorders of bone development. University of London. Francis Galton Laboratory for National Eugenics. *Eugenics Laboratory Memoir, 22,* 1925.

DYSCHONDROPLASIA

CLEVELAND, M.: Chondrodysplasia. *Surg., Gynec. & Obst., 47:*338, 1928.

DANNENBERG, J. T., ANTON, J. I., and SPIEGEL, M. D.: Madelung's deformity. *Am. J. Roentgenol., 42:*671, 1939.

EHRENFRIED, A.: Hereditary deforming chondrodysplasia. Multiple cartilaginous exostoses. *J. A. M. A., 68:*502, 1917.

FAIRBANK, H. A. T.: Generalized diseases of the skeleton. *Proc. Roy. Soc. Med., 28:* 1611, 1935.

HUNTER, D. and WILES, P.: Dyschondroplasia (Ollier's disease). *Brit. J. Surg., 22:*507, 1934-35.

KEITH, SIR A.: The nature of the structural alteration in the disorder known as multiple exostoses. *J. Anat., 54:*101, 1920.

MAHORNER, H. P.: Dyschondroplasia. *J. Pediat., 10:*1, 1937.

OLLIER, M.: De la dyschondroplasie. *Bull. Soc. de Chir. de Lyon., 3*:22, 1899-1900.
PHEMISTER, D. B.: Operative arrestment of longitudinal growth of bones in the treatment of deformities. *J. Bone & Joint Surg., 15*:1, 1933.
SANDERSON, G. H. and SMITH, F. S.: Chondrodysplasia (Ollier's disease). *J. Bone & Joint Surg., 20*:61, 1938.
SLOANE, D., SLOANE, M. F., and GOLD, A. M.: Dyschondroplastic bow legs. *J. Bone & Joint Surg., 18*:183, 1936.

LIPOCHONDRODYSTROPHY

ENGLE, D.: Dysostosis multiplex; Pfaundler-Hurler syndrome; report of 2 cases. *Arch. Dis. Child., 14*:217, 1939.
HARVEY, R. M.: Hurler-Pfaundler syndrome (Gargoylism). *Am. J. Roentgenol., 48*:732, 1942.
HEMHOLZ, H. F. and HARRINGTON, E. R.: Syndrome characterized by congenital clouding of the cornea and other anomalies. *Am. J. Dis. Child., 41*:793, 1931.
HURLER, G.: Ueber einen Typ multiplex Arbartungen, vorwiegend am skelettsystem. *Ztschr. f. Kinderh., 24*:220, 1920.

ACHONDROPLISIA

JONES, HUGHES, E. W. A.: Studies in achondroplasia. *J. Anat., 66*:565, 1932.
KAUFMANN, E.: *Chondrodystrophia foetalis, Untersuchungen über die sogenannte foetale Rachitis.* Berlin, 1882.
LANDANER, W. and DUNN, L. C.: *J. Genetics, 23*:397, 1930.
McCALLUM, W. G.: *Bull. Johns Hopkins Hosp., 26*:182, 1915.
PAROTT, J.: *Bull. Soc. d'antrop. de Paris, 1*:296, 1878.
SHELLING, D. H.: Achondroplasia in *Brennemann's Practice of Pediatrics.* Vol. IV, Chap. 28. W. F. Prior, Inc., 1945.

OSTEOCHONDROSIS DEFORMANS TIBIAE

BARBER, C. G.: Osteochondrosis deformans tibiae. *Am. J. Roentgenol., 42*:498, 1939.
BLOUNT, W. P.: Tibia vara; osteochondrosis deformans tibiae. *J. Bone & Joint Surg., 19*:1, 1937.
SLOANE, D., SLOANE, M. F., and GOLD, A. M.: Dyschondroplastic bow legs. *J. Bone & Joint Surg., 18*:183, 1936.

CHONDRO-OSTEODYSTROPHY

BRAILSFORD, J. F.: Chondro-osteodystrophy. Roentgenographic and clinical features of child with dislocation of vertebrae. *Am. J. Surg., 7*:404, 1929.
JACOBSEN, A. W.: Hereditary osteochondro dystrophia Deformans. Family with twenty members affected in five generations. *J. A. M. A., 113*:121, 1939.
MEYER, H. F. and BRENNEMANN, J.: A rare and osseous dystrophy (Morquio). *Am. J. Dis. Child., 43*:123, 1932.
MORQUIO, L.: Sur une forme de dystrophie osseouse familiale. *Arch. de méd. d. enf., 32*:129, 1929.
POHL, J. F.: Chondro-osteodystrophy (Morquio's disease). *J. Bone & Joint Surg., 12*:187, 1939.
RUGGLES, H. E.: Dwarfism due to disordered epiphyseal development. *Am. J. Roentgenol., 25*:91, 1931.
RUSSO, P. E.: Chondro-osteodystrophy; Morquio's disease: Case observed during pregnancy. *Radiology, 41*:42, 1943.

DYSOSTOSIS CLEIDOCRANIALIS

CYRIAX, E. F.: A case of cleido-cranial dysostosis. *Edinburgh Med. J., 30*:600, 1923.
FITCHET, S. M.: Cleidocranial dysostosis: Hereditary and familial. *J. Bone & Joint Surg., 11*:838, 1929.

MARIE, P. and SAINTON, P.: Observation d' Hydrocéphalie hereditaire. (pére at fils) par Vice de Développement du Crane et due cervean. *Bull et mém. Soc. Méd. d. Hóp de Paris, 14*:706, 1897; *15*:436, 1898.

MOREIRA, G.: Cleidocranial dysostosis as hereditary disease. *Brazil-med., 41*:273, 1927.

OSTEOPOIKILOSIS

ALBERS-SCHONBERG, H.: Eine seltene bisher nicht bekannte structuranomalie des skelettes. *Fortschr. a. d. Geb. d. Röntgenstrahlen, 23*:174, 1915.

VOORHOEVE, N.: L'image radiologique non encore décrite d'une anomalie du squelette. *Acta. radiol., 3*:407, 1924.

OSTEOGENESIS IMPERFECTA

BRAILSFORD, J. F.: Osteogenesis imperfecta. *Brit. J. Radiol., 16*:129, 1943.

KNAGGS, R .L.: Osteogenesis imperfecta. *Brit. J. Surg., 11*:737, 1924.

LOVETT, R. W. and NICHOLS, E. H.: Osteogenesis imperfecta; with report of a case, with autopsy and histological examination. *Brit. M. J., 2*:915, 1906.

RIESEMAN, F. R. and YATER, W. M.: Osteogenesis imperfecta. Its incidence and manifestations in seven families. *Arch. Int. Med., 67*:950, 1941.

VROLIK: Tabul. ad. illust. embryo-genesin hominis et mammalium. Tab. 91, Amsterdam, 1845.

WEBER, M.: Osteogenesis imperfecta congenita: Study of its histopathogenesis. *Arch. Path., 9*:984, 1930.

OSTEOPETROSIS

ALBERS-SCHONBERG, H.: Röntgenbilder einer seltenen Knockenerkrankung. Munchen Med. Wchnschr., *51*:365, 1904. *Fortschr. a. d. Geb. d. Röntgenstrahlen, 11*:261, 1907.

CLIFTON, W. M., FRANK, A., and FREEMAN, S.: Osteopetrosis (Marble bones). *Am. J. Dis. Child., 56*:1020, 1938.

KARSHNER, R. G.: Osteopetrosis. *Am. J. Roentgenol. 16*:405, 1926.

KERR, H. D.: A case of osteopetrosis complicated by osteogenic sarcoma. *Am. J. Roentgenol., 35*:212, 1936.

PIRIE, A. H.: The development of marble bones. *Am. J. Roentgenol., 24*:147, 1930.

POUNDERS, C.: Congenital osteosclerosis (marble bone). *Am. Int. Med., 8*:966, 1935.

CHAPTER XV

Extraskeletal Calcification and Ossification

Contents

It is necessary to distinguish extra-skeletal calcification from extra-skeletal ossification. While the distinction is not always possible clinically, it can be made both roentgenographically and pathologically. However, the two processes, calcification and ossification, are not necessarily independent since, in many instances, the deposition of calcium salts precedes the formation of bone.

Foci of extraskeletal calcification and ossification generally develop at sites of soft tissue degeneration and necrosis; exceptions are calcinosis universalis and myocitis ossificans progressiva in which calcification and ossification occur in apparently normal tissues.

EXTRASKELETAL CALCIFICATION

Many theories have been formulated to explain the deposition of calcium salts in foci of soft tissue necrosis. It has been suggested that necrotic tissues liberate fatty substances which combine with calcium salts to form calcium soaps. Calcium salts enter the necrotic areas from the blood stream by osmosis, the attraction presumably being an alkaline reaction of the necrotic tissue. When an alkaline reaction develops in such organs as the kidneys and lungs, widespread calcium deposits may result without the presence of necrosis.

A discussion of phosphatase and the part it plays in the calcification process was presented in Chapter I. Calcification in the kidney and urinary bladder is associated with increased phosphatase activity, but there is no proof that phosphatase is an important factor when calcium salts are deposited in many of the necrotic soft tissues.

Asami and Dock ligated the renal artery and vein of the kidney in rabbits and observed that bone and calcium deposition took place independently in different parts of the kidney. Bone formation was most active adjacent to the epithelium of the renal pelvis.

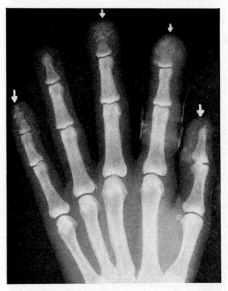

Huggins, in experiments with dogs, found that bone forms when specimens of bladder, ureter, and renal pelvis epithelium, are transplanted to fascia lata, the rectus abdominis muscle sheath, or to subcutaneous tissue. He also observed bone formation in fascia transplanted to the bladder of the dog provided the urine was diverted following the transplant.

FIGURE 316. Calcinosis circumscripta (so-called "calcium gout").

CALCINOSIS

Calcinosis, a rare entity first described by Weber in 1878, is characterized by calcium plaques and nodules in the skin and subcutaneous tissue. Verse and Brooks divided the cases into two types, which they termed *calcinosis circumscripta* and *calcinosis universalis*.

Calcinosis Circumscripta

This, the benign form, occurs principally in adult women. The calcium deposits are generally limited to the skin and subcutaneous tissues of the fingers (Fig. 316). While the deposits may involve entire fingers and other areas in the extremities, they are ordinarily confined to the tissues overlying the terminal phalanges. A superficial resemblance to the tophi of gout is responsible for the term calcium gout or kalkgicht of German authors. Actually there is no known relation between calcinosis and gout.

Calcinosis circumscripta frequently is associated with *scleroderma* and *Raynaud's disease*. Trophic changes created in the extremities by these diseases unquestionably play an important part in creating extraskeletal calcium deposits.

In the roentgenogram the deposits of calcium are seen as multiple, closely approximated nodules. Plaques, spikes, and streaks are exceptional.

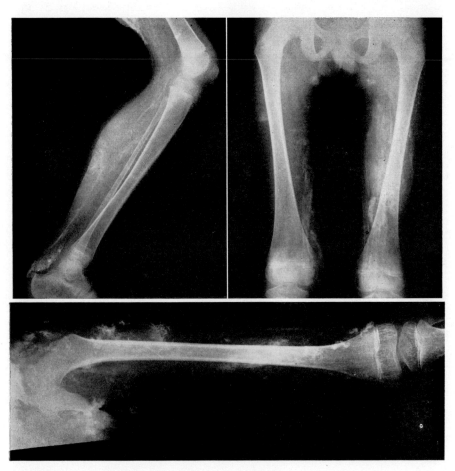

FIGURE 317. Calcinosis

Calcinosis Universalis

Generalized calcinosis is a rare disease characterized by numerous widespread calcium deposits which in addition to involving skin and subcutaneous tissues may involve fascias and muscle sheaths. The disease is manifest principally in the extremities and buttocks, but trunk and head lesions are not unusual.

Calcinosis universalis is a disease of children. When the calcium deposition is extensive, invalidism and death may occur. The etiology is unknown, and there is no known form of effective therapy.

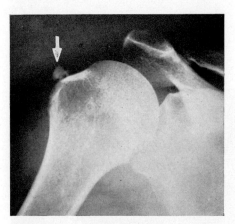

FIGURE 318. Calcareous tendinitis. Deposition of calcium in the supraspinatus tendon.

Wilens and Derby reported a case of calcinosis universalis in 1926. Their patient was a boy whose symptoms began between the ages of two and three years. Multiple superficial tender swellings gradually developed in all extremities and the buttocks. The swellings represented calcium deposits, which became visible at several points when the overlying skin ulcerated.

Bauer, Marble, and Bennett studied this same case and reported their findings in 1931. They found normal blood calcium and phosphorus but at the same time noted a pronounced capacity for retaining absorbed calcium and phosphorus. Histological studies of early lesions revealed finely divided calcium granules deposited at the periphery of normal-appearing fat cells. Later, with an increased deposition of calcium, the fat cells became filled and obscured by the calcium. Fibrous encapsulation of the calcium nodules and plaques gradually took place. Numerous foreign body giant cells were clustered around the calcium masses. No degeneration, necrosis, inflammation, or hemorrhage was observed that could have served as a basis for the calcification. Indeed, nothing in the histologic picture reflected etiologic factors. Presumably the disease represents a disturbance of calcium and phosphorus metabolism.

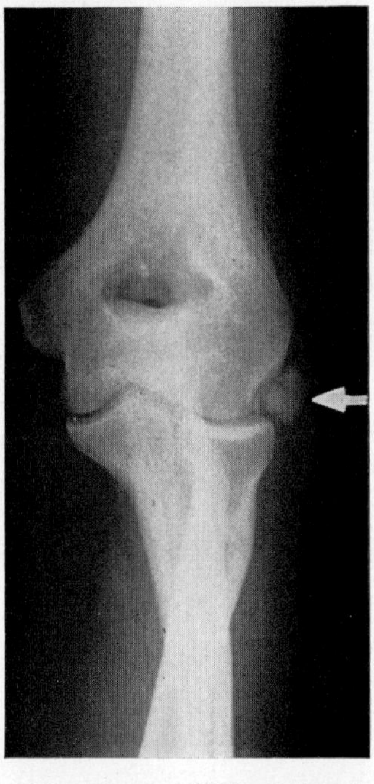

CALCAREOUS TENDINITIS

FIGURE 319. Calcium deposit in the radio-capitellar joint capsule and overlying structures.

Calcium deposits occur at sites of degeneration or necrosis in the following sites: the supraspinatus tendon (Fig. 318), the flexor carpi ulnaris, the tendons attaching to the greater trochanter of the femur, the tendons adjacent to the metacarpo-phalangeal joints (Cooper), and around the radio-capitellar joint (Fig. 319). Amorphous calcium carbonate and calcium phosphate are deposited, usually in a circumscribed small quantity, at the site of degeneration or frank necrosis in the tendon substance. The calcium deposit, which long exhibits a paste-like consistency, is, in time, either spontaneously absorbed or solidified to stone-like density.

The best known and most common location of calcifying tendinitis is in the supraspinatus tendon. In gliding beneath the acromion and over the humeral head this tendon is subjected to considerable pressure

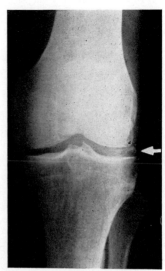

FIGURE 320. Calcification of the lateral meniscus.

and friction. These forces create areas of degeneration and necrosis in the tendon, and, once the calcium is deposited, accentuate the pain by further compressing the already tense and painful focus of calcification. Occasionally the calcium is extruded from the tendon over the floor of the subdeltoid bursa. Pain is relieved once the tense calcium deposit is released through rupture, or perforation by a needle or scalpel.

CALCIFICATION OF MENISCI

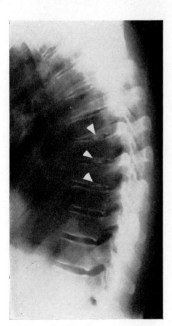

Calcification of menisci is rare, but is believed to take place at sites of degeneration and necrosis (Fig. 320). The entire meniscus may be outlined by the rim of calcium salts. Watson-Jones has described a case in which ossification followed meniscus calcification. Menisci and intervertebral discs are extraosseous, but not extraskeletal. Calcification of these structures is discussed here for convenience.

CALCIFICATION OF INTERVERTEBRAL DISCS

FIGURE 321. Calcification of intervertebral discs.

Calcification of intertebral discs, a rare finding, first described by Calve and Galland, may involve the nucleus pulposis, the annulus fibrosis, or both (Fig. 321). Transformation to bone is said not to occur.

CALCIFICATION ASSOCIATED WITH TOXIC DOSES OF VITAMIN D

There have been instances in which the administration of massive doses of vitamin D have produced foci of degeneration and calcification at widespread points in blood vessels, muscles, skin, and subcutaneous tissue (Fig. 322). Generalized mobilization of skeletal minerals takes

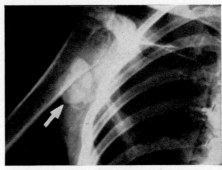
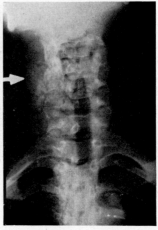

FIGURE 322. Metastatic calcification associated with hypervitaminosis D. A. *(Left)* Axillary calcium deposit. B. *(Right)* Deposit of calcium in the neck.

place simultaneously, and during the resulting excretion of large quantities of calcium in the urine, calcium deposits frequently appear in both the parenchyma and pelvis of the kidneys. The picture is similar to that seen in some cases of hyperparathyroidism.

CALCIFICATION OF CHRONIC GRANULOMATOUS ABSCESSES

A tuberculous abscess is a familiar site of calcification (Fig. 275). During the healing stage a massive calcium deposition may completely replace the contents of the abscess.

CALCIFICATION OF SOFT TISSUE TUMORS

Fibromata and hemangiomata (Fig. 323) are the tumors that most frequently exhibit calcium deposits. In fibromata the calcium is laid down at sites of degeneration and necrosis. In hemangiomata the calcium is laid down within organized thrombi formed in tumor vessels. Phleboliths form in the same manner. Calcification of patent arteriosclerotic vessels is confined to the vessel walls, whereas calcification within most thrombosed vessels is limited to the thrombus.

EXTRASKELETAL OSSIFICATION
(Heterotopic bone formation)

Myocitis ossificans, the most spectacular of the several types of heteotopic bone formation, exists in two strikingly different forms, known as myocitis ossificans progressiva and myocitis ossificans circumscripta.

Myocitis Ossificans Progressiva

The progressive form of myocitis ossificans, a rare disease first described by Patin in 1692, begins during the first decade of life and may spread until most of the skeletal muscles have been replaced by bone. The incidence in boys has been slightly greater than in girls, and nearly all reported cases have been in Caucasians. No prominent hereditary factor has been noted. Nothing is known of the etiology although trauma is believed to be an aggravating factor.

A curious characteristic of the disease is its frequent association with congenital deformities of the fingers and toes, principally the thumbs and first toes. Microdactyly and brachydactyly reflect the defective metatarsals or metacarpals, and abbreviated fused

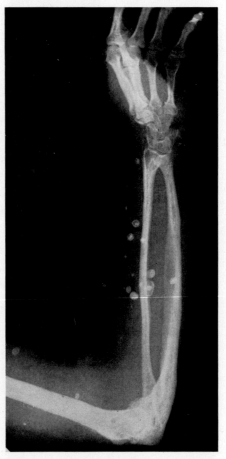

FIGURE 323. Calcium deposits in an extensive hemangioma.

phalanges. Defective stature and sex differentiation have not been unusual.

In most of the reported cases the paraspinal muscles have been the first involved. Muscles of the thighs, scapulae and arms have also had a high incidence of early involvement. Pain and swelling develop over the sites of ossification during early stages. In advanced stages bony bridges often extend between the humerus and scapula, and between

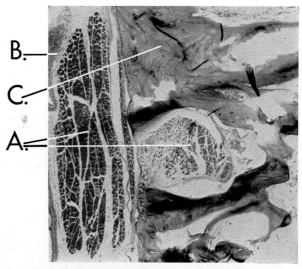

FIGURE 324. Myocitis ossificans, late stage. A. Muscle. B. Lamellated bone.

the scapula and ribs. Ossification may extend to overlying fascia, to tendons, and to ligaments. In only one known instance, a case reported by Rosenstirn, has there been ossification of subcutaneous tissue.

Pathologic Anatomy

Grossly, small and large masses of bone replace areas of skeletal

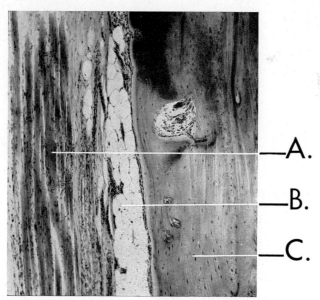

FIGURE 325. Compact bone in a section of myocitis ossificans. A. Muscle fibers. B. Zone of fat and cellular fibrous tissue. C. Compact bone.

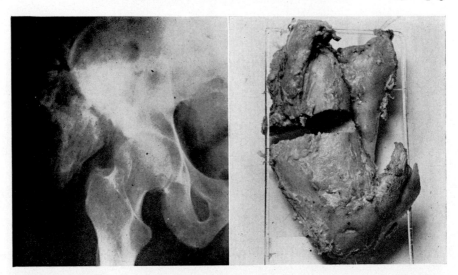

FIGURE 326. Massive myocitis ossificans in the right gluteal muscle of a 48 year old male. A. *(Left)* Roentgenogram. B. *(Right)* Surgical specimen, removed one year following a fall on the right hip.

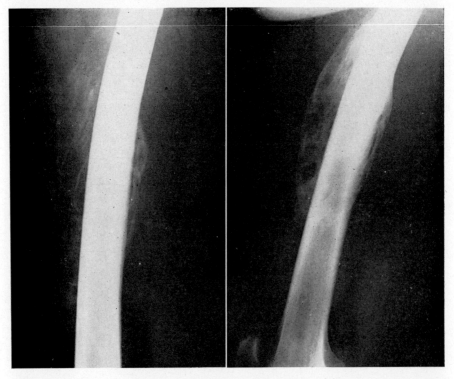

FIGURE 327. Myocitis ossificans, following a "charley horse" of the right thigh incurred in college football. A. *(Left)* Six weeks following injury. B. *(Right)* Twelve weeks following injury.

muscles. A stage of calcium deposition does not precede the formation
of bone. At the outset the bone is fibrous in character and is relatively

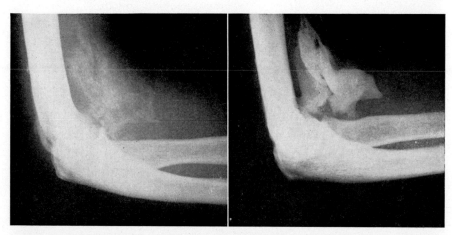

FIGURE 328. Anticubital myocitis ossificans complicating a dislocation of the elbow in a
24 year old male. The elbow dislocation, which resulted from a fall on the outstretched
hands, was reduced 30 minutes after the injury. A. *(Left)* Six weeks after the injury. The
elbow was passively stretched daily during the first two weeks post-injury. B. *(Right)*
Five months post-injury.

soft. Fibrous bone is gradually replaced by mature lamellar cancellous
and compact bone.

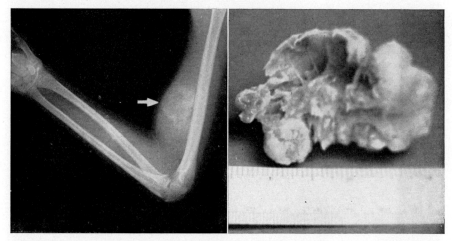

FIGURE 329. Myocitis ossificans of the anterior arm muscles. A. *(Left)* Roentgenogram.
B. *(Right)* Surgical specimen.

Histologic studies disclose the interesting fact that the formation of
new bone takes place in fibrous connective tissue elements in the muscles and not in the muscle fibers themselves. Fibroblastic proliferation

in the fibrous tissue strands and the sheets within and around the muscle is followed by ossification.

Muscle fibers at sites of ossification undergo atrophy and fibrous tissue replacement. There is no metaplasia of muscle to bone. Grieg has suggested that the entity be renamed fibrositis ossificans progressiva.

Treatment: No therapy yet employed has proved of lasting benefit. A recurrence of the bone formations has regularly taken place after masses of bone have been excised. Waiting until the bone is mature, as is practiced successfully with traumatic myocitis ossificans, has not prevented recurrence of the ossification.

Diagnosis: Once the disease is well established the diagnosis is obvious.

Traumatic Myocitis Ossificans

(Myocitis ossifications circumscripta)

Traumatic, or circumscribed, myocitis ossificans, a relatively common entity, is characterized by the ossification of organized traumatic hematomata in and adjacent to skeletal muscles. The muscles most frequently involved

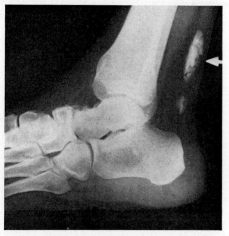

FIGURE 330. Heterotopic ossification of the tendo-Achilles. Male age 50 who had had two operations on the tendo-Achilles during childhood.

are the quadriceps femoris and the brachialis anticus. Ossification in the quadriceps generally follows a heavy blow to the anterior aspect of the thigh ("charleyhorse" of football players) (Fig. 327); ossification in the brachialis anticus is usually a complication of posterior dislocation of the elbow joint (Fig. 328).

Pathogenesis

While the injury and the hematoma may be limited to a muscle, it is the rule that adjacent periosteum is also traumatized. Organization of a muscle hematoma close to a bone appears to mobilize calcium from the bone, a condition which favors calcification and ossification. In the young fibrous tissue of the organized hematoma, fibrous bone trabeculae take shape and join together to form primitive cancellous bone. At this stage the bone is poorly calcified and presents no sharp line of demarcation either grossly or roentgenographically. As the bone matures it is transformed to mature lamellar bone, becomes smooth in outline, and increasingly dense (Figs. 324 & 325). Occasionally the mass of fibrous bone is absorbed and not replaced by lamellar bone. A small or extensive attachment, fibrous or bony, to the adjacent skeletal bone is almost invariable.

Fields of cartilage often appear in areas of myocitis ossificans during the early immature stage. Ossification of the cartilage takes place by direct metaplasia or by a primitive form of enchondral ossification.

As Watson-Jones and Roberts have pointed out, ossification of subperiosteal hematomata and of partially or completely avulsed tendons, aponeuroses and ligaments should not be classified as myocitis ossificans.

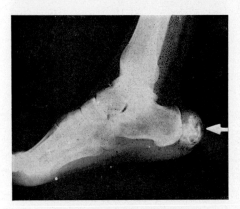

FIGURE 331. Heterotopic bone formed posterior to the tuber os calcis.

Differential Diagnosis

During its period of evolution, myocitis ossificans circumscripta may resemble an osteogenic sarcoma. In myocitis ossificans there are no destructive changes in the adjacent portion of the skeleton. During a period of observation the immature myocitic bone tends to become somewhat smaller and more clearly outlined. An advancing osteogenic sarcoma steadily enlarges and possesses a poorly defined margin.

Treatment

The early aspiration of muscle hematomata will often prevent myocitic ossification. The early reduction of dislocations and fractures, and the repair of avulsed periosteum, tendons and ligaments also tends to reduce heterotopic ossification.

In many instances the bony mass limits the mobility of the host muscle, and when located in a muscle overlying a joint such as the brachialis anticus, the mass may act as a mechanical block to joint motion. In these instances an excision of the heterotopic bone is indicated. But it is mandatory to defer the operation until the heterotopic bone is "mature," as indicated by the presence of a sharp and smooth outline.

PELLIGRINI-STIEDAS DISEASE

This disease, described by Pelligrini in 1905 and Stieda in 1908, is characterized by a circumscribed deposit of calcium or bone directly over or just below the adductor tubercle of the femur (Fig. 322).

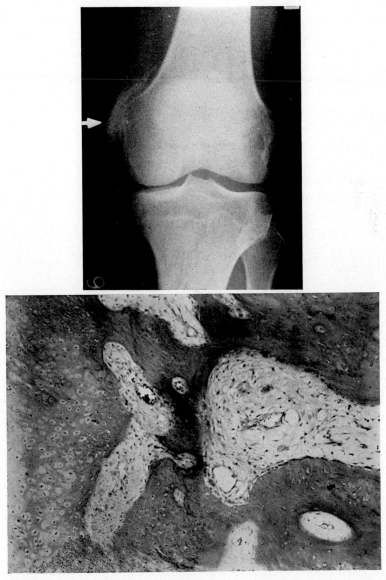

FIGURE 332. Pelligrini-Stieda's disease. A. *(Above)* Roentgenogram right knee. B. *(Below)* Photomicrograph showing cartilage and bone elements in the tissue overlying the adductor tubercle (arrow).

Etiology

Just as in myocitis ossificans, there are factors in the etiology that remain to be clarified. There is also uncertainty in many cases regarding the exact location of the mass or nodule. Traumatic factors are considered to be the most important, and include avulsion of a small fragment of bone or periosteum from the adductor tubercle, contusions to the adductor tubercle, sprain of the proximal end of the tibio-collateral ligament, and injuries to a bursa overlying the tubercle. Nachlas and Olpp contend that none of these are the etiologic factors. It is their opinion that the traumatic factor is represented by friction between the tubercle and a "membrane" which moves over the tubercle during knee joint motions. The membrane, according to their dissections, lies beneath the fascia and envelops the entire medial femoral condyle area. An area of degeneration or necrosis is said to be the response to trauma and the basis for the calcification and subsequent ossification. Pelligrini, Kulowski, and Finder conclude that the lesion is in the tibio-collateral ligament, and is the response to a sprain that avulses fibers of the ligament and periosteum. Considerable evidence is at hand to indicate that the lesion can develop both in relation to the ligament and independent of the ligament.

Pathogenesis

The conclusion is warranted that traumatic degeneration and necrosis represent the initial lesion, wherever its location. Calcification takes place and the calcium deposit may long remain unchanged. In most instances, however, the deposit is invaded by blood vessels and the lesion ossified. Ossification occurs first in the core of the lesion and spreads to the periphery which is generally composed of hyalin and fibrocartilage.

The calcified mass may be from one to many centimeters in diameter. While a small disc-shaped lesion is most common, numerous cases have been reported in which the mass of bone or calcium measured many centimeters across. A narrow space usually separates the lesion from the adductor tubercle. This is particularly true of the smaller lesions; large masses frequently fuse to the medial condyle of the femur.

During its evolution the lesion may contain little calcium and have a poorly defined margin. When the lesion becomes mature and stabilized, it is more dense and is sharply circumscribed. In this latter state it may remain for many years and cause no significant disability.

OSSIFICATION OF THE TENDO-ACHILLES

True heterotopic ossification of a tendon is rare. Whereas tendon calcification is most often observed in the supraspinatus, tendon ossication is most common in the tendo-Achilles.

In most known cases, a tendo-Achilles tenotomy has preceded the ossification by a period of many years (Fig. 330). Only seldom has the ossification been associated with disabling pain.

Deposits of amorphous calcium have not been observed in the Achilles tendon. This is difficult to explain. Presumably a sub-clinical calcium deposit precedes the formation of the osseous mass.

REFERENCES

ASAMI, G. and DOCK, W.: Experimental studies on heteroplastic bone formation. *J. Exper. Med., 32*:745, 1920.

BAUER, W., MARBLE, A., and BENNETT, G. A.: Further studies in a case of calcification of subcutaneous tissue (calcinosis universalis) in a child. *Am. J. M. Sc., 182*:237, 1931.

BROOKS, W. D. W.: Calcinosis. *Quart. J. Med., 3*:293, 1934.

COOPER, W.: Calcareous tendinitis in the metacarpophalangeal region. *J. Bone & Joint Surg., 24*:114, 1942.

FINDER, J. G.: Calcification of the tibial collateral ligament. *J. A. M. A., 102*:1373, 1933.

GRIEG, D. M.: *The Pathology of Bone.* Edinburgh, 1931.

HUGGINS, C. B.: Experimental osteogenesis. *Proc. Soc. Exper. Biol. & Med., 27*:349, 1930.

HUGGINS, C. B.: The formation of bone under the influence of epithelium of the urinary tract. *Arch. Surg., 22*:377, 1931.

KULOWSKI, J.: Post-traumatic para-articular ossification of the knee joint. *Am. J. Roentgenol., 47*:392, 1942.

MATHER, J. H.: Progressive myocitis ossificans. *Brit. J. Radiol., 4*:207, 1931.

MULLIGAN, R. M.: Metastatic Calcification. *Arch. Path., 43*:177, 1947.

NACHLAS, I. W. and OLPP, J. L.: Para-articular calcification (Pelligrini-Stieda) in affections of the knee. *Surg. Gynec. & Obst., 18*:206, 1945.

PELLIGRINI, A.: Traumatic calcification of the collateral tibial ligament of the left knee joint. *Clin. Med., 2*:433, 1905.

PHEMISTER, D. B.: Ossification in kidney stones attached to the renal pelvis. *Am. J. Surg., 78*:239, 1923.

ROSENSTIRN, J.: Contribution to the study of myocitis ossificans. *Am. J. Surg., 68*:485, 1918.

STIEDA, A.: Ueber eive typische Verletzungam unteren Femurende. *Arch. f. klin. Chir., 85*:815 1908.

VERSE, M.: Ueber calcinosis universalis. *Beitr. z. path. Anat. u.z. allg. Path., 53*:212, 1912.

WATSON-JONES, R. and ROBERTS, R. E.: Calcification, decalcification and ossification. *Brit. J. Surg., 21*:461, 1934.

WEBER, H.: *Korresp. Bl. f. Schw Aerzte.* Basel, *8*:623, 1878.

WILENS, G. and DERBY, J.: Calcification of subcutaneous tissue in a child. *Am. J. Dis. Child., 31*:34, 1926.

CHAPTER XVI

Osseous Lesions in the
Reticulo-Endothelioses

Contents

In this discussion of the reticulo-endothelial hyperplasias, both the granulomatous and lipoid storage lesions will be included. The fact that the etiology is unknown and that our concept of this group of entities is unsettled and constantly changing, scarcely needs to be mentioned. With so many unanswered questions surrounding this subject it is difficult to present a satisfactory classification; however the following tentative classification is suggested:

RETICULO-ENDOTHELIOSES

A. Classification based upon distribution of lesions
  I. Reticulo-endothelioses localized to bones
    1. Eosinophilic granuloma
    2. Solitary xanthoma

II. Generalized reticulo-endothelioses
   1. Hand-Christian's disease
   2. Letterer-Siwe's disease
   3. Gaucher's disease
   4. Nieman-Pick's disease

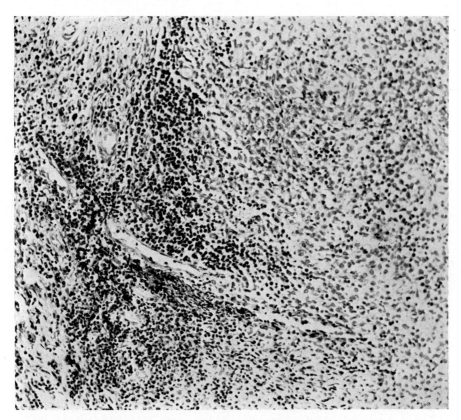

FIGURE 333. Eosinophilic granuloma. Cells with dark staining nuclei are principally eosinophils; most of the pale staining cells are histiocytes. (Courtesy, A. Purdy Stout, M.D.)

B. Classification based upon the lipoid factor
  I. Non-lipoid (granulomatous) reticulo-endothelioses
    1. Eosinophilic granuloma
    2. Hand-Christian's disease
    3. Letter-Siwe's disease
  II. Primary lipoidoses (Lipoid storage)
    1. Gaucher's disease
    2. Nieman-Pick's disease
    3. Solitary xanthoma

EOSINOPHILIC GRANULOMA

In 1929, Finzi reported a case of localized reticulo-endotheliosis which he termed "myeloma with prevalence of eosinophils." Mignon, in 1930, published a case of "granulations tumor" of the skull. Schairer described a similar case in 1938 and termed it "Osteomyelitis with eosinophil reaction." It was in 1940 that this entity suddenly attained a prominent place in medical literature through the reports of Otani

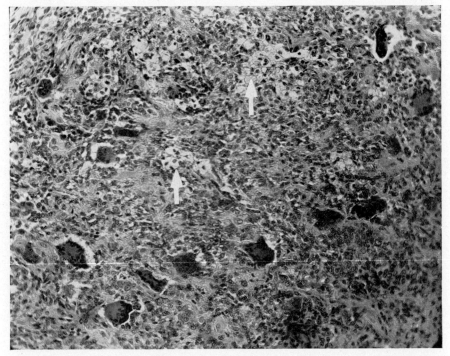

FIGURE 334. Eosinophic granuloma in a healing stage. The eosinophils are missing; lipophages (arrows) and multinucleated giant cells have entered the microscopic picture.

and Ehrlich, Jaffe and Lichtenstein, and Hatcher. All reports emphasized the granulomatous and benign character of the osseous lesions, and the prominent infiltration of eosinophilic leucocytes. Otani and Ehrlich studied seven cases and termed the entity "solitary granuloma of bone." In the reports of Jaffe and Lichtenstein, and Hatcher the prominence of the eosinophils led them independently to employ the term "eosinophilic granuloma of bone." This is the term that is now the most widely used. Farber in 1941, less impressed with the eosinophils, devised the term "destructive granuloma of bone." As a fortunate result of these reports the entity is now being widely recog-

nized and its true benign character appreciated. There is little doubt
that many of these cases in the past have been erroneously treated as
malignancies.

PATHOLOGIC ANATOMY

The earlier reports stated that the skeletal changes were represented
by a solitary lesion; in subsequent reports it became evident that the
lesions in the bones are often multiple. In Green and Farber's report
of ten cases, four disclosed a solitary lesion and six multiple lesions. Of
the multiple lesions the average
number was 16 and the maximum number was 25.

The distribution is similar to
that of multiple myeloma and
metastatic malignancies. In addition to the long tubular bones
the ribs, vertebrae and skull are
the usual sites. Involvement of
the bones of the hands or feet is
rare. Lesions are not confined to
any one portion of the bone, but
occur in diaphyses and metaphyses and occasionally in epiphyses.

Macroscopically the osseous lesions are round or oval and purely destructive in character. The
tissue filling the bony defects is

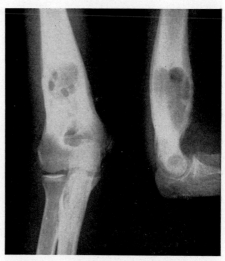

FIGURE 335. Eosinophilic granuloma of the
lower humerus of a 16 year old female (solitary lesion).

friable but firm, and is reddish-gray, yellowish, or yellow-streaked. In
the healing stage the tissue tends to be fibrous in character and a light
gray color. Pathologic fractures are relatively common and superimpose
on the lesions the elements of hemorrhage, necrosis, fibrosis, and new
bone formation.

Microscopically the tissue is granulomatous (reticulo-endothelial)
and is profusely infiltrated with leucocytes, the majority of which are
eosinophils (Fig. 333). Hatcher described the tissue as having a fibroblastic stroma with many macrophages, multinucleated cells, and foci
of necrosis. "Most striking were the focal collections of eosinophilic
polymorphonuclear leucocytes in the granulation tissue." The histiocytes
(macrophages, reticulocytes, reticular cells) represent the primary cells,
not the eosinophiles.

The multinucleated giant cells, when present, are most numerous near areas of hemorrhage or necrosis. They function as phagocytes and contain fragments of eosinophils, red blood cells and debris. Large mononucleated phagocytes (giant histiocytes) generally are more numerous than the multinuclear type. These cells have sharply outlined cell walls and large nuclei containing a delicate nuclear membrane and finely divided chromatin material, resembling the nuclei of the stromal cells. Stromal cell cytoplasm frequently is foamy in character. Histologically there are few lymphocytes or plasma cells. Mitotic figures are rarely seen. As the lesion matures, vacuolated mononuclear cells (lipophages) tend to become more numerous.

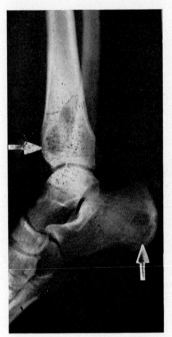

In older lesions that undergo healing, the eosinophils gradually diminish in number and ultimately disappear (Green & Farber). The xanthomatous element becomes the most prominent for a time (Fig. 334). Fibroblastic proliferation is accelerated and fibrous tissue steadily replaces the other elements of the lesion. Ultimately the fibrous tissue ossifies, completing the healing process.

Jaffe and Lichtenstein studied two rib lesions and noted healing by resolution. It is their contention that eosinophilic granulomata can heal by resolution without passing through a lipogranulomatous stage.

FIGURE 336. Multiple eosinophilic granulomas of the lower extremity (arrows).

ROENTGENOLOGIC CORRELATION

The purely osteolytic character of the lesions is clearly portrayed in roentgenograms. Cortices may be expanded, and the formation of periosteal bone in the periosteum overlying the lesion is the rule. There are no pathognomonic X-ray changes; in fact, the lesions somewhat resemble those of metastatic carcinoma, multiple myeloma, and Ewing's tumor. In the skull the lesions tend to involve the inner table more than the outer; however, there have been instances where the reverse was true, and it is common for both tables to be destroyed by the granuloma.

Since most of the long bone lesions are central and purely destructive, pathologic fractures are common. Healing frequently takes place in the fracture and may simultaneously promote the healing of the granuloma.

Identification of an eosinophilic granuloma radiographically calls for roentgenograms of the entire skeleton. Solitary lesions are less frequently observed when the entire skeleton is routinely examined.

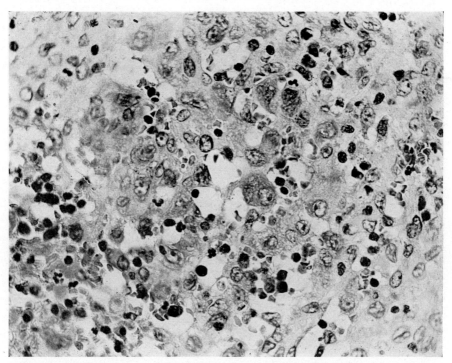

FIGURE 337. Hand-Christian's disease. Photomicrograph demonstrating histiocytes, lipophages, and scattered eosinophils. (Courtesy, A. Purdy Stout, M.D.)

CLINICAL CORRELATION

Gross and Jacox reviewed 16 cases and noted that in all except three the patient was younger than 21 years. Eleven had skull lesions, of which five were frontal. Long bones were involved in five instances, the ribs in five, and a scapula in one. The duration of symptoms varied from ten days to two months. Pain was a prominent symptom in seven cases. There have been no instances of diabetes insipidus, mental changes, or dwarfism.

Thus far no deaths have occurred in patients known to have an eosinophilic granulomata, so no autopsies have been reported. For this reason the question of the existence of associated visceral lesions remains unanswered. It is presumed that if they exist at all they are minimal. Sternal punctures have revealed instances of eosinophilia in the sternal marrow, which is assumed to be evidence of systemic involvement. An eosinophilia in the blood stream, varying from 4 percent to 11 percent, was recorded in seven of the 16 cases reviewed by Gross and Jacox.

Diagnosis

While admitting that the histologic changes vary widely in different stages of the lesions, routine biopsies are definitely indicated in order to establish the diagnosis.

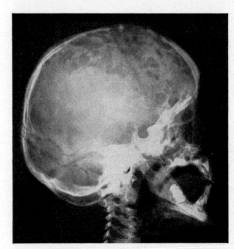

FIGURE 338. Hand-Chrisitan's disease. Skull lesions in a five year old male. The lesions became resistant to roentgenotherapy at the end of one year.

Differential Diagnosis

Eosinophilic granulomata must be differentiated from myelomata fibrous dysplasia, giant cell tumors, solitary bone cysts, tuberculous and syphilitic osteomyelitis, and Ewing's tumors.

Prognosis

When a definite diagnosis of eosinophilic granuloma is established the prognosis is excellent. However, until it is certain that the bone lesions are not part of a Hand-Christian's or Letterer-Siwe's disease the prognosis should be guarded. It is frequently impossible to differentiate these three syndromes from each other histologically.

HAND-CHRISTIAN'S DISEASE

TERMINOLOGY

Terms used in referring to this disease include Schüller-Christian's disease, xanthomatosis, lipogranulomatosis, lipoidosis, and lipoid histiocytosis.

When he was a resident physician in 1893, Hand reported the first case of lipogranulomatosis. The patient was age 3 and had a pneumonia, a polyuria, a geographic skull, and exophthalmos. A diagnosis of tuberculosis was made but was corrected in 1921 when Hand, after reading Shüller's and Christian's articles, reported a second case.

Schüller reported three cases in 1915 in a general discussion of skull defects; Christian's case, a five year old girl, was described in 1919.

Since Rowland's article in 1928 the disease has generally been classified with the disturbances of lipoid metabolism. However, Hand-Christian's disease is no longer believed to a lipoid storage disease of the type represented by Gaucher's and Nieman-Pick's diseases; it is a granulomatous disease in which variable amounts of cholesterol is secondarily deposited. Experimental cholesterol storage lesions do not

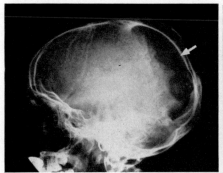
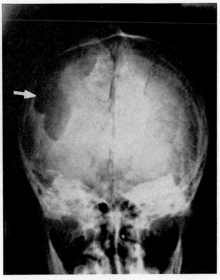

FIGURE 339. Hand-Christian's disease with an extensive skull defect (arrow).

precipitate the formation of granulomata; neither do the soft tissue cholesterol deposits in familial xanthomatosis create granulomatous reactions.

PATHOLOGIC ANATOMY

Macroscopically the lesions are composed of firm, yellowish, friable, "putty-like" tissue which fills skeletal and soft tissue defects.

Almost any area of the skeleton may become the site of typical lesions. In the *calvarium,* lipogranulomata form between the dura and the skull, destroying rounded circumscribed areas of the bone (Figs. 338 & 339). The map-like outline of the bony defects gave rise to the descriptive term "geographic skull." Deposits also form on the outer surface of the skull, destroying the outer table at the outset. At the *base of the skull* the granulomata generally begin in the region of the sella turcica, and it is believed to be the resultant pressure exerted upon the pituitary gland that causes the dwarfism occasionally observed.

The lesion may extend anteriorly to enter the orbital fissures. Lipo-granulomatous deposits in the orbits are responsible for the exophthalmos not infrequently associated with Hand-Christian's disease. Encroachment upon the hypothalmus is said to cause the diabetes insipidus.

Lesions in the mandible are the cause of loose decaying teeth. In a few instances mastoid lesions have led to middle ear inflammation. Any portion of the long bones, ribs, clavicles, vertebrae, and pelvis may become the site of characteristic osteolytic lesions.

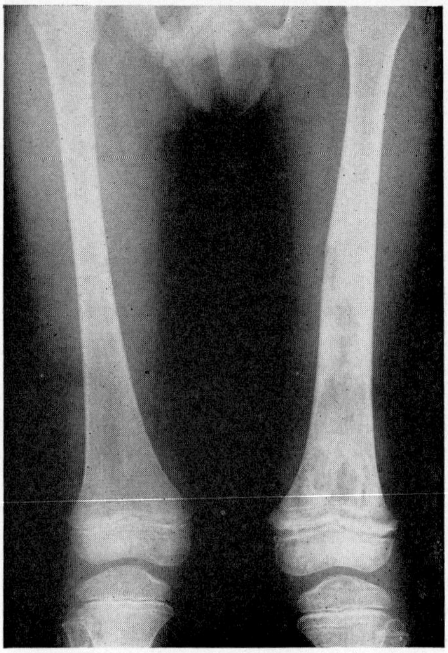

FIGURE 340. Hand-Christian's disease with involvement of the left femur.

Visceral lesions have been identified in the majority of the reported cases; the more frequent sites have been the lungs, pleura, liver, spleen, lymph glands, thymus, heart, and brain.

Microscopically the skeletal lesions are similar to those of eosinophilic granuloma; this is particularly true during the early stages of the lesions (Fig. 337). The cholesterol element is reflected by the numerous foam cells that become evident in later stages. Just as in eosinophilic granulomata, the lipoid laden histocytes gradually disappear during the healing stage. Eosinophilic leucocytes are numerous early, diminish with cholesterinization of the lesion, and disappear during healing. Throughout the sequence of events the reticulum cell proliferation is the most significant feature.

ROENTGENOLOGIC CORRELATION

In the roentgenogram the individual skeletal lesions of Hand-Christian's disease cannot be differentiated from those of eosinophilic granuloma. Differentiation is based on associated clinical symptoms, the presence of visceral lesions, and the course of the disease.

CLINICAL CORRELATION

Hand-Christian's disease is neither rare, nor limited to children and young adults, as formerly believed. With more biopsies and a wider understanding of the disease many more cases are being observed. No age group is immune but the incidence is highest in male children.

As Walgreen, Mallory, and others have pointed out, every degree of variation exists between Hand-Christian's disease and eosinophilic granuloma, and between Hand-Christian's disease and Letterer-Siwe's disease. There is increasing evidence that these three diseases represent varied clinical expressions of the same basic disorder.

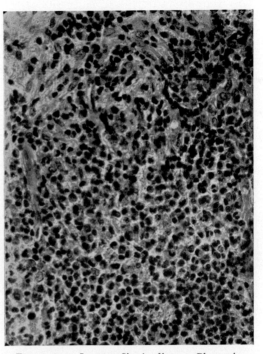

FIGURE 341. Letterer-Siwe's disease. Photomicrograph of a typical field showing numerous eosinophils infiltrated among the histiocytes.

Symptoms

Pressure and impingement created by the lipogranulomata dictate much of the symptomatology. The triad of symptoms formerly held necessary as a basis for diagnosis are diabetes insipidus, exophthalmos, and defects in the membranous bones of the skull. This symptom triad is not present in most cases and when seen denotes a late stage of the disease. An enlarged spleen and generalized lymphadenopathy are also late symptoms. Visceral symptoms are not present in many cases; in fact, some cases are claimed to possess no symptom producing visceral lesions at anytime in their course.

Pain, swelling, and tenderness frequently exist at sites of bone lesions, particularly when the involved bones are superficial. A low grade fever and a moderately elevated leucocyte count are not unusual. A slight eosinophilia is the only alteration seen in the differential blood count. A moderate increase in blood cholesterol is present at times, but is not essential to the diagnosis and is not anything approaching a consistent finding.

Prognosis

Approximately two-thirds of the cases are fatal. In general, the younger the patient the more catastrophic the disease. The course is chronic, often extending over a period of several years, and subject to exaccerbations and remissions.

Treatment

Roentgentherapy deserves a trial.

LETTERER-SIWE'S DISEASE

Letterer-Siwe's disease is a non-lipoid reticulo-endotheliosis which appears to be identical with infectious reticulo-endotheliosis. The reticulo-endothelial hyperplasia is invariably generalized and invariably fatal.

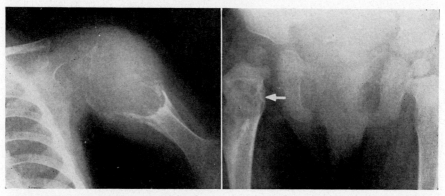

FIGURE 342. Letterer-Siwe's disease in a female age 14 months. Large masses developed in the left arm and neck three months prior to death. Roentgen therapy to the left humerus and right femur was not beneficial. A. *(Left)* Roentgenogram to show the extensive involvement of the left humerus. B. *(Right)* Roentgenogram to show the lesion of the right femur.

An acute course is characteristic, and this feature sets the disease apart from Hand-Christian's disease which generally runs a chronic course.

AGE INCIDENCE

Letterer-Siwe's disease is a disease of infants; it is rare after the age of two years. Wallgren states that Letterer-Siwe's disease is merely Hand-Christian's disease in infants.

SYMPTOMS

Fever, skin rashes, purpura, generalized lymphadenopathy, splenomegaly, multiple hemorrhages, and skeletal defects are characteristic. The skeletal lesions cannot be differentiated from those of Hand-Christian's disease (Fig. 342).

PATHOLOGIC ANATOMY

Macroscopically the multiple reticulo-endothelial granulomata have characteristics similar to those of Hand-Christian's disease except for a wider dissemination in most instances. Bone lesions cannot be differentiated from those of the other non-lipoid reticulo-endothelioses.

Microscopically the lesions resemble those of eosinophilic granulomata in their early stage. Eosinophils and histiocytes are numerous, but foam cells are conspicuous for their paucity or absence (Fig. 341). The virtual absence of cholesterinization of the lesions is explained on the basis of the brief duration of the disease. A protracted chronic course is necessary for the deposition of cholesterol.

GAUCHER'S DISEASE

Philip Charles Ernst Gaucher described the disease which bears his name in 1882. While generally referred to as Gaucher's disease the entity is known by several other terms which include primary idiopathic splenomegaly, Gaucher's large celled splenomegaly, and cerebroside lipoidosis. It is a rare, familial, constitutional disease of the reticuloendothelial system in which the cerebroside, kerasin, is deposited in the reticular cells of the spleen, liver, bone marrow, and lymph glands. Epstein and Lorenz in 1930 were the first

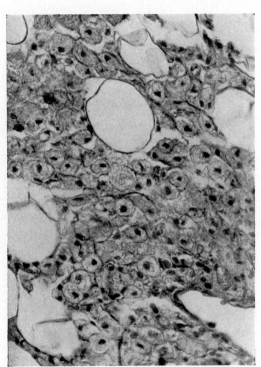

FIGURE 343. Gaucher's disease. Photomicrograph demonstrating a typical mass of closely packed reticular cells. (Courtesy, A. Purdy Stout, M.D.)

to identify the lipoid stored in the lesions to be kerasin. Since then Cushing and Stout, and others have confirmed this observation. Ludwig Pick gave the first detailed description of the skeletal changes.

PATHOLOGIC ANATOMY

Grossly, the massive splenomegaly is the most outstanding change. The liver and deep lymph glands are also enlarged, but to a lesser degree. Skeletal lesions deserve emphasis; Thannhauser stated, "The involvement of the skeletal system is as constant in Gaucher's disease as involvement of the spleen. It is one of the main features, not secondary, of the disease." Changes are generalized throughout the skeleton, but are particularly prominent in the femora, vertebrae, and sternum. Accumulations of Gaucher cells (lipoid laden histiocytes) create areas of osteoresorption and, at times, cortical expansion. Expansion of the lower femoral metaphyses is responsible for the club-shaped contour described by roentgenologists. Sections through the bones disclose numerous white and pale yellow circumscribed deposits of Gaucher cells. Reddish areas denote sites of hemorrhage and gray areas, sites of necrosis. Involved vertebrae become so weakend and porotic that they

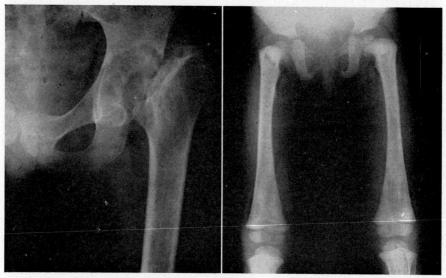

FIGURE 344. *(Left)* Gaucher's disease. Antero-posterior roentgenograms of the left hip of a 33 year old female exhibiting destruction of the head and neck of the femur. (Courtesy, A. Purdy Stout, M.D.)

FIGURE 345. *(Right)* Gaucher's disease in a child. Antero-posterior roentgenogram of the femora showing bilateral metaphyseal involvement.

are subject to pathological compression fractures. The periosteum is uninvolved.

Joints, the knee and hip in particular, may be invaded by direct extension; this usually is achieved by collapse of one of the bones making up the joint. According to Schein and Arkin there have been 16 cases of Gaucher's disease reported in which the hip joint was involved. Only one case, that of Cushing and Stout, was explored surgically. In that case, a female age 33, the head and neck of the femur were extensively destroyed and were excised along with six loose fragments (Fig. 344). Aseptic necrosis had taken place in the femoral head.

Microscopically the principle feature is the so-called Gaucher cell.

which is a large pale reticular cell filled with kerasin (Fig. 343). Masses of these cells closely packed, fill the lesions. Areas of necrosis, hemorrhage, and fibroblastic proliferation frequently interrupt the monotonous sheets of Gaucher cells.

Roentgenologic Correlation

The roentgenogram reflects the osteoporosis and thin cortices of involved areas of the skeleton. Areas presenting a "moth eaten" appearance are not unusual; the small or large radiolucent areas represent sites in which osseous tissue is replaced by masses of Gaucher cells.

Reactive osteosclerosis may develop at the margins of some of the older bone lesions. Skull lesions are not unusual. Melamed and Chester observed a case in which there was destruction of many vertebrae. Broadening of the metaphyses of the long bones is an important roentgenographic feature (Fig. 345).

Clinical Correlation

Gaucher's disease exists in two forms: the acute infan-

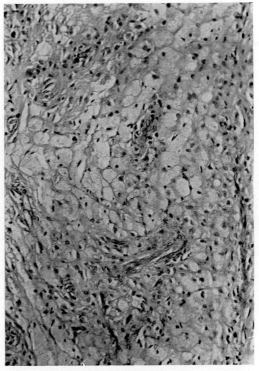

FIGURE 346. Solitary Xanthoma. Photomicrograph of a field of lipophages.

tile form and the adult form. The infantile form has its onset the first six months of life, runs an acute course, and is usually fatal by the end of the second year. Differentiation from Nieman-Peck's disease is often difficult and may be definite only after a chemical analysis of the lipoid contained in the lesions. The adult form generally starts insidiously between childhood and young adulthood. The survey of Cushing and Stout disclosed that 58 percent of the cases had the onset of symptoms during the first decade; the onset in the remaining 42 percent, was between the ages of 10 and 38.

There is no sex or racial predominance, although some statistics have indicated that the disease favors white females. A familial factor exists in more than one-third of the reported cases (Thannhauser). Leuco-penia, a low grade fever, malaise, and bone pain are the rule. Bone pain may become severe. Areas of patchy pigmentation, yellowish brown in color, may involve the skin.

Diagnosis

A sternal puncture is employed when the diagnosis is in question. Blood chemistry is normal; the kerasin does not accumulate in the blood stream.

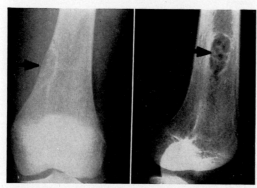

Prognosis

The prognosis is good in adults, fair in adolescents, and poor in infants and young children.

Treatment

FIGURE 347. Solitary xanthoma of the lower femur (arrows).

Roentgentherapy is not beneficial. Splenectomy frequently is resorted to when the spleen becomes massive. Pack and Silverstone believe that bone involvement becomes more extensive after splenectomy.

NIEMAN-PICK'S DISEASE

Nieman-Pick's disease is a generalized reticulo-endotheliosis in which the diamino-phosphatide, sphingomyelin, is the lipoid stored in the foam cells. Enormous lipoid accumulations are stored in the histio-cytes of all organs in the body.

The disease develops principally in Jewish infants, runs an acute course, and is rapidly fatal. There is no hereditary factor.

Localized skeletal defects are not seen, but the bone marrow, like all other tissues of the body, contains large numbers of xanthomatous cells.

SOLITARY SKELETAL XANTHOMA

Gross and Jacox found reports of seven cases of solitary skeletal xanthomata. Eosinophils were not mentioned in the descriptions of the microscopic changes. The lesions were described as lipoid granulomata, and as pure xanthomata (Fig. 346). Differentiation histologically of solitary or multiple xanthoma of bone from eosinophilic granulomata depends principally upon the presence of eosinophils in the latter.

The solitary xanthoma reported by Berman and Sinberg was in an Italian boy age 12 and involved an area one inch in diameter in the lower one-third of the left femur. No recurrence of the lesion followed surgical excision.

REFERENCES

EOSINOPHILIC GRANULOMA

FARBER, S.: The nature of solitary or eosinophilic granuloma of bone. *Am. J. Path.,* *17*:625, 1941.

FINZI, O.: Mieloma con prevalenza delle cellule eosinofile, circoscritto all' osso frontale in un giovane di 15 anni. *Univera Med., 91*:239, 1929.

GREEN, W. T. and FARBER, S.: "Eosinophilic or solitary granuloma" of bone. *J. Bone & Joint Surg., 30*:499, 1942.

GROSS, P. and JACOX, H. W.: Eosinophilic granuloma and certain other reticulo-endothelial hyperplasias of bone. *Am. J. M. Sc., 203*:673, 1942.

HATCHER, C. H.: Eosinophilic granuloma of bone. *Arch. Path., 30*:828, 1940.

JAFFE, H. L. and LICHTENSTEIN, L.:Eosinophilic granuloma of bone. *Arch. Path., 37*:99, 1944.

LICHTENSTEIN, L. and JAFFE, H. L.: Eosinophilic granuloma of bone. *Am. J. Path., 16*:595, 1940.

MALLORY, T. B.: Eosinophilic granuloma of bone. Case 26362. *New England J. Med., 223*:149, 1940.

MIGNON, F.: *Fortschr. a. d. Geb. d. Röntgenstrahlen, 42*:749, 1930.

OTANI, S. and EHRLICH, J. C.: Solitary granuloma of bone. *Am. J. Path., 16*:479, 1940.

SCHAIRER, E.: Osteomyelitis mit eosinophiler Reaktion. *Zentralbl. f. allg. Path. u. path. Anat., 71*:113, 1938.

HAND-SCHULLER-CHRISTIAN AND LETTERER-SIWE'S DISEASES

ABT, A. F. and DENENHOLZ, E. J.: Letterer-Siwe's disease. *Am. J. Dis. Child., 51*:499, 1936.

BURMAN, M. S. and SINBERG, S. E.: Solitary xanthoma (lipoid granulomatosis) of bone. *Arch. Surg., 37*:1017, 1938.

CHRISTIAN, H. A.: Defects in membranous bones, exophthalmos and diabetes insipidus; an unusual syndrome of dyspituitarism. *M. Clin. N. Am., 3*:849, 1920.

FOOT, N. C., and OLCOTT, C. T.: Report of a case of nonlipoid histiocytosis (Reticuloendotheliosis). *Am. J. Path., 10*:81, 1934.

FREUND, M. and RIPPS, M. L.: Hand-Schuller-Christian disease. A case in which lymphadenopathy was a predominant feature. *Am. J. Dis. Child., 61*:759, 1941.

FRASER, J.: Skeletal lipoid granulomatosis (Hand-Schuller-Christian disease). *Brit. J. Surg., 22*:800, 1935.

HAND, A.: Defects of membranous bones, exophthalmos and polyuria in childhood. Is it dyspituitarism? *Am. J. M. Sc., 162*:509, 1921.

HAND, A.: Polyuria and tuberculosis. *Arch. Pediat., 10*: 673, 1893.

LETTERER, E.: Alenkamische Retikulose. *Frankfurt. Ztschr. f. Path., 30*:377, 1924; *Klin. Wchnschr., 13*:1046, 1934.

ROWLAND, R. S.: Xanthomatosis and reticulo-endothelial system. *Arch. Int. Med., 42*:611, 1928.

SCHULLER, A.: Uber eigenartige Schadel-defekte im Jugendalter. *Fortschr. a. d. Geb. d. Röntgenstrahlen, 23*:12, 1915; *Wien Med. Wochenschr., 71*:510, 1921.

SCHULTZ, A., WERMBTER, F., and PUHL, H.: Eigentumliche granulomartige Systemerkrankung des hamatopoetischen apparates. *Virchows Arch. f. path. Anat., 252*:519, 1924.

Siwe, S.: Die Reticuloendotheliose—ein neues. Krankheitsbild unter den Hepato-splenomegalien. *Ztschr. f. Kinderh., 55*:212, 1933.

Snapper, I. and Pariesel, C.: Xanthomatosis generalizata ossium. *Quart. J. Med., 2*:407, 1933.

Sosman, M. C.:Xanthomatosis (Schüller-Christian disease; Lipoid Histiocytosis). *J. A. M. A., 98*:110, 1932.

Thannhauser, S. J.: Lipidoses. Disease of Cellular Lipid Metabolism. Oxford Univ. Press, New York, 1940.

Wallgren, A.: Systemic reticuloendothelial granuloma. *Am. J. Dis. Child., 60*:471, 1940.

GAUCHER'S DISEASE

Aballi, A. J. and Kato, K.: Gaucher's disease in early infancy. Review of literature and report of case with neurological symptoms. *J. Pediat., 13*:364, 1938.

Cushing, E. H. and Stout, A. P.: Gaucher's disease. *Arch. Surg., 12*:539, 1926.

Epstein, E., and Lorenz, K.: Phosphatidzellverfettung der milz in Uiemann-Pick-scher Krankheit in Vergleich mit Lipoidosis in marbus Gaucher und Schuller-Christian'schen Krankheit. *Ztschr. f. physiol. Chem., 192*:145, 1930.

Foot, N. C. and Ladd, W. E.: Case of Gaucher's splenomegaly. *Am. J. Dis. Child., 21*:426, 1921.

Gaucher, P. C. E.: *De l'epithelioma primitif de la rate.* These de Paris, 1882.

Kato, K.: Changes of bone in Gaucher's disease. *Tr. Am. Pediat. Soc., 43*:43, 1931.

Kirklin, B. R. and Hefke, H. W.: Roentgenologically demonstrable changes in bone in Gaucher's disease. *Am. J. Roentgenol., 24*:258, 1930.

Melamed, S. and Chester, W.: Osseous form of Gaucher's disease. Case report. *Arch. Int. Med., 61*:798, 1938.

Milch, H. and Pomeranz, M.: Bone changes in Gaucher's splenomegaly. *Am. J. Surg., 89*:552, 1929.

Pach, G. T. and Silverstone, S. M.: Gaucher's disease. Report of a case improved after splenectomy. *Am. J. Surg., 41*:77, 1938.

Pick, L.: *Die skelettform des morbus Gaucher.* Fischer, Jena, 1927.

Pick, L.: Zur pathologischen Anatomie des morbus Gaucher. *Med. Klin., 18*:1408, 1922.

Reiss, O. and Kato, K.: Gaucher's disease. Clinical study with special references to roentgenography of bones. *Am. J. Dis. Child., 43*:365, 1932.

Schein, A. J. and Arkin, A. M.: Hip joint involvement in Gaucher's disease. *J. Bone & Joint Surg., 24*:396, 1942.

Welt, S., Rosenthal, N. and Oppenheimer, B. S.: Gaucher's splenomegaly with especial reference to skeletal changes. *J. A. M. A., 92*:637, 1929.

CHAPTER XVII

Bone Changes Produced by Lead, Bismuth, Phosphorus, Radium, and Fluorine

Contents

LEAD

In plumbism much of the lead taken into the body is deposited in the skeletal system. This phenomenon may take place at all ages, but the lead causes no visible changes in the structure of the bones except during the growing years. During growth an osteosclerotic disc known as the "lead line" forms on the metaphyseal side of epiphyseal plates (Figs. 348 and 349).

ETIOLOGY

A review of the reported cases of plumbism discloses that the sources of the lead have been numerous. Lead projectiles imbedded in bone or soft tissue have resulted in plumbism through slow disintegration and absorption. Senturia demonstrated that lead fragments may gradually lose their definition in roentgenograms, and through erosion and disintegration slowly deposit enough lead in the circulation to produce plumbism.

Other sources of lead poisoning are lead dust inhaled and ingested in industry, lead paint, water from lead pipes, lead medications, and cosmetics containing lead compounds. Caffey reported two cases of lead poisoning in infants that acquired the lead by chewing off the lead paint on woodwork and beds. Kato stated that numerous cases of lead poisoning developed when Japanese infants ingested leaded face powder used by their mothers. Several cases of lead meningitis were cited in Kato's report.

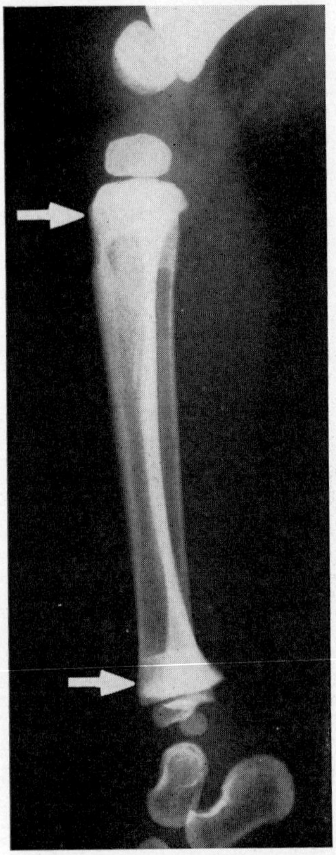

PATHOLOGIC ANATOMY

Caffey studied the lower femoral epiphysis and metaphysis of an infant that expired from plumbism. Histologically the "lead line" was found to consist of small closely packed trabeculae. However, the photomicrograph disclosed that in this juxta epiphyseal zone of sclerosis the trabeculae were composed principally of calcified cartilage derived from the zone of provisional calcification. Only a narrow margin of most of the trabeculae was formed of bone. Farther into the metaphysis the intratrabecular islands of calcified cartilage were smaller and more nearly normal in size. Within the "lead line" the greatly increased number of trabeculae diminished the size of the marrow spaces. Microscopic changes from ingestion of excessive bismuth and phosphorus are similar to those of lead-poisoning.

FIGURE 348. Lead poisoning. Arrows point to unusually wide "lead lines" indicating that lead absorption took place over a period of many months.

Distribution of Lead in Bones

Aub has shown that lead is concentrated in the bone substance proper; marrow stores only traces of the lead. The bone ends were found to contain larger deposits of lead than diaphyses; Vogt reported a case in which 0.527 mg. of lead per gram of bone existed in the epiphyseo-metaphyseal regions.

ROENTGENOLOGIC CORRELATION

The metaphyseal discs of calcified cartilage and bone ("lead lines") are clearly portrayed in roentgenograms. Aub, and Vogt contended that the radio-opacity of the "lead lines" was due principally to the deposition of lead. Histologic studies have disclosed a sufficient concentration of calcified cartilage and bone to account for most of the radio-opacity. Hodges, Phemister, and Brunschwig support the belief that the lead contributes little to the radio-opacity of the "lead lines."

Lead absorption over a brief period during growth produces a thin "lead line" (Fig. 349); lead absorbed over a long period creates a wide "lead line" (Fig. 348). When no further lead is absorbed the discs cease to increase in width but persist in approximately the dimensions attained. As growth at the epiphyseal plate continues, the discs are left behind as monuments to the period of plumbism.

In adults the lead is diffusely distributed through the bones, and creates neither histologic nor roentgenologic changes.

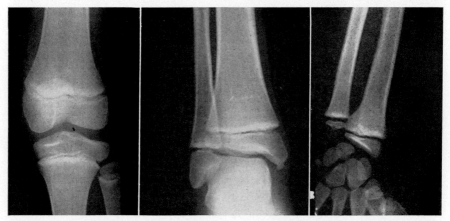

FIGURE 349. Lead poisoning. The narrow juxtaepiphyseal zones of osteosclerosis ("lead lines") indicate a brief period of lead absorption.

CLINICAL CORRELATION

The "lead line" in the gums adjacent to the teeth is a prominent clinical feature and, according to Aub et al, is the result of fine black amorphous granules deposited in the connective tissue at the base of the mucous membrane epithelium. Widespread caries of the teeth is the rule.

Other manifestations may include stippling of red blood cells, excessive lead in the urine, wrist drop, and encephalopathy.

BISMUTH

Bismuth is capable of producing changes in the growing skeleton that are similar to those noted in plumbism. Caffey, after studying the bone changes in lead poisoning, investigated the reaction of the skeleton to bismuth. He concluded that the distribution in the bones and the pathologic and roentgenologic changes were similar. Metaphyseal "bismuth lines" are similar to "lead lines." Vogt also observed "bismuth lines," as did Park and his associates.

Bismuth used in the treatment of syphilis is the principle cause of "bismuth lines" in the growing skeleton. Such changes were observed in the newborn when the mother had received bismuth therapy. Infants and children receiving several courses of bismuth developed a transverse metaphyseal line with each course.

Caffey administered bismuth to puppies and observed skeletal changes similar to those seen in infants. He found a definite correlation between the quantity of bismuth administered and the width of the reactive transverse metaphyseal lines.

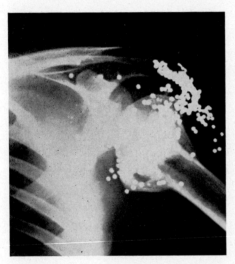

FIGURE 350. Lead shot deposited in the left shoulder for a period of many years, caused lead poisoning.

Histologic studies revealed the same densely packed trabeculae seen in lead and phosphorus lines. Most of the trabeculae were composed of calcified cartilages with thin "fringes" of bone. Both osteoblastic and osteoclastic activity were below normal. After formation of the trabeculae at the enchondral line by the apposition of a layer of bone around a core of calcified cartilage, the process of replacement of the core of calcified cartilage by bone failed to take place, thus causing the intratrabecular islands of calcified cartilage to persist abnormally long.

PHOSPHORUS

Wegner, in 1872, noted increased bone formation on the metaphyseal side of epiphyseal plates during and after the administration of phosphorus. In 1918 Phemister observed that juxta-epiphyseal phosphorus lines were broadest at the sites of the most rapidly growing epiphyses. Normal growth is resumed when the administration of phosphorus is discontinued. The epiphyses grow away from the transverse lines, but the lines remain visible in roentgenograms for several or many years. Very small doses of yellow phosphorus, once used in the treatment of rickets, produced transverse metaphyseal lines. Larger doses produced skeletal deossification.

Transverse lines in late stages, after the epiphyses have grown away from them, consist of thin or thick transverse bony trabeculae that joint up to form an osseous disc. Such discs may be intact or interrupted, prominent or scarcely visible, single or multiple, and may be located close to epiphyses or in diaphyses. It is not possible to differentiate histologically or radiographically the transverse lines of phosphorus, lead, and bismuth.

During the many years that yellow phosphorus was employed in the manufacture of matches, the employees handling the phosphorus were subject to phosphorus poisoning. Most prominent of the manifestations were periostitis and osteomyelitis of the mandible. Such cases have been rare since non-poisonous red phosphorus was substituted for yellow phosphorus.

RADIUM

ETIOLOGY

After Blum's and Hoffman's reports, Martland, Conlon and Knef (1925) de-

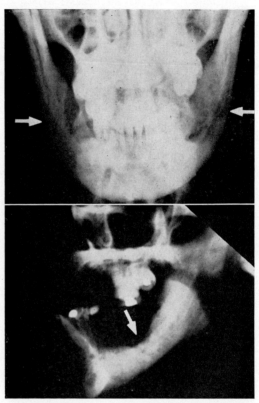

FIGURE 351. Radium poisoning in a female age 40 acquired from painting radium watch dials. Mandible became extensively involved (arrows). Radium radiations detected in urine, feces, and expired air.

scribed in detail several cases of radium-poisoning among painters of luminous clock dials. It was common practice among the radium-dial painters to tip their brushes with their lips. In the course of three to seven years of painting 250 to 300 dials daily, sufficient radium was ingested to create a high incidence of clinical symptoms. Measurements were made of the gamma ray emanations given off by the body in the exhaled air.

Medications containing radium have been employed for a wide

variety of entities, and in several cases have been responsible for sarcomatous changes. Norgaard described a case in which ten micrograms of radium chloride were injected into a knee joint for the treatment of arthritis. Eight years later a fibrosarcoma was discovered which involved the knee joint together with the upper tibial epiphysis and metaphysis.

Hatcher reviewed 24 cases in which a bone sarcoma followed radium or roentgen-ray radiation. Seventeen of the twenty-four cases were irradiated for tuberculous arthritis. In three cases the sarcoma developed at the site of a previous tumor for which the irradiation therapy was given. The irradiation sarcomata were clinically and histologically different from the original tumors. Three to eleven years were required for a sarcoma to develop from radium or roentgen-ray radiations.

Pathologic Changes

While the mandible has been the most frequent site of the skeletal lesions of radium poisoning, any part of the skeleton may become involved. The constant emanations, particularly the gamma and beta rays, from as little as .01 mg. of radium in the body may lead to osseous necrosis, osteitis, and frequently also to malignant changes (sarcoma). The osteitis and periostitis of the mandible ("radium jaw") are similar to the jaw lesions of yellow phosphorus poisoning.

In 1926 Phemister produced areas of osseous necrosis in dogs by implanting radium in the skeleton. The rate of creeping substitution was slowed because of damage to overlying soft tissues by the radiation. It was noted that large areas of necrotic bone, when used in weight-bearing, did not sequestrate but were slowly replaced by creeping substitution. When not used in weight-bearing, the necrotic bone was sequestrated, then slowly absorbed.

Evans and associates studied radium metabolism in rats and found that the bones became more fragile from radium rays. Fracture healing was satisfactory but a pronounced concentration of radium was deposited in the callus. Hypercalcification was observed in the ends of the long bones.

All of the recorded cases of radium-poisoning have been in adults (Martland). If chronic radium-poisoning were to occur in a child, it would likely produce a transverse metaphyseal zone of sclerosis. Both Thomas and Bruner, and Evans, Harris, and Bunker reported experimental radium poisoning in young rats in which they observed transverse metaphyseal zones of hypercalcification.

Clinical Correlation

Radium poison exists in acute and chronic forms depending upon the quantity of radium deposited in the body. Large doses of radium in the body produce acute poisoning which is rapidly fatal. Small quantities of radium in the body cause chronic poisoning which may

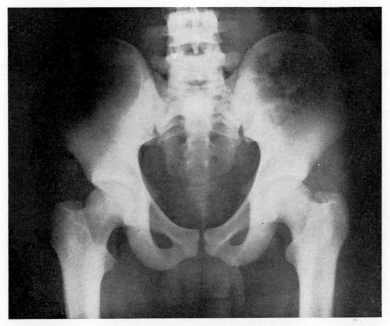

FIGURE 352. Fluorine poisoning. Permanent diffuse osteosclerosis as a consequence of chronic fluorine poisoning. (Courtesy, *U. S. Army Institute of Pathology*, Acc. No. 86050.)

run a course lasting 20 years or more, that frequently terminates as osteogenic sarcoma.

The body can resist much greater doses of radium (radium or roentgen-ray) from external sources than from deposits of radio-active substances, including radio-active isotopes, inside the body. According to Rajewsky the principal source of damage from radio-active deposits is from the alpha particles not from gamma rays which are the rays generally employed in radiation therapy.

Radium has been used internally in the treatment of Hodgkin's disease. Steven's patient was benefited by the radium but developed radium-poisoning. Stevens then used Aub's treatment of lead poisoning, which consists of a calcium-restricted diet plus ammonium chloride, thyroid extract, and parathormone; improvement is said to have followed this therapy.

FLUORINE

The ingestion of small quantities of fluorine over a period of several years leads to a great increase in the hardness and density of the skeleton (Fig. 352).

ETIOLOGY

Moller and Gudjonsson reported fluorosis in miners of cryolite. Cryolite is a double fluoride of sodium and aluminum and contains 54 percent fluorine. It was shown that the fluorosis resulted from the cryolite dust that was swallowed, and not from the dust that was inhaled; absorption of cryolite takes place only through the intestinal tract.

In Bishop's patient fluorosis developed from working in phosphate rock, a substance with a high fluorine content.

Fruit and vegetable insecticides containing fluorine compounds have caused fluorosis when the sprayed foods were consumed.

Drinking water in various parts of the world, particularly in India, contains sufficient fluorine to produce mottling of the teeth in the young.

PATHOLOGIC CHANGES

Generalized intrinsic bone proliferation is the basis for the pronounced increase in skeletal density. Cortices are thickened, principally at the expense of the medullary canals, through endosteal bone apposition. Periosteal bone formation is irregular and in severe cases leads to numerous excrescences. Moller described calcification and ossification of many ligaments including the vertebral longitudinal ligaments. Bony bridges spanned vertebral bodies in several of the advanced cases.

In Moller's series skull changes were observed in only the most severe cases. Bishop's patient had no skull changes.

The involved bones weighed up to three times their normal weight, and presented chalky white surfaces. An analysis of the fluorine content of the bones disclosed that bones with the greatest density possessed the largest quantity of calcium and magnesium fluoride. However, it is the reactive osteosclerosis that is responsible for the hardness and milky-white radio-opacity, not the fluorine proper. The bone remains permanently dense; deossification to normal density does not occur.

Mottling of teeth takes place when fluorosis occurs during enamel development. Hypoplasia of the enamel structure is responsible for the mottled appearance.

Microscopic changes

Ash and Angevine noted large trabeculae with a granular appearance and lamellae with irregularities, poor definition, and a tendency to undergo fragmentation. Moller saw an "irregular organic matrix and a varying but excessive deposition of calcium."

DIFFERENTIAL DIAGNOSIS

The uniform increase in density of the long bones helps differentiate fluorosis from entities such as osteopetrosis and melorheostosis. No areas of osteolysis or circumscribed osteosclerosis occur in fluorosis; neither is there bowing of the long bones and flattening of vertebral bodies. Coarse trabeculation is not seen; this fact helps differentiate fluorosis from Paget's disease.

REFERENCES

AUB, J. C., EVANS, R. D., GALLAGHER, D. M., and TIBBETTS, D. M.: Effects of treatment on radium and calcium metabolism in the human body. *Ann. Int. Med., 11*:1443, 1938.

AUB, J. C., FAIRHALL, L. T., MINOT, A. S., and RESNIKOFF, P.: Lead Poisoning. (a monograph). *Medicine, 4*:1, 1925.

BISHOP, P. A.: Bone changes in chronic fluorine intoxication; roentgenographic study. *Am. J. Roentgenol., 35*:577, 1936.

BLUM, T.: Osteomyelitis of the mandible and maxilla. *J. Am. Dent. A., 11*:802, 1924.

BRANDL, J., and TAPPEINER, H.: Uber die Ablagerung von Fluorverbindungen un Organismus nach Futterung nut Fluornatorium. *Ztschr. f. Biol., 10*:518, 1891.

CAFFEY, J.: Changes in growing skeleton after administration of bismuth. *Am. J. Dis. Child., 53*:56, 1937.

CAFFEY, J.: Clinical and experimental lead poisoning. Some roentgenologic and anatomic changes in growing bones. *Radiology, 17*:957 1931.

DE EDS, F.: Chronic fluorine intoxication; a review. *Medicine, 12*:1, 1933.

EDITORIAL: Chronic fluorine intoxication. *J. A. M. A., 123*:150, 1943.

ELIOT, M. M., SOUTHER, S. P., and PARK, E. A.: Transverse lines in x-ray plates of long bones of children. *Bull. Johns Hopkins Hosp., 41*:364, 1927.

EVANS, R. D., HARRIS, R. S., and BUNKER, J. W. M.: Radium metabolism in rats and the production of osteogenic sarcoma by experimental radium poisoning. *Am. J. Roentgenol., 52*:353, 1944.

HATCHER, C. H.: Development of sarcoma in bone subjected to roentgen or radium irradiation. *J. Bone & Joint Surg., 27*:179, 1945.

HOFFMAN, F. L.: Radium necrosis. *J. A. M. A., 85*:961, 1925.

KATO, K.: Lead meningitis in infants. *Am. J. Dis. Child., 44*:569, 1932.

LEAKE, J. P.: Radium poisoning. *J. A. M. A., 99*:1077, 1932.

LINSMAN, J. F. and McMURRAY, C. A.: Fluoride osteosclerosis from drinking water. *Radiology, 40*:474, 1843.

MARTLAND, H.: Radium poisoning. *Cecil's Textbook of Medicine.* W. B. Saunders Co., Philadelphia, 1944.

MARTLAND, H. S., CONLON, P., and KUEF, J. P.: Some unrecognized dangers of the use and handling of radioactive substances. *J. A. M. A., 85*:1769, 1925.

MOLLER, F. P.: Chronic fluorine poisoning, seen from the roentgenological stand-point. *Brit. J. Radiol., 12*:13, 1939.

MOLLER, P. F. and GUDJONSSON, S. V.: Massive fluorosis of bones and ligaments. *Acta radiol., 13*:269, 1932.

NORGAARD, F.: The development of fibrosarcoma as a result of the intra-articular injection of radium chloride for therapeutic purposes. *Am. J. Cancer, 37*:329, 1939.

PARK, E. A., JACKSON, D., and KAJDI, L.: Shadows produced by lead in X-ray pictures of growing skeleton. *Am. J. Dis. Child., 41*:485, 1931.

PHEMISTER, D. B., MILLER, E. M., and BONAR, B. E.: Effect of phosphorus in rickets. *J. A. M. A., 70*:850, 1921.

PHEMISTER, D. B.: Radium necrosis of bone. *Am. J. Roentgenol., 16*:340, 1926.

RAJDWSKI, B.: Researches in the problem of radium poisoning and tolerance dose of radium. *Radiology, 32*:57, 1939.

ROHOLM, K.: *Fluorine Intoxication.* H. K. Lewis, London, 1937.

SENTURIA, H. R.: The roentgen findings in increased lead absorption due to retained projectives. *Am. J. Roentgenol., 47*:381, 1942.

STEVENS, R. H.: Radium poisoning. *Radiology, 39*:39, 1942.

VOGT, E. C.: A roentgen sign of plumbism. *Am. J. Roentgenol., 24*:550, 1930.

WEGNER, G.: *Virchows Arch. f. path. Anat., 55*:9, 1872.

WILKIE, J.: Two cases of fluorine osteosclerosis. *Brit. J. Radiol., 13*:213, 1940.

CHAPTER XVIII

Benign Tumors of Bones

Contents

CLASSIFICATION

The classification of benign tumors of bones is based upon their histologic structure, the principal component tissue dictating the name of the tumor. This is not an entirely satisfactory basis for classification but will have to suffice until more is known of the etiology of these neoplasms.

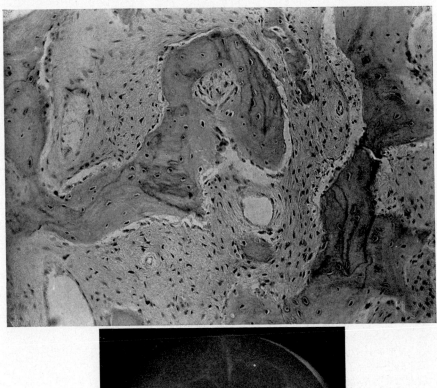

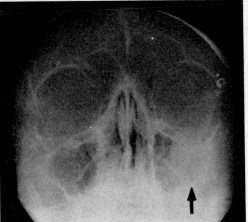

FIGURE 353. A. *(Above)* Osteoma, spongy type, removed from the antrum. Most of the traceculae showed a lamellated structure. B. *(Below)* Roentgenogram of tumor (arrow).

In the majority of instances the proper classification of a given benign tumor is relatively simple. However, it is not always a simple matter to distinguish certain benign from malignant tumors of bones;

nor is it always possible to differentiate, on a microscopic basis, between bone of traumatic origin and neoplastic bone.

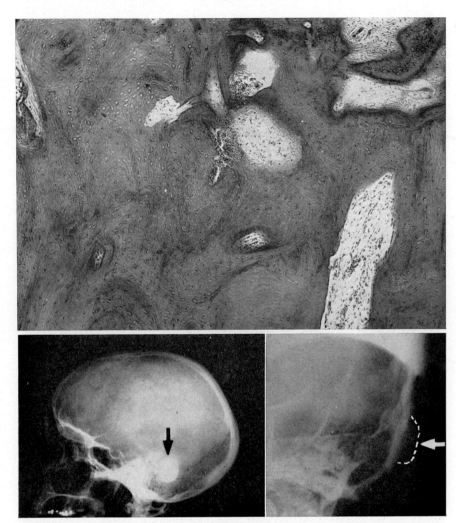

FIGURE 354. A. *(Above)* Osteoma, eburnated type. The tumor projected from the outer table of the skull. B. *(Below)* Lateral and antero-posterior roentgenograms of the tumor (arrow).

THE CLASSIFICATION OF PRIMARY BENIGN TUMORS OF BONES

NAME OF TUMOR	PRINCIPAL TISSUES FORMED BY TUMOR
1. Osteoma	Lamellated bone
2. Chondroma	Cartilage
3. Osteochondroma (Exostosis)	Cartilage and bone
4. Chondroblastoma	Chondroblastic tissue and calcified cartilage

5. Osteoid osteoma   Osteoid and primitive bone
6. Benign giant-cell
    tumor   Undetermined
7. Fibroma   Fibrous tissue
8. Hemangioma   Blood vessels
9. Adamantinoma   Odontogenic tissues (Adamantine epithelium)
10. Odontoma   Odontogenic tissues (combinations of enamel,
                                dentine and cementum)
11. Lipoma   Adipose tissue
12. Myxoma   Myxomatous connective tissue

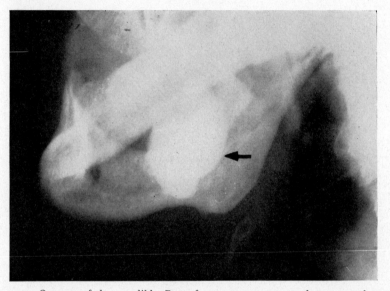

FIGURE 355. Osteoma of the mandible. Part of tumor was spongy and part was eburnated.

OSTEOMA

An osteoma, most benign of bone tumors, is a true neoplasm forming on the basis of intramembranous ossification. As would be anticipated most osteomas develop on the skull and in those of the facial bones that are of membranous origin (Figs. 353, 354, & 355). While the majority of these tumors are diagnosed in childhood a few do not make their presence known until adult life.

Osteomas are not rare, but they are not nearly so common as osteochondromas. Growth is slow, and they rarely, if ever, undergo maligant changes. From a broad base the tumor generally projects from either table of the skull, into the orbit, or into the frontal, ethmoid, or maxillary sinuses. A bosselated or lobulated periphery is the rule and it is not unusual for lobes of the tumor to break off and undergo aseptic

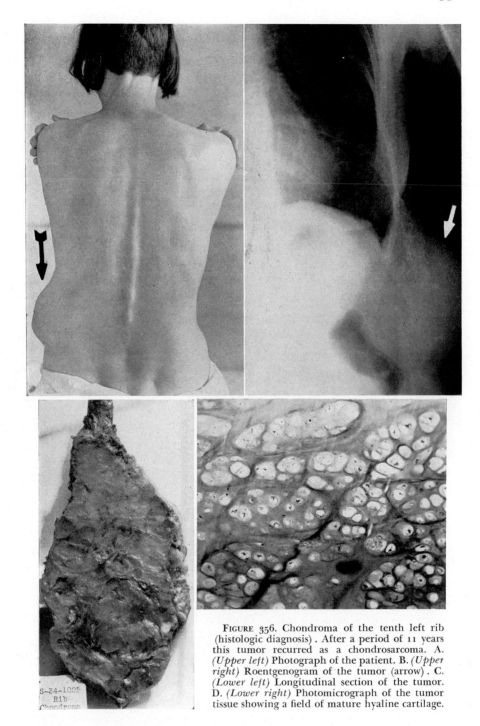

FIGURE 356. Chondroma of the tenth left rib (histologic diagnosis). After a period of 11 years this tumor recurred as a chondrosarcoma. A. *(Upper left)* Photograph of the patient. B. *(Upper right)* Roentgenogram of the tumor (arrow). C. *(Lower left)* Longitudinal section of the tumor. D. *(Lower right)* Photomicrograph of the tumor tissue showing a field of mature hyaline cartilage.

necrosis. In roentgenograms of an osteoma in a paranasal sinus (Fig. 353B) the tumor generally presents a greater degree of radio-opacity than would pus; the irregular outline of the tumor also aids in the differentiation. When growing from the inner table of the skull, osteomas must be differentiated from meningeal osteophytes, and from traumatic and inflammatory hyperostoses.

Osteomas seldom produce symptoms. When they are the cause of significant symptoms, or when they create cosmetic distortion, they should be excised.

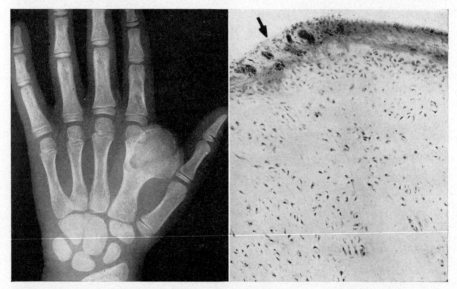

FIGURE 357. Enchondroma of the second metacarpal. A. *(Left)* Roentgenogram. B. *(Right)* The arrow points to the capsule which is functioning as a perichondrium.

PATHOLOGIC ANATOMY

Osteomas are composed entirely of lamellated cancellous bone or, in occasional instances, of compact bone, and are enveloped by a thin fibrous membrane which serves as a periosteum. Enlargement of the tumor takes place, not by intrinsic growth as seen in chondromas, but only by peripheral bone apposition beneath the tumor capsule. At the termination of growth, a plate of lamellar bone forms at the periphery, sharply outlining the tumor grossly and roentgenographically.

Typical osteomas are divisible on the basis of their density into two types, spongy and eburnated.

Spongy Type

As the name implies, the spongy type of osteoma is made up of cancellous bone, the trabeculae of which, while they vary from thin to thick, are composed of lamellated bone (Fig. 353A). When fibrous tissue predominates and the bony trabeculae are the primitive fibrous type, the tumor is an ossifying fibroma. Marrow elements of an osteoma usually are fibrous but in exceptional cases are mixed fatty and hematogenous. The histogenesis is simply that of fibrous bone and its replacement by lamellar bone. In general the less the density the more rapid the growth and the larger the tumor.

Eburnated Type

The word eburnated describes the ivory-like density of this type of osteoma. In cross-section the tumor resembles compact bone in density, but histologic sections do not usually reveal numerous haversian canals (Fig. 354A). It is the central portion of the tumor that is the oldest and the most dense. Growth of an eburnated osteoma is very slow, and only rarely does the size exceed

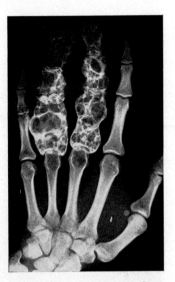

FIGURE 358. Multiple enchondromas of the middle and ring fingers in a 28 year old male.

one inch in diameter. Alternating periods of growth and quiescence in the tumor are reflected by the pattern of blue cement lines in the trabeculae and haversian systems.

CHONDROMA

Chondromas are benign cartilage tumors. They are more frequently solitary than multiple, and while they usually remain of small size, they may grow to large dimensions. Whereas osteochondromas develop at the periphery of host bones, chondromas generally occupy a central position; thus the name enchondroma. Chondromas are most common in the short tubular bones, the more frequent sites being the phalanges of the hands and feet, the metacarpals, metatarsals, rib cartilages, sternum, and vertebrae (Figs. 356 to 359). Only rarely are the long bones involved. The incidence is almost equally divided between the sexes. While the diagnosis is generally made during the first three decades, there are rather numerous instances where the tumor is not detected until late adult life. The peak incidence in the Geschichter and Copeland series was between the ages of 20 and 30 years. Nearly all chondromas are believed to form during the growing years even though the diagnosis is long delayed.

PATHOLOGIC ANATOMY

Chondromas tend to be rounded and possess a grooved surface which makes them bosselated or lobulated, depending upon the depth of the grooves. Palpation discloses a firm rubbery compressability except in

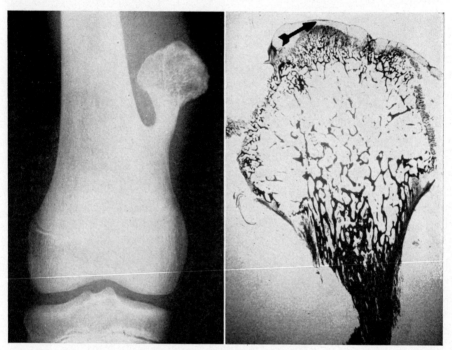

FIGURE 359. Osteochondroma of the lower femoral metaphysis. A. *(Left)* Roentgenogram. B. *(Right)* Histologic section of the tumor.

those cases where a hardness results from an ossified surface layer. As a reaction to trauma, including pathologic fracture, inflammation, or malignant change, the overlying bone or soft tissues may become securely fixed to the tumor. At the site of a chondroma the host bone may be expanded either in a circumscribed area or in the entire circumference. Distortion, perforations, and pathologic fractures are relatively common.

Cross-section of a chondroma frequently reveals a multilobulated structure and the pale, blue, opalescent, wet, glistening appearance of hyaline cartilage. Cystic and gelatinous areas are common. Areas of degeneration are detected by their yellow or brown discoloration, and areas of calcification, by their white or bluish-gray appearance. While most chondromas are composed principally of hyalin cartilage, many have areas in which the matrical substance is fibrillated or mucinous in character. The tumor capsule, a thin membrane intimately attached to the surface, follows all grooves and crevices and functions as a perichondrium (Fig. 357B). Fine septa of white fibrous tissue pass through

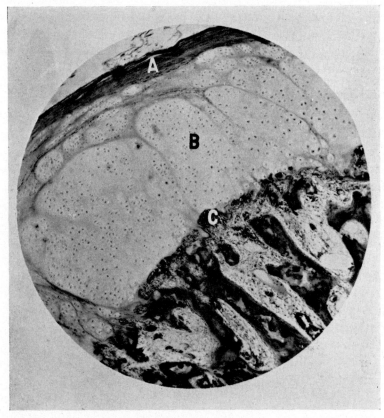

FIGURE 359. (Continued) C. Photomicrograph of the tumor's cartilaginous cap (at the site of the arrow, Figure 359B.). A. Perichondrium. B. Non-calcified hyaline cartilage. C. Enchondral line showing active growths as indicated by the presence of intratrabecular islands of calcified cartilage.

the tumor in many directions, dividing it into incomplete lobes. Except when areas of calcification or ossification are encountered the mass cuts very much like rubber.

Nutrient vessels of the tumor consist of a system of lymphatics extending centrally from the periphery, and of blood vessels extending along the interlobular fibrous septa. Growth for the most part takes place at the periphery beneath the capsule which possesses the mother tissue of a perichondrium. Intrinsic growth is a factor in some cases and is achieved through proliferation of chondrocytes within their lacunae. Little of the *etiology* is understood. An hereditary factor has been observed, and there have been instances of solitary chondroma in which there was convincing evidence of a traumatic factor. Cohnheim's cell rest theory is accepted by many investigators as the best explanation of chondroma. McMaster found isolated islands of cartilage in the skeleton following rickets, and it is his belief that these nests of chondrocytes are capable of developing into chondromas. Geschickter and Copeland contend that most skeletal chondromas represent histogenetically supernumerary joint cartilages.

Microscopic Features

Histologically, chondromas are composed principally of mature hyaline cartilage and to a minor degree of cartilage in various stages of differentiation from embryonic to mature. When the cartilage is foetal in type the chondrocytes are numerous and often stellate in shape. In the fields of mature cartilage one to several chondrocytes lie in each of the numerous, well-formed lacunae. No purposeful, orderly arrangement of the cells and matrix is seen. In growing chondromas the least mature cells are seen at the periphery beneath the perichondrium, and the most mature cells at the center. When myxomatous areas are present they generally lie near the periphery.

Hyalinization often apears in areas of the matrix and in the fibrous septa. Ossification is rather often observed but seldom represents a prominent feature. Microscopic patches of ossification sometimes develop at sites of calcification and are on the basis of either direct metaplasia or enchondral ossification. A ring of osteoid or bone occasionally forms at the periphery of quiescent chondromas.

MALIGNANT TRANSFORMATION

Malignant changes are by no means rare and consist of a transformation to a chondrosarcoma or chondromyxosarcoma. Reactivation of growth in a chondroma during adult life should arouse suspicion of malignant changes. Such changes are more common in the sternal, vertebral, and pelvic chondromas. Notwithstanding the fact that chondromas of phalanges generally show immature, aggressive-appearing chondrocytes, malignant changes are very rare.

ROENTGENOGRAPHIC CORRELATION

In roentgenograms, skeletal chondromas frequently resemble bone cysts, particularly so in bones of the hands and feet. It should be remembered that chondromas are far more common than cysts in bones of the hands and feet.

CLINICAL CORRELATION

Most chondromas produce no symptoms and therefore are not diagnosed unless they ultimately cause deformation or a pathologic fracture.

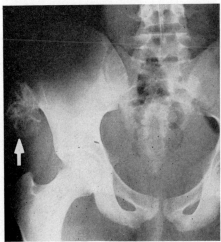

FIGURE 360. Osteochondroma of the right ilium in a boy age 12. A. *(Above)* Roentgenogram. B. *(Below)* Histologic section of a portion of the tumor at its cap. Arrow points to a tendon inserting at the margin of the tumor.

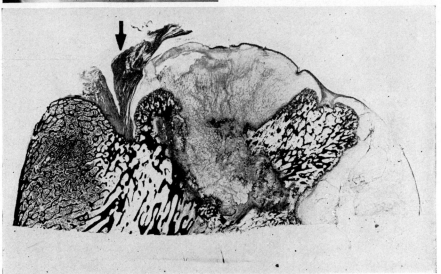

Very large chondromas may press on vital structures. Many of these enormous tumors are in reality slow-growing chondrosarcomas.

Ten to 25 per cent of the chondromas removed surgically are said to recur. It is essential to remove all of the capsule with the tumor if recurrences are to be avoided. Bone grafts placed in bony defects created by removal of chondromas facilitate reossification.

Ollier's dyschondroplasia may present the picture of multiple chondromas; however, Ollier's disease is better classified with the dysplasias, and was discussed in Chapter XIV.

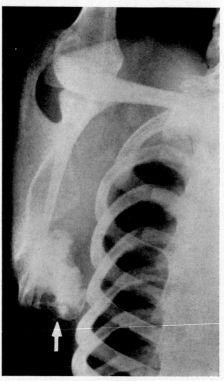

FIGURE 361. Osteochondroma of the scapula (arrow) in a female age 20.

OSTEOCHONDROMA

The osteochondroma, most common of all bone tumors, is composed of a bony base, a crown of hyaline cartilage, and an overlying thin fibrous capsule. While any metaphysis may be the site of an osteochondroma, the more frequent sites in the approximate order of their frequency are the lower femur, upper tibia, upper femur, upper and lower humerus, lower tibia, pelvis and vertebrae (Figs. 359 to 362). Since osteochondromas are primarily tumors of childhood the majority are diagnosed during the first two decades.

Growth of the tumor takes place, for the most part, only so long as the adjacent epiphyseal plate of the host bone remains open. In an adult the location of an individual osteochondroma on its host bone depends principally upon the age of the patient at the time the tumor first developed. Thus, if the osteochondroma appears during early childhood it would, by adulthood, be located on the diaphysis at a considerable distance from the epiphysis. In the rare instances when an osteochondroma forms on an epiphysis, the tumor always remains in the same position with relation to the epiphysis regardless of the time of origin.

While osteochondromas may be solitary or multiple, the multiple type generally represents the entity known as hereditary multiple exostoses described in Chapter XIV. No hereditary factor has ever been observed in solitary osteochondromas.

Pathologic Anatomy

For descriptive purposes it is clarifying to divide the osteochondroma into three parts: a fibrous capsule (which includes a perichondrium), a cartilaginous cap, and a bony base.

Fibrous capsule

This, the confining membrane of the tumor, is composed of dense fibrous tissue and measures from a few micra to a millimeter in thickness. The deep layer of the capsule is intimately fused to the underly-

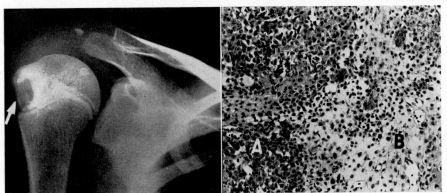

FIGURE 362. Chondroblastoma. A. *(Left)* Roentgenogram. B. *(Right)* Photomicrograph.

ing cartilaginous cap and serves as a perichondrium. Within the perichondrium there resides the mother tissue of the tumor for it is here that the chondrocytes are created. When cellular proliferation in the mother tissue is active, growth of the tumor is active, and when no further cartilage cells are formed, growth of the tumor ceases. In the surgical excision of an osteochondroma it is important that the fibrous capsule be carefully removed with the tumor.

Histologically, the capsule has relatively few cells, and these are elongated fibrocytes lying in the plane of the tumor surface. Collagenous fibers, clearly visible in the superficial layers, gradually disappear from view in the deeper layers where the capsule blends with the cartilage cap.

Cartilaginous Cap

A grooved, bosselated layer of hyalin cartilage crowns the tumor and varies in thickness from a millimeter to one or more centimeters. Except for a thin zone of calcified matrix at the chondro-osseous junction, the cartilage is non-calcified. During growth of the tumor, the

chondrocytes in the superficial layer are immature; in the deeper layers the chondrocytes are fully matured. The termination of tumor
growth is marked by the cessation of enchondral ossification, a pronounced thinning or disappearance of the zone of the non-calcified
cartilage, and the appearance of a thin subchondral plate of lamellated
bone which resembles articular cortex of adult joints.

Histogenesis

To understand the steps in enchondral ossification is to understand
the histogenesis of osteochondromas (Chapter I). In most instances the
enchondral ossification in osteochondromas is similar to that seen at
normal epiphyseal plates. However, the zone of columns in the cartilage cap is frequently poorly defined. Just as in normal growth of
the long bones, the greater the distance that intratrabecular islands
of calcified cartilage matrix are detected from the enchondral line, the
more rapid the rate of growth.

Osseous Portion

The osseous portion of osteochondromas varies from broad and
short to long and pedunculated, and the attachment to the host bone
may be by a base wider than the crown or, by a stem-like pedicle. When
pedunculated the pedicle deviates toward the center of the diaphysis
and away from the epiphysis. This is in response to growth of the host
bone and to compression of the tumor by overlying soft tissues. Larger
osteochondromas possess a marrow cavity that communicates directly
with the marrow canal of the host bone. Cortex and periosteum of the
host bone are continuous with similar structures of the tumor.

The marrow spaces of the tumor are usually filled with fibrous tissue
but may contain fat and hematogenous cells particularly when the
tumor communicates with the marrow of the host bone.

While the major portion of an osteochondroma is composed of
cancellous bone, there is a peripheral cortical wall that reaches its
maximum thickness and density at the junction of the tumor with
the host bone. Except for the new trabeculae forming at the enchondral
line during growth, all bone of the tumor is lamellated in structure.

ETIOLOGY

The cause and origin of osteochondromas is unsettled. It was long
held that this tumor represented a fragment of an epiphyseal plate
It was a popular contention that a small area at the periphery of the
epiphyseal plate became pinched off and continued growing. It was

pointed out, in support of this explanation, that the enchondral line both of the adjacent epiphyseal plate and the osteochondroma became quiescent at about the same time in the process of skeletal growth.

Cartilaginous cell rests have been observed at both intraosseous and subperiosteal locations in metaphyses, thus leading to the belief that Cohnheim's cell rest theory is a likely explanation of osteochondromas.

Geschickter and Copeland have emphasized the fact of the origin of many osteochondromas at sites of tendon anchorage. It is their conviction that an osteochondroma represents an overgrowth of a tubercle intended for the insertion of a major tendon; they believe the overgrowth is made possible by the presence of a periosteal defect adjacent to the tubercle.

The tendon attachments steadily migrate during growth requiring a complex series of adaptive changes. It is conceivable that a fragment of mesenchyme could be left behind to grow independently and build a tumor.

ROENTGENOGRAPHIC CORRELATION

Roentgenograms of osteochondromas reflect their location, size, approximate rate of growth, and the presence of a malignant transformation.

Since the fibrous tissue capsule overlying the cartilaginous cap contains no bone or calcium it is not visualized in roentgenograms. The extent to which the cartilaginous cap is visualized varies widely because of the broad variation in width of the zone of calcified cartilage.

CLINICAL CORRELATION

Since most osteochondromas produce no symptoms they are commonly discovered during roentgenologic and physical examinations for other conditions.

Symptoms occasionally arise from pressure of the tumor on nerves or other vital structures. Friction and pressure on the crown of an osteochondroma is capable of creating a painful adventitious bursa. The more superficial and exposed tumors may receive numerous traumata and the fracture of the pedicle of such osteochondromas is not unusual. Such fractures often heal, but in some instances the tumor becomes permanently freed from the host bone.

Treatment consists of excision of those osteochondromas that impinge upon vital structures, are subjected to multiple contusions, have disabling adventitious bursitis, produce objectionable cosmetic defects, and particularly of those that show evidence of malignant transformation. Routine removal of these tumors is probably justified.

During the excision of an osteochondroma care should be taken to include the layer of fibrous capsule adjacent to the cartilaginous crown. This precaution assures the removal of all mother tissue of the tumor. It has been urged by some investigators that the periosteum of the tumor and adjacent portion of the host bone be included in the excision. This concept is based upon the theory that subperiosteal islands of cartilage may be present that could later give rise to a recurrence of the tumor.

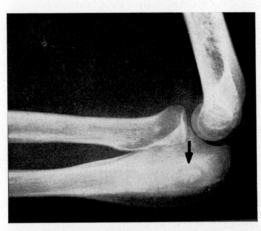

FIGURE 363. Osteoid osteoma in an olecranon of a boy age 10. A. Lateral roentgenogram. Arrow points to the tumor. Note the reactive periosteal bone. B. (*Opposite page*) Photomicrograph of a typical field. The dark staining trabeculae are bone, the pale staining trabeculae are osteoid.

MALIGNANT TRANSFORMATION

Chondrosarcoma develops in the cartilaginous cap in an incidence that is given variously from 1 to 7 percent. Details of the characteristics of this transformation are given in Chapter XIX under the heading of *Chondrosarcoma*. Reactivated growth and calcification in the cap of an osteochondroma in a patient past 20 years of age should be looked upon as a malignant transformation until proved otherwise.

BENIGN CHONDROBLASTOMA

This tumor, originally described by Ewing (1928) as a benign calcifying giant cell tumor, was later (1931) reported in detail by Codman who termed it an epiphyseal chondromatous giant cell tumor. In 1942 Jaffe and Lichtenstein reviewed the subject and reported 9 new cases. They recommended the term benign chondroblastoma of bone, emphasized the benign character of the tumor, and separated it from the category of the giant cell tumor.

PATHOLOGIC ANATOMY

These tumors appear in epiphyses during the growing period (Fig. 362). In the nine cases reported by Codman the tumor was in the upper humeral epiphysis. In the nine cases reported by Jaffe and Lichtenstein four of the tumors were in the lower femur, three in the

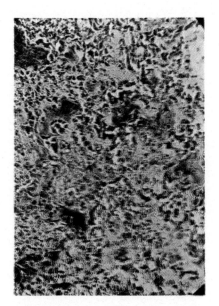

FIGURE 363. *(Continued)* B. See opposite
page for description.

upper tibia, one in the lower tibia and one in the upper humerus. All originated in epiphyses, but in six there was extension into the adjacent metaphysis. All lesions were round or oval and varied from one to 6 cm. in diameter. The tumor mass is firm and gritty and is sharply demarcated from the adjacent bone. Growth of the tumor is slow.

Histopathology

Stromal cells are round or polyhedral, medium sized, have relatively large nuclei, and a poorly defined narrow rim of cytoplasm. Numerous multinucleated giant cells infiltrate the stroma and consist of tumor giant cells with an average of three nuclei, and phagocytic giant cells with many nuclei. Few or many masses of calcium granules and foci of calcified cartilage are scattered through the tumor tissue. Jaffe and Lichtenstein have pointed out that the fragments of calcified cartilage

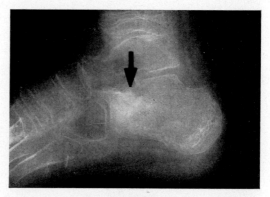

FIGURE 364. Osteoid osteoma of the os calcis (arrow).

are necrotic. Malignant transformations are not seen; there are never more than widely scattered mitotic figures.

ROENTGENOLOGIC CORRELATION

The mottling that characterizes the roentgenogram is due to the foci of calcium crystals and calcified cartilage. A well defined bony wall marks the boundary of the tumor. The tumor may be central or peripheral in its position within the epiphysis. Seldom does the tumor attain sufficient size to expand the epiphysis.

CLINICAL CORRELATION

Benign chondroblastomas predominate in males. Six of Codman's patients and all of Jaffe and Lichtenstein's were males. The latter authors' patients varied from 13 to 17 years of age. Slowly increasing pain characterizes these tumors.

Therapy: Radiation therapy will cure these neoplasms but since a biopsy is imperative, the tumor may as well be curetted out at the time of the biopsy. Simple curettage is not followed by recurrences.

Differential Diagnosis

Chondroblastomas must be differentiated from giant-cell tumors, osteoblastic sarcomas, and chondrosarcomas. While the epiphyseal location is in common with that of the giant cell tumor, the chondroblastoma differs in that it exists in young patients, is a small lesion, and shows mottling rather than soap-bubble trabeculations in the roentgenogram. The age incidence is the same as that of osteogenic sarcomas but the chondroblastoma is epiphyseal in origin, grows very slowly and does not tend to perforate the overlying cortex. It has not been uncommon for the chondroblastoma to be misinterpreted as a chondrosarcoma, both roentgenologically and microscopically. This is an unfortunate error if it leads to radical surgical therapy.

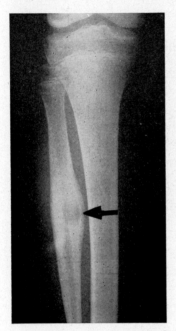

FIGURE 365. Osteoid osteoma of the fibula. (Courtesy, *U. S. Army Institute of Pathology*, Acc. No. 160444.)

OSTEOID OSTEOMA

This interesting entity, described by Jaffe in 1932, has stimulated considerable speculation regarding its character. Although it is the concensus that the lesion represents a neoplasm, as suggested by Jaffe, some observers hold that the so-called osteoid osteoma is either a dysplasia, an ossifying fibroma, or the end-stage of an inflammatory process.

Osteoid osteomas have occurred at all ages, but the majority of cases have been in adolescents and young adults. The lesions are monocentric, and, while an area of cancellous bone is the preferred site, a few have appeared directly in the cortex of long bones. This type of osteoma has been observed at such widespread sites as the phalanges of the hands and feet, astragalus, os calcis, ilium, tibia, femur, and ulna (Figs. 363 to 366).

Grossly the lesion is rounded, moderately dense, 5 mm. to 20 mm. in diameter, and is enveloped by a narrow translucent zone which sharply outlines the firm pea-sized tumor body. When located near the periphery of the host bone, the process prompts the formation of a circumscribed area of periosteal bone. Such bone is reactive, non-neoplastic, and is thickest directly over the tumor, tapering off proximally and distally.

Microscopic changes in the central mass or tumor proper are characterized by cellular fibrous tissue in which osteoid trabeculae actively form. For some reason not evident from histologic studies most of the trabeculae fail to calcify. It is this consistent tendency for the trabeculae to remain in the osteoid state that caused Jaffe to employ the term

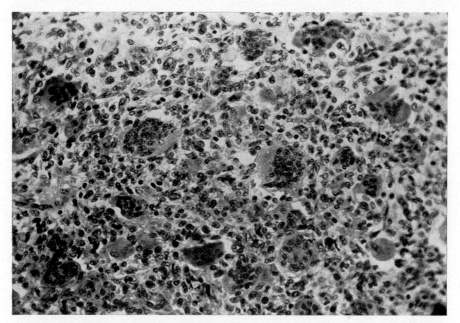

FIGURE 366. Giant-cell tumor. Grade I. Benign: The giant cells, large and numerous, have multiple nuclei similar to the nuclei of the stromal cells. Stromal cells are uniform, show no atypism and only rare mitotic figures. Solitary fields of Grade I give no assurance that the tumor is benign. The entire tumor must be composed of Grade I tissue to pronounce the tumor benign.

osteoid osteoma. In the combined osteoblastic and osteoclastic activity seen in most microscopic fields, the osteoblastic phase predominates. Bony trabeculae are scattered through the tumor and, with hematoxylin-eosin stain, present a striking contrast along side the pale pink staining osteoid trabeculae. Trabeculae vary in size and shape, but do not undergo transformation to lamellar bone. No trabeculae appear in the narrow zone of moderately dense and cellular fibrous tissue that envelopes the central mass.

The cause of the overlying periosteal bone is not always evident. In some instances the tumor causes an erosion and perforation of the cortex. The resulting subperiosteal hematoma and the reparative re-

sponse are soon manifest by the formation of periosteal bone. No inflammatory cells are seen in the periosteal reaction or in the tumor
proper; neither are there signs of aseptic necrosis.

Roentgenographically the small tumor mass is clearly defined, partly
as a result of the peripheral translucent zone of fibrous tissue. It is
not uncommon for osteoid osteomas to be erroneously diagnosed as

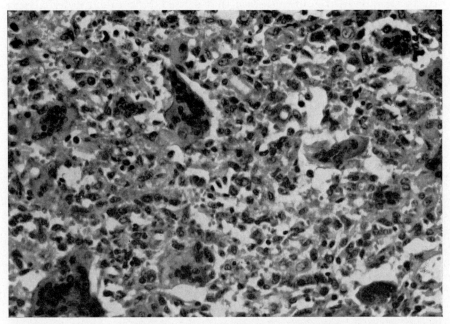

FIGURE 367. Giant-cell tumor. Grade II: (Neither entirely benign nor frankly malignant.)
Both the nuclei of the giant cells and the stromal cells show atypism, and scattered mitotic
figures. Stromal cells are more compact and the giant cells somewhat less numerous than
in Grade I. (Courtesy, *U. S. Army Institute of Pathology*, Acc. No. 30642.)

pyogenic osteomyelitis, and for the tumor to be referred to as a sequestrum.

The treatment is surgical and consists of excision of the tumor mass.
No recurrences have been reported following simple enucleation of
the tumor.

GIANT CELL TUMOR

SYNONYMS

Osteoclastoma, myeloid sarcoma, giant-cell sarcoma, tumeur à myeloplaxes, Riesenzell tumor, chronic hemorrhagic osteomyelitis.

HISTORICAL

For more than a century the giant-cell tumor of bone has called

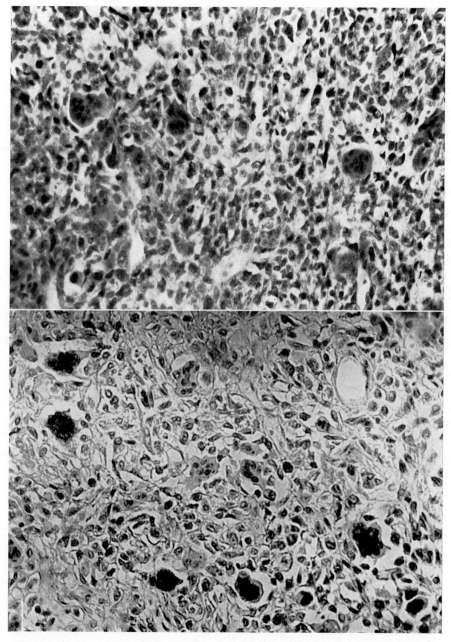

FIGURE 368. A. *(Above)* Giant-cell tumor. Grade III: (Frankly malignant.) The stroma is sarcomatous resembling fibrosarcoma, stromal cells are large, atypism is diffuse, and mitotic figures numerous. Giant cells are smaller, fewer in number, and tend to show the same anaplastic changes seen in the stromal cells. These tumors are painful. Severe pain in a giant cell tumor is an ominous sign. B. *(Below)* From a pulmonary metastasis of a malignant giant cell tumor.

forth unending investigations and speculation regarding its true character. To this day there is a group of investigators who deny that this lesion is a neoplasm; to this group the lesion is a post-traumatic reparative granuloma.

Warren (1837) described giant-cell tumors of the femur, tibia and jaws. In 1845 Lebert separated carcinomas from sarcomas and described giant-cell tumors, noting their large giant cells and benign character. Paget (1853) employed the term "myeloid tumors" to designate what we now call giant-cell tumors. It was Paget's opinion that this lesion is a benign neoplasm which, in some instances, undergoes malignant transformation. Virchow did not concur, contending that most giant-cell tumors are malignant.

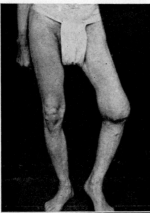

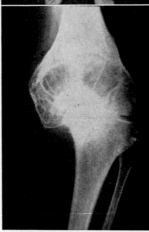

FIGURE 369. Giant-cell tumor of the lower femur with collapse of the articular cortex and loss of the medial cartilage space (40 years duration—age of patient, 75 years).

Nélation (1863) gave the first comprehensive report of both the gross and microscopic characteristics of giant-cell tumors; however his follow-up study was brief and incomplete. Gross accurately analyzed a series of 70 cases in 1879 but the widespread practice of treating these tumors by amputation persisted. During the second and third decades of this century, Bloodgood waged a country-wide crusade for the recognition of giant-cell tumors as benign lesions. He urged that the term giant-cell tumor replace the older term, giant-cell sarcoma.

In more recent years the subject of the giant-cell tumor has been elucidated by such investigators as Ewing, Stewart, Stout, Jaffe, Lichtenstein and Portis, and Geschickter and Copeland.

ETIOLOGY

The etiology of giant-cell tumors, although extensively investigated, remains unknown. Etiologic theories explain the lesion as a reparative response to trauma, as a neoplasm, as a hyperparathyroid disturbance, and as a chronic inflammation.

Trauma

Mallory, Konjetzny, Pommer, and Lubarsch looked upon the giant-cell tumor, not as a neoplasm, but as an exaggerated reparative response to trauma. An area of traumatic osseous necrosis and associated hematoma is said to become the site of an excessive concentration of osteoclasts, endothelial monocytes, and granulation tissue. Konjetzny's ex-

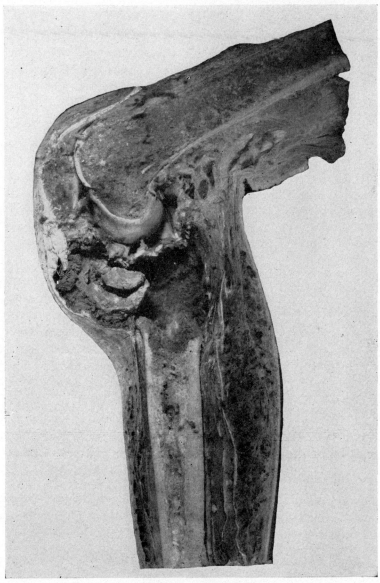

FIGURE 370. Giant-cell tumor of the upper tibia with collapse of the tibial plateau. (Courtesy, *Army Institute of Pathology*, Acc. No. 30642.)

perimental intramedullary hematomas developed a superficial histologic resemblance to giant-cell tumors during their reparative stage.

Even among investigators who consider the giant-cell tumor to be a true blastoma there are many who believe that trauma in some manner plays an important part in the etiology. Geschickter and Copeland contend that, following trauma to the epiphyseal cortex, there is abnormal hyperplasia of osteoclasts during the process of osteoclastic resorption of the necrotic bone and calcified cartilage.

Neoplasm

The majority of oncologists in this country have viewed the giant-cell tumor as a neoplasm. Those who have thus expressed themselves include Stewart, Coley, Ewing, Bloodgood, Jaffe, Stout, and Geschickter and Copeland.

Hyperparathyroid disturbance: Not a small number of investigators consider the solitary giant-cell tumor to be identical with the brown tumors of hyperparathyroidism. It cannot be denied in some instances that there is a resemblance histologically. However, there are several important differences which have been adequate to convince most observers that brown tumors and giant-cell tumors must be classified separately. A form of parathyroid gland disturbance, not manifest as generalized osteitis fibrosa, has been visualized by Weinmann and Sicher as being the cause of the solitary benign giant-cell tumor.

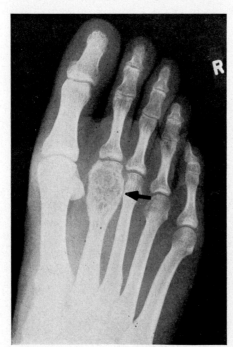

FIGURE 371. *(Continued)* C. Roentgenogram of Figure 371B.

Chronic Inflammation

Giant-cell tumors have been diagnosed as chronic hemorrhagic osteomyelitis in the belief that the underlying pathologic change was a chronic inflammation. This theory is no longer held.

PATHOLOGIC ANATOMY

Skeletal Distribution

An outstanding characteristic of the giant-cell tumor is its disposi-

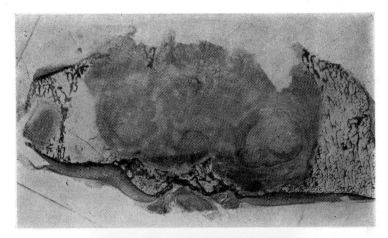

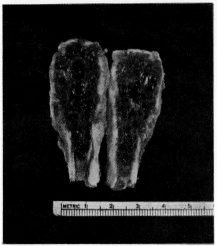

FIGURE 371. A. *(Above)* Giant cell tumor of the upper tibial epiphysis. Histologic section of entire tumor. B. *(Below)* Giant cell tumor of second metatarsal.

tion to develop within epiphyses of the long tubular bones, particularly the distal epiphyses of the femur and radius, and the proximal epiphysis of the tibia (Figs. 369 to 374). No bone that develops on the basis of enchondral ossification is immune. Other locations of the tumor include the pelvis, vertebrae, humeri, and the metatarsals. When giant-cell tumors have developed in the skull it generally has been in those

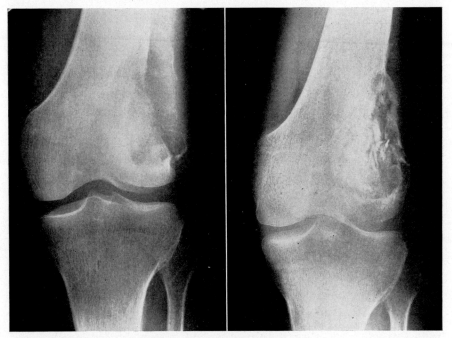

FIGURE 372. Giant-cell tumor of the lateral femoral condyle. A. *(Left)* Pre-operative roentgenogram. B. *(Right)* Roentgenogram taken six months after curettage and insertion of bone chips.

bones that were preformed of cartilage, the most frequent site being in the mandible.

Gross Pathology

A giant-cell tumor is soft, friable, and vascular. The striking multi-colored appearance of the tumor on cross section is the result of small areas of hemorrhage in various states of organization. Blood and blood pigments are responsible for the coloring of the red, brown, and green areas. Areas of fibrosis are gray to white, and areas of necrosis are usually yellow. Fibrous or fibro-osseous strands extend from the periphery across the tumor in numerous directions partitioning the tumor mass into many segments. Except for trabeculae of fibrous bone in the fibrous strands or areas of fibrosis where the bone is protected from the tumor tissue, bone does not form within the tumor. It is rare for the stroma of the tumor to form even microscopic areas of bone. If a material amount of bone is being formed by or in the tumor tissue the lesion is probably an ossifying fibroma, fibrous dysplasia, or an osteoblastic sarcoma.

Several small cysts or a large solitary cyst may be identified within the tumor and probably represent areas of liquid necrosis. Small cysts are common in younger tumors, and large cysts more often observed after radiation therapy.

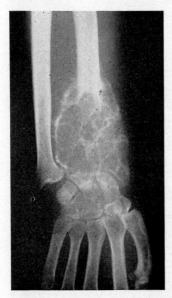

FIGURE 373. Giant-cell tumor of the distal radius showing the much-described "soap bubble" trabeculations.

A capsule does not envelop giant-cell tumors; tumor tissue simply ends abruptly at its marrow or bony margin. Reactive marrow fibrosis is generally found in a narrow zone adjacent to the tumor, but this should not be mistaken for tumor capsule.

The overlying bony cortex is ordinarily described as expanded. This should not be interpreted to mean that the cortex is stretched to accommodate the enlarging tumor. Actually the old cortex is absorbed and the thin "expanded" margin of bone over the tumor represents periosteal new bone layed down in response to tumor growth, and presumably to preserve continuity in the host bone. Penetration and destruction of all overlying bone has occurred in some of the larger and more aggressive tumors.

Pathologic fractures occur in about one-sixth of the cases; it seems surprising that this incidence is not higher.

Microscopic Pathology

GIANT CELLS: The histopathology of giant-cell tumors has long intrigued investigators (Figs. 366 to 369). Numerous large multinucleated giant-cells form the most prominent part of the picture. The largest and most numerous giant cells ever observed are seen in giant-cell tumors. Ten to two-hundred nuclei fill the central portion or the entire cell, and in general, the larger the number of nuclei the larger the cell. Giant-cell nuclei resemble the stromal cell nuclei. It is usually true that the more numerous the giant-cells, the greater the proportion of round cells to spindle cells in the stroma. It is widely believed that the giant-cells originate by a fusion of a group of stromal cells. There are numerous exceptions, but most of the giant-cells of fibrous osteitis, osteoblastic sarcoma, and brown tumors are smaller than those of giant-cell tumors.

Until recently the giant cells were considered to be the more important part of the tumor. Jaffe and others have drawn attention to evidence that it is the stroma that holds the key to the tumor's true character.

STROMA: The stroma cells deserve to be examined with much care. Their nuclei are round or oval and there is a central nucleolus. The cytoplasm forms only a narrow peripheral zone which is polygonal, oval, or spindle-shaped and frequently has a poorly defined cell wall. There is wide variation in the proportion of rounded to spindle cells, but in most instances the spindle cells are dominant. Little collagenous differentiation is seen.

Grading of the stroma: Grading to indicate the degree of benignancy or aggressiveness of giant-cell tumors has been proposed by Ewing, Goforth, Jaffe et al., and Stewart et al. While no method of grading is entirely reliable, much worth-while information can be gained. The

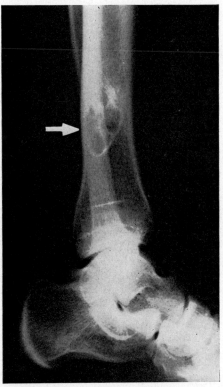

FIGURE 374. Non-osteogenic fibroma of the tibia. A. Lateral roentgenogram of an 18 year old male. This tumor was originally diagnosed as a solitary xanthoma.

three grades outlined by Jaffe, Lichtenstein, and Portis will be reviewed here. Since it is a common experience to identify more than one grade in different fields of the same tumor, it is recommended that "the most ominous-appearing field" be used as the basis for formulating treatment and rendering a prognosis.

Grade I: This group is said to make up about one-half of the giant-cell tumors. There are numerous large giant-cells in virtually all fields and their nuclei are similar to the nuclei of the stromal cells (Fig. 366). The stromal cells are predominantly spindle-shaped, are not compact, show very few mitoses, and no atypism. Stromal cells should be examined under high power.

Grade I giant-cell tumors are clearly benign but when not completely removed tend to recur. With proper local initial treatment the prognosis is good.

Grade II: This group is neither entirely benign nor frankly malignant (Fig. 367). There is a decided tendency toward recurrence, and recurrent masses may ultimately undergo malignant transformation.

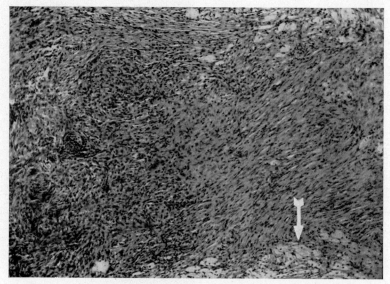

FIGURE 374. *(Continued)* Photomicrograph of a typical field. Nests of foam cells (arrow) frequently are a part of the microscopic picture.

Stromal cells are quite compact and may present a whorled arrangement. There is definite atypism varying from slight to a point just short of the degree characteristic of frank malignancy. Scattered mitoses are seen and a few of the stroma cells have either two nuclei or enlarged nuclei. Nuclei of the giant-cells show the same atypism observed in the stromal cell nuclei.

Grade III: This is the small group of giant-cell tumors in which the stroma is sarcomatous and is "frankly and obviously malignant" (Fig. 368). Stromal cells are large, show diffuse atypism, and many mitotic figures. The giant cells are diminished in number, contain few nuclei and show the same anaplastic changes seen in the stromal cells.

Cases have been reported in which the giant-cell tumor transformed slowly from Grade I or Grade II to Grade III; in other reported instances the tumor has been malignant from the outset.

Histological Differential Diagnosis

Giant-cell tumors must be differentiated from lesions characterized by a fibroblastic stroma infiltrated by multinucleated giant cells. These lesions include the brown tumors of hyperparathyroidism, fibrous dysplasia, eosinophilic granuloma, and the lining membrane of solitary bone cysts.

Fibrous dysplasia: Fibrous bone and a more fibrous (more collagenous) stroma are a consistent part of fibrous dysplasia, neither of which appear to any appreciable degree in giant-cell tumors. Giant cells, when present in fibrous dysplasia, are smaller and more scattered than those of giant-cell tumors.

Eosinophilic granuloma: This and others of the group of reticulo-endothelioses may possess areas of a fibroblastic stroma infiltrated by fairly large multinucleated giant-cells. However, in most areas the eosinophils, reticulocytes and foam cells clearly distinguish these lesions from giant-cell tumors. It deserves to be emphasized that when a lesion presents numerous fields of a fibroblastic stroma that contain few or no giant-cells, that lesion very likely is not giant-cell tumor, even though other fields may show numerous giant-cells.

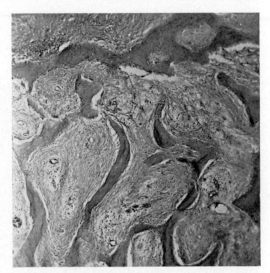

FIGURE 375. Ossifying fibroma. Photomicrograph of a histologic section of a small maxillary fibroma. The fibrous tissue of the tumor is producing fibrous bone trabeculae.

Solitary bone cysts: The lining membrane of a solitary bone cyst may possess a fibrous or fibroblastic stroma and scattered giant-cells. The stroma cells are generally smaller than those of a giant-cell tumor, and there is more collagen. Giant-cells are less numerous in the lining of a solitary cyst and it is quite common for the lining membrane to show a zone of primitive bone trabeculae.

Osteoblastic sarcoma: The osteoid and tumor bone in an osteoblastic sarcoma is usually the most important point upon which this tumor is differentiated from a malignant giant-cell tumor. Both tumors may have scattered small tumor giant-cells and a few large multinucleated phagocytic giant cells.

ROENTGENOGRAPHIC CORRELATION

Contrary to widespread belief, there are no pathognomonic roent-genographic portrayals of giant-cell tumors. The much described "soap-bubble" tumor of adult epiphyses generally proves to be a giant-cell tumor, but there have been abundant instances when an entirely dif-ferent lesion was responsible for the "soap-bubble" trabeculations. Other tumors that have caused such an appearance include chondromas, angiomas, and fibrous dysplasia.

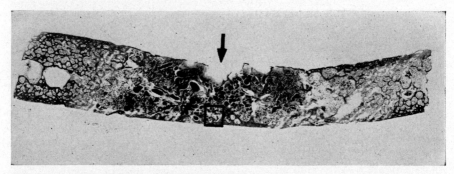

FIGURE 376. Cavernous hemangioma of the skull. A. Histologic section of the tumor (arrow).

When a giant-cell tumor is visualized by the roentgen-ray prior to late stages, the tumor is found to occupy an eccentric position, not central. A number of giant-cell tumors have been followed from the time of their incipiency until they came to occupy much of the host epiphysis. These cases established the subcortical origin of the tumor. Extension of the tumor mass along lines of least resistance takes the tumor across the cancellous bone of the epiphysis ultimately to occupy virtually the entire epiphysis. Breaks in the peripheral cortex usher the tumor into adjacent soft tissues; breaks in the articular cortex ad-mit the tumor to the joint. Extension into the metaphysis is the rule in sizeable tumors, and this is understandable since this tumor seldom develops until after epiphyseal plates have entirely disappeared.

In a few instances osteolytic carcinoma metastases have developed in epiphyses and resembled giant-cell tumors. Metastases seldom occur in epiphyses, are purely osteolytic, do not expand the cortex, and tend to be multiple.

By the time large brown tumors make their roentgenographic ap-pearance in hyperparathyroidism, there is substantial and often ad-vanced generalized osteoporosis. Skeletal changes in giant-cell tumors are limited to the site of the solitary tumor.

Pathologic fractures occurred in 14 percent of the cases in the series analyzed by Geschickter and Copeland. In the roentgenogram these fractures are found to vary from narrow nondisplaced infractions of the thin overlying cortex to complete collapse and telescoping of the host epiphysis.

CLINICAL CORRELATION

The great majority of giant-cell tumors develop in individuals past 20 years of age, the peak incidence taking place in the third decade. The sex incidence is equally divided.

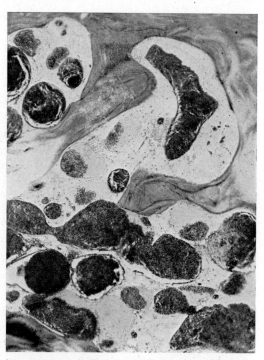

Growth of the tumor is slow, and significant pain may be delayed until the area of osseous destruction has attained considerable size. Expansion of the host bone with palpable enlargement is a relatively late manifestation. A pathologic fracture may be the patient's first warning of the lesion's existence.

As already mentioned, a history of previous trauma to the site of the tumor is encountered so frequently that many investigators have concluded that trauma is the principal etiologic fac-

FIGURE 376. *(Continued)* B. Photomicrograph of the area in the square marked on A.

tor. However, many patients with a giant-cell tumor give no convincing history of having experienced specific trauma. If trauma were the principal cause of this lesion, there should be instances in which giant-cell tumors followed a fracture of epiphyses.

Therapy

Proper treatment for a given giant-cell tumor can be outlined only after a careful study of the histopathology of the tumor. Such a study can seldom be carried out on the material available from a punch biopsy. A thorough local excision by curettage followed by packing the cavity with bone chips is the treatment of choice when the tumor is at an easily accessible location, as is usually the case. In giant-cell tumors of the lower one-third of the femur, Johnson and Lyford recommend curettage followed by telescoping of the tumor site to diminish the size of the cavity and thereby hasten solid bony bridging. Giant-cell tumors of the radius, lower ulna, upper fibula, and bones of the hands and feet are best treated by excision of the entire area of involvement or the entire bone. Replacement of the area of resection is frequently indicated. If a detailed microscopic study of tissue reveals

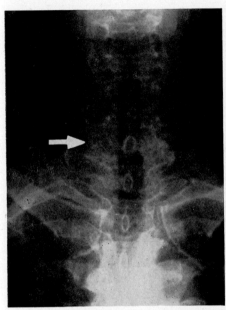

a grade II tumor, a recurrence of the growth must be anticipated. Such a recurrent tumor often requires either a more radical local excision or an amputation. If the histologic analysis discloses areas of frankly malignant stroma, an amputation must be considered whenever the tumor is in an extremity.

Intense roentgen therapy is most useful in the treatment of those patients in whom the tumor is surgically inaccessible. Roentgen radiation in small and inadequate dosage is condemned on the basis of considerable evidence that, far from killing all of the tumor cells, the radiation actually stimulates many of the

FIGURE 377. Hemangioma of the body of the 7th cervical vertebra (arrow).

cells into more active growth and aggressiveness. The administration of roentgen radiation on the basis of the roentgenographic findings alone cannot be justified. An adequate biopsy is essential.

INTRAOSSEOUS FIBROMA

Two types of intraosseous fibroma will be described: (1) Non-osteogenic fibroma, and (2) Ossifying fibroma. Both are benign connective tissue tumors. The entity now known as non-osteogenic fibroma was described in 1942 by Jaffe and Lichtenstein. They have clarified the status of this lesion and have drawn it out of such categories as osteitis fibrosa, solitary xanthoma, xanthic variant of giant-cell tumor, and fibrous osteomyelitis.

Ossifying fibromas rarely occur outside the jaws so are observed principally by dentists and oral surgeons. Lesions in other parts of the skeleton that resemble the ossifying fibroma histologically usually prove to be fibrous dysplasia. It has been claimed that some of the jaw lesions diagnosed as ossifying fibroma are in reality fibrous dysplasia. Schlumberger contends that an ossifying fibroma is indistinguishable histologically from fibrous dysplasia.

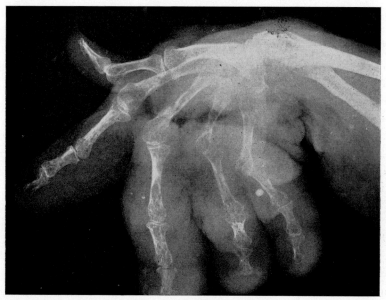

FIGURE 378. Hemangioma of the hand and forearm involving both the soft tissues and the bones.

Both non-osteogenic and ossifying fibromas are entirely benign, and a recurrence has not followed a complete removal of the tumor.

Non-Osteogenic Fibroma

These lesions, as pointed out by Jaffe and Lichtenstein, develop in the shafts of the long bones more frequently in the lower extremities than in the upper and show a preference for the metaphyseal level of the shaft (Fig. 374). In the ten cases presented, the ages were between eight and 16 years and the sexes equally divided.

Grossly

The tumor is loculated, produces an eccentric area of involvement— only rarely producing a fusiform cortical expansion—and is filled with a friable or moderately dense yellowish fibrous tissue. Bony trabeculae form the walls of most of the loculations that are seen both on gross and roentgen examination. Loculations, while nearly always present, are neither as small nor as numerous as those seen in metaphyseal hemangiomas.

Histologically

A non-osteogenic fibroma is characterized by a stroma of relatively small spindle shaped connective tissue cells that have a tendency to form "whorled bundles." Multinucleated giant-cells are seen in many fields, but most of these cells have relatively few nuclei and are located in largest numbers around areas of hemorrhage, signifying a phagocytic function. In approximately one-half of the Jaffe and Lichtenstein series there were groups of foam cells. It is the presence of these lipoid laden cells that has caused these tumors to be classified as solitary xanthomas; and these cells plus the multinucleated giant-cells have been responsible for the diagnosis of xanthic variant of giant-cell tumor. Inflammatory cells have not been observed in this tumor but, notwithstanding this fact, there have been occasions when this tumor has been attributed to an end-stage of a bone abscess.

Ossifying Fibroma

Ossifying fibroma, a term first used by Phemister and Grimson, refers to a rather rare cellular fibroma in which fibrous bone trabeculae are interspersed throughout the tumor tissue (Fig. 375). These tumors occur almost exclusively in the mandible and maxilla, are slow-growing and generally small. While fibromas, both ossifying and non-ossifying, tend to be more cellular than normal connective tissue, the area occupied by the cells seldom is greater than that occupied by the collagenous fibers. When there is little collagen and dense cellularity, a fibrosarcoma must be suspected.

Whereas the bone in an osteoma is of a mature lamellated character, the bone in an ossifying fibroma is fibrous and primitive. The bone trabeculae of an ossifying fibroma may be either small and scattered or continuous and united into a network of cancellous bone.

HEMANGIOMA OF BONE

Hemangioma of bone, a rare tumor clinically, is relatively common pathologically. While observed principally in the vertebral bodies and the skull it also occurs in the metaphyses of the long tubular bones (Figs. 376 to 379). Unlike giant-cell tumors, they do not invade epiphyses and joints. That these tumors frequently exist without causing clinical symptoms is indicated by Topfer's study in which he sectioned

2154 vertebral columns and found hemangiomas in 257 instances (11.93 percent). Most of the tumors were solitary, and nearly all were in vertebral bodies. Bucy and Capp in 1930 collected 47 clinical cases

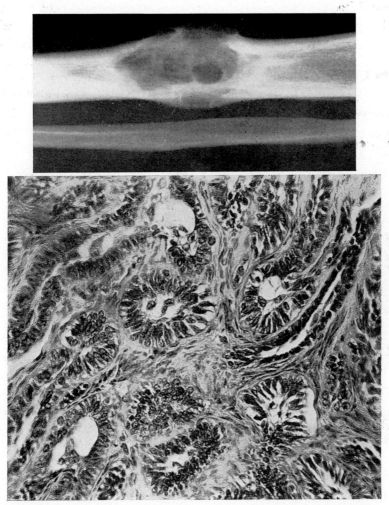

FIGURE 379. Adamantinoma of the tibia. A. *(Above)* Antero-posterior roentgenogram of the middle one-third of the tibia and fibula. B. *(Below)* Photomicrograph of a typical field of enameloblastic epithelium.

of primary hemanigioma of the bones. Ackerman and Hart in 1942 reported a rare case in which there were multiple skeletal hemangiomas of a lower extremity.

PATHOLOGY

Hemangiomas are composed of masses of blood vessels held in a widely variable fibrous stroma (Fig. 376A). Bone adjacent to the tumor is slowly absorbed as the tumor grows. Reactive bony trabeculae generally form and are manifest by many small but dense loculations as in hemangiomas of long bones, or by coarse longitudinal bars when a vertebral body is extensively involved. In rare instances "sun ray" reactive bony trabeculae have been a prominent feature particularly when

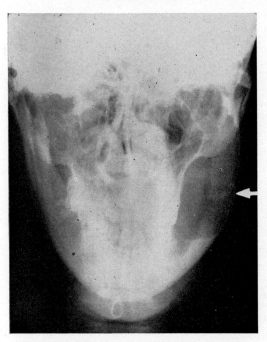

FIGURE 380. Adamantinoma of the mandible (arrow).

a hemangioma involved one of the flat bones. It is the patterns of reactive bone that are responsible for most of the roentgenographic features of these tumors. In rare cases vertebral bodies have undergone pathologic compression from the extensive destruction of both cancellous and compact bone. Extension of the tumor into the vertebral canal has led to spinal cord compression in several of the reported cases. Skull hemangiomas frequently have their origin in adjacent meninges.

Excision of the tumor tissue may be complicated by profuse hemorrhage. Bailey and Bucy reviewed five cases in which a vertebral hemangioma was explored surgically. In three of these cases the patient expired from operative hemorrhage.

Microscopically

The blood vessels form the most prominent portion of the tumor and are cavernous or capillary in type, the former being much the more common. Cavernous vessel spaces generally are filled with blood, lined by a single layer of endothelial cells, and have a scanty, loose connective tissue stroma. A dense fibrous stroma is occasionally associated with capillary hemangiomas. No mitotic figures are seen. A capsule does not form to demarcate the tumor. Scattered groups of fat and foam cells may be identified. Reactive bony trabeculae generally show both osteoblastic and osteoclastic activity at their borders.

THERAPY

Bucy and Capp recommended resection or cauterization when possible, reserving roentgen therapy for the inaccessible tumors. They warned that the spinal cord could be damaged by radiation therapy to vertebral hemangiomas. Radical surgery such as amputation is never

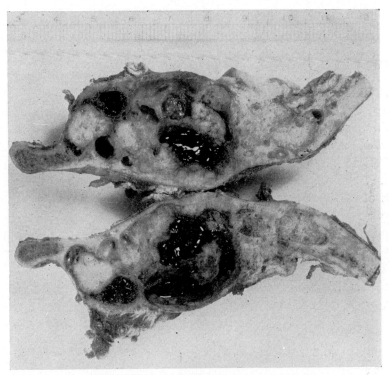

FIGURE 381. Adamantinoma of the mandible. Bisected specimen. (Courtesy, A. Purdy Stout, New York.)

indicated. In the Ackermann and Hart case roentgen therapy caused active osteoblastic activity and replacement of most of the tumor tissue by bone.

ADAMANTINOMA

SYNONYMS

Ameloblastoma (Churchill), adamantoblastoma (Thoma), adamantine epithelioma, epithelial odontoma.

The two most important tumors of dental origin are the adamantinomas and the odontomas. These tumors possess distinctive features that set them apart from all other tumors that occur in the skeletal system. Malassey, in 1885, described adamantinomas and attributed the origin of many of the odontogenic neoplasms to what he termed the "débris paradentaires," also known as epithelial debris of Malassey or simply paradental epithelium. These terms refer to groups of epithelial cells in the foetus that lie at the periphery of the sites at which the teeth are forming. Opinions now vary regarding the proportion of adamantinomas that originate from the débris paradentaires," as compared to those originating from the oral epithelium and from the enamel organ.

PATHOLOGY

A typical adamantinoma is a benign, slow growing central tumor located in the mandible or maxilla in the region of the molar teeth of a middle-aged or young adult (Figs. 380 & 381). The tumor is composed not of enamel as the name implies, but principally of enamel epithelium, and may be cystic or solid, the former being the more common. Over a period of many years the tumor may greatly expand the walls of the involved maxilla, but until the tumor mass becomes very large, a confining bony wall envelops it; after perforation, the adjacent soft tissues are compressed but not invaded. The path of extension may lead the tumor into an antrum, an orbit, or even into the cranial vault.

In several instances adamantinomas have been observed in the tibia (Fig. 379), femur, ovary, and hypophyseal stalk. As yet, no tenable theory has been proposed to explain the presence of the tumor in these locations.

Cystic adamantinomas tend to be more common in the mandible, and the solid type is more often observed in the maxilla. Cysts are unilocular, have smooth walls or walls possessing multiple epithelial papillae.

In the tibia, the tumor is generally diaphyseal, multicystic and is eccentrically positioned.

Histopathology

Epithelial cells constitute the most prominent feature of the microscopic picture (Fig. 379B). These cells differentiate toward either enameloblastic epithelium or squamous epithelium. A vascular fibrous stroma may enclose multiple islands of epithelial cells, or islands of reticulated cells may be surrounded by a layer of columnar enameloblasts. Enameloblasts may form alveoli, small masses, or columns.

Malignant Changes

In rare instances adamantinomas have become malignant and metastasized. Malignant changes take place more frequently in the solid type, and the changes are manifest both in the epithelium and the connective tissue stroma. Recurrences after incomplete removal of the tu-

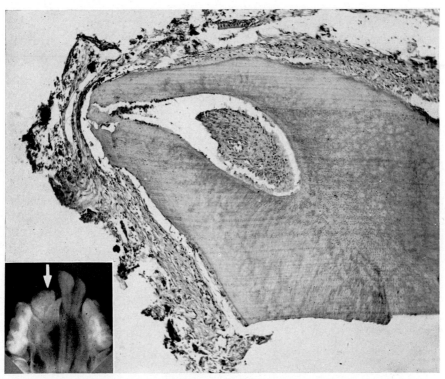

FIGURE 382. Odontoma of the maxilla. Photomicrograph of a denticle from the tumor shown in the roentgenographic insert. (Courtesy, A. Purdy Stout, New York.)

mor tend to undergo malignant transformation. Excision of the original tumor should be thorough in order to prevent dangerous recurrences. Kegel condemns the simple curettage of these tumors on the basis of the high rate of recurrence following this procedure; he recommends a more radical excision.

ODONTOMA

An odontoma is a rare benign dental tumor in which mesenchymal rather than epithelial elements predominate (Figs. 382 & 383). This tumor, nearly always mandibular in location, appears during the first and second decades prior to completion of the second dentition. The origin is from both mesenchymal and epithelial components of the tooth germ, and rarely, as in the case of cementomas, from a portion of the dental follicle. In a sense an odontoma is simply the manifestation of a distorted development of the germ of one or more teeth. It is exceptional for an odontoma to become large and painful. These tumors frequently exist undetected for many years.

PATHOLOGY

Odontomas may be hard or soft, the hard or calcified type acquiring

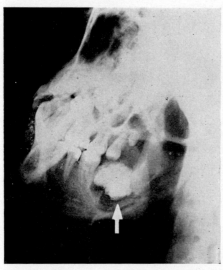

its hardness from variable proportions of enamel, dentine, cementum, and bone. While most hard odontomas contain all of the calcified dental tissues, there are instances in which only one of these tissues forms the tumor, *e.g.*, cementoma, enameloma, and dentinoma. A so-called calcified mixed odontoma contains both rudimentary and well-defined teeth. Teeth may project in all directions from the hard, irregular tumor surface. When the tumor is somewhat less highly differentiated, the enamel, dentine, and cementum may exist in the form of irregular purposeless masses.

FIGURE 383. Odontoma of the mandible. Roentgenogram of the mandible and the tumor (arrow). (Courtesy, *Army Institute of Pathology*, Acc. No. 84173.)

In soft odontomas the tissue is less highly differentiated, and tends to be fibromatous in character with only minimal tooth elements and epithelium. Odontogenic fibrosarcomas are also observed, and are highly malignant.

Soft odontomas have been known to recur after surgical excision, whereas no recurrences have been observed after removal of hard odontomas.

LIPOMA

In only a few instances has a lipoma been identified in a bone. According to Haas these reported lipomas produced no characteristic signs or symptoms. Bartlett has reported two cases of lipoma of the periosteum.

Histologically the picture is that of normal fatty tissue.

MYXOMA OF BONE

Primary myxoma of bone has been reported but there is a reasonable doubt that such a tumor exists. Examination of a small portion of a chondroma has led to the diagnosis of myxoma in instances when only a myxomatous area of the chondroma was studied. Geschickter and Copeland contend that a chondromyxoma goes through a myxomatous stage in its transition from primitive connective tissue to cartilage. It has been long believed that the myxomatous areas in a chondroma represent a regressive or degenerative change in the cartilage.

Myxomatous areas are gelatinous in appearance, resembling Wharton's jelly in the umbilical cord, both grossly and microscopically.

Histologically it is characterized by stellate-shaped cells with dendritic processes in a homogenous mucoid material that takes a pale basophilic stain. While the cell processes may be long and anastomosing, collagenous bundles are absent.

Whenever myxomatous tissue is identified in association with a skeletal lesion great care should be taken to make certain that the tissue is not part of a chondromyxosarcoma, before pronouncing it benign.

REFERENCES

ACKERMANN, A. J. and HART, M. S.: Multiple primary hemangioma of the bones of the extremity. *Am. J. Roentgenol., 48*:47, 1942.

BAILEY, P. and BUCY, P. C.: Cavernous hemangioma of vertebrae. *J. A. M. A., 92*:1748, 1929.

BARTLETT, E. I.: Periosteal lipoma. *Arch. Surg., 21*:1015, 1930.

BELL, A. L.: A case of adamantinoma of the femur. *Brit. J. Surg., 30*:81, 1942.

BLOODGOOD, J. C.: Bone tumors. *Ann. Surg., 80*:817, 1924.

BLOODGOOD, J. C.: The conservative treatment of giant-cell sarcoma. *Ann. Surg., 56*:210, 1912; *69*:345, 1919; *Am. J. Surg., 37*:105, 1923.

BUCY, P. C. and CAPP, C. S.: Primary hemangioma of bone. *Am. J. Roentgenol., 22*:1, 1930.

CHURCHILL, H. R.: Histological differentiation between certain dentigerous cysts and ameloblastoma. *Dental Cosmos, 74*:1173, 1934.

CODMAN, E. A.: Epiphyseal chondromatous giant-cell tumors of upper end of humerus. *Surg., Gynec. & Obst., 52*:543, 1931.

COLEY, WILLIAM B.: Malignant changes in the so-called benign giant-cell tumor. *Am. J. Surg., 28*:768, 1935.

EWING, J.: *Neoplastic Diseases.* W. B. Saunders Co., Philadelphia, 1942.

FINCH, E. F. and GLEAVE, H. H.: A case of osteoclastoma with pulmonary metastasis. *J. Path. & Bact., 29*:399, 1926.

GESCHICKTER, C. F. and MASSERITZ, I. H.: Primary hemangioma involving bones of the extremities. *J. Bone & Joint Surg., 20*:888, 1938.

GESCHICKTER, C. F. and COPELAND, M. M.: Tumors of the bone. *Am. J. Cancer,* 1936.

GESCHICKTER, C. F. and COPELAND, M. M.: Recurrent and so-called metastatic giant-cell tumor. *Arch. Surg., 20*:713, 1930.

GOFORTH, J. L.: Giant-cell tumor of bone. *Arch. Surg., 13*:846, 1926.

HAAS, S. L.: Lipoma of bones. *Dean Lewis Practice of Surgery,* Vol. II, page 15. W. F. Prior Co., 1927.

Hempstead, B. E.: Osteomas of paranasal sinuses and the mastoid process. *J. A. M. A.,* *111*:1273, 1938.

Hitzrot, J. M.: Hemangioma cavernosum of bone. *Ann. Surg., 65*:476, 1917.

Jaffe, H. L.: Osteoid osteoma. *Arch. Surg., 31*:709, 1935.

Jaffe, H. L., Lichtenstein, L., and Portis, R.: Giant-cell tumors of bone. *Arch Path., 30*:993, 1940.

Jaffe, H. L. and Lichtenstein, L.: Non-osteogenic fibroma of bone. *Am. J. Path., 18*:205, 1942.

Jaffe, H. L. and Lichtenstein, L.: Benign chondroblastoma of bone. A reinterpretation of the so-called calcifying or chondromatous giant-cell tumor. *Am. J. Path., 18*:969, 1942.

Jaffe, H. L. and Lichtenstein, L.: Osteoid osteoma. Further experience with this benign tumor of bone. *J. Bone & Joint Surg., 22*:645, 1940.

Jansen, M.: Dissociation of bone growth (exostoses and enchondromata) or Ollier's dyschondroplasia and associated phenomena in *Rob't. Jones Birthday Volume.* Oxford Univ. Press, London, 1928.

Johnson, R. W. and Lyford, J.: Treatment of giant-cell tumor in lower third of femur by curettage and telescoping fragment of bone. *J. Bone & Joint Surg., 27*:557, 1945.

Kegel, R. F. C.: Adamantine epithelioma. *Arch. Surg., 25*:498, 1932.

Konjetzny, C. E.: Die sogenannte "lokalisierte ostitis fibrosa." *Arch. f. klin. Chir., 121*:467, 1922.

Lebert, H.: *Physiologie pathologique.* Balliére, Paris 2:120, 1853.

Lubarsch, O.: Lokalisierte ostitis fibrosa. *Arch. f. klin. Chir., 121*:147, 1922.

Luck, J. V.: Correlation of roentgenogram and pathologic changes in ossifying and chondrifying primary osteogenic neoplasms. *Radiology, 40*:253, 1943.

Malassey, M. L.: Sur le rôle des débris epithélieux paradentaires. *Arch. de physiol., 6*:379, 1855.

Mallory, F. B.: Giant-cell sarcoma. *J. Med. Res., 24*:463, 1911.

Myerding, H. W.: Giant-cell tumor of the femur. *S. Clin. N. Am., 15*:1207, 1935.

Myerding, H. W.: Exostosis. *Radiology, 8*:282, 1927.

Nelaton, E.: *Tumeurs á myeloplaxes.* Paris, 1860.

Orr, J. W.: Malignant osteoclastoma. *J. Path. & Bact., 34*:265, 1931.

Paget, J.: *Lectures on Surgical Pathology,* 3rd ed. page 544. Lindsay and Blakiston. Philadelphia, 1871.

Phemister, D. B. and Grimson, K. S.: Fibrous osteoma of the jaws. *Ann. Surg., 105*:564, 1937.

Platt, H.: Giant-cell tumor of bone. *Surg., Gynec. & Obst., 60*:318, 1935.

Pommer, G.: Zur kenntnis der progressiven. Hämaton und Phleamasieveränderungen der Röhrenknochen. *Arch. f. Orthop., 17*:17, 1919.

Schlumberger, H. G.: Fibrous dysplasia of single bones. (Monostotic fibrous dysplasia.) *Mil. Surg., 99*:504, 1946.

Schramm, G.: Pathogenesis of cartilaginous exostosis and enchondromas. *Arch. f. orthop. u. Unfall-Chir., 27*:421, 1929.

Stewart, F. W., Coley, B. L., and Farrow, J. H.: Malignant giant-cell tumor of bone. *Am. J. Path., 14*:515, 1938.

Stone, W. S. and Ewing, J.: An unusual alteration in the natural history of a giant cell tumor of bone. *Arch. Surg., 7*:280, 1923.

Thoma, K. H.: *Clinical Pathology of the Jaws.* Charles C Thomas, Springfield, 1934.

Topfer, D.: Uber ein infiltriend wachsendes Hamangiom. *Frankfurt Ztsch. f. Path., 36*:337, 1928.

Weinmann, J. P. and Sicher, H.: *Bone and Bones.* Fundamentals of bone biology. C. V. Mosby Co., St. Louis, 1947.

Worth, H. M.: Tumors of the jaw. *Brit. J. Radiol., 10*:223, 1937.

CHAPTER XIX

Malignant Primary Tumors of Bones

Contents

HISTORICAL

"The malignant tumors of bone constitute one of the most important departments of oncology"—Ewing.

Much progress has been made in recent years in the organization and understanding of this long neglected subject.

It was not until 1845 that Lebert, in a histologic study, separated skeletal carcinomatous metastases from the bone sarcomas. In Europe all of the primary bone malignancies long were grouped together under the term osteosarcoma.

Much was accomplished by the oncologist, Ewing, and the surgeon, Bloodgood, in their efforts to better coordinate the laboratory and clinical aspects of bone tumors. Perhaps the greatest contribution to the organization and understanding of this subject has been Codman's Registry of Bone Sarcoma, created in 1920 by the American College of Surgeons. The vast material of the Registry has been extensively studied by such investigators as Codman, Ewing, Kolodny, Geschickter and Copeland, and MacDonald and Budd.

Etiology

Notwithstanding the magnitude of the numerous investigations on this subject, the etiology of the malignant bone tumors remains unknown. Our knowledge of the etiology has lagged far behind our knowledge of the gross and histologic structure of these tumors. Of the numerous etiologic theories, some are tenable and possess practical value, others are pure scholastic invention.

The explanation of bone tumors on the basis of cell rests of embryonic and adult cells has been popular. But after a careful analysis of the evidence, Ewing stated: "It must be admitted that the existence of isolated cell groups as the source of many sarcomas has not been proved."

Growth restraint was assumed by Kolodny to exist and to be an important specific factor in preventing neoplastic proliferation. Insufficient growth restraint is sometimes seen in reparative proceses to the end that the repair becomes intensely accelerated beyond the purposeful response associated with normal tissue repair.

The existence of a constitutional predisposition has been strongly suggested on occasion. Hereditary etiologic factors have unquestionably been observed in certain tumors.

Evidence that bone sarcomas are the direct or indirect result of parasitic invaders is controversial and unconvincing. Thus far, microorganisms have not been cultured from the skeletal malignancies.

Brunschwig and Bissell produced osteogenic sarcomas experimentally by using radium, X-radiation, and carcinogenic chemicals. It has been shown experimentally that many of the carcinogenic chemicals produce a carcinoma when applied to an epithelial surface, and a sarcoma when placed beneath the epithelium. Radium poisoning as a basis for the development of osteogenic sarcoma was described in Chapter XVIII.

Trauma is widely believed to be an aggravating or precipitating factor in the etiology of many bone malignancies. According to Moore, 22 to 40 percent of the patients with a bone sarcoma give a history of recent trauma. Haas has set down the following criteria which in his opinion must be present in the case in order to consider the traumatic factor to be of etiologic significance:

1. Definite proof of a trauma of sufficient degree to produce tissue injury in the region in which the tumor was found.

2. No gross lesion found at the time of the accident and no previous injury or disease in the same region.

3. Sufficient time must have elapsed from the time of the injury to allow for the growth of the tumor to the size it had attained when first recognized. The period would be less in a superficial bone than it would be in a deep bone.

4. Definite signs of tissue disturbances should persist from the time of injury to the time of development of the tumor.

Let us hope that the etiology of malignancies will become known in the not too distant future. In all probability, neoplasms of different types will prove to have different etiologic factors.

PATHOGENESIS

ORIGIN

The site of origin of a primary skeletal malignancy may be clearly evident, particularly in early stages, or, as is so frequently true in advanced stages, the site of origin can only be surmised. Tumors of peripheral origin tend to extend into the medullary canal and central tumors tend to expand and perforate the overlying cortex. The tissue of origin of a given tumor may be reflected in the tumor cells and in their arrangement. In poorly differentiated tumors, however, the tissue of origin may be deeply obscured.

GROWTH

Growth of most primary bone malignancies, particularly the chondrosarcomas, is by expansion, not by infiltration that characterizes carcinomas.

Numerous observers have noted that osteogenic sarcomas have alternating periods of aggressive growth and relative quiescence. Reviews of the Registry's osteogenic sarcomas disclosed that the period from the onset of symptoms to the time of surgery was greater in the "cured" cases than in the "uncured." This observation was interpreted by Ferguson to mean that amputations carried out early were performed, in most instances, during an actively growing period of the tumor, thus favoring a fatal course. He recommended that amputations be deferred until a period of quiescence. There were numerous objectors to the Ferguson interpretation. MacDonald and Budd "prefer to believe" that the more highly malignant osteogenic sarcomas grow more rapidly and therefore produce earlier symptoms and undergo early metastasis.

BLOOD SUPPLY

Most sarcomas have an abundant blood supply, an exception being the sclerosing areas of osteosarcomas. Primary bone tumors build upon a scaffold of blood vessels. These vessels are acquired from invaded tissues and from the tumor tissue. Tumor cells frequently may be seen lining blood vessels and sinusoids. Both the pattern and the path of the tumor are determined in great part by the blood vessels acquired or produced by the tumor.

In bone-forming tumors the greater the vascularity the less dense the tumor bone. A vascular bone tumor also causes increased vascularity of the adjacent area of the host bone, and thereby causes localized deossification of the host bone. Hemorrhages into the tumor tissue are commonplace and may give rise to hematomas and areas of degeneration and necrosis. Hematomas and areas of necrosis are replaced by either fibrous connective tissue or tumor tissue.

The path of the tumors' spread is both along and within blood vessels. With blood vessels forming the most important part of the stroma it is remarkable that hematogenous metastases do not occur earlier and more frequently than is observed. Primary malignant bone tumors do not possess a network of lymphatics. In only occasional instances have these tumors spread along lymph channels.

ROENTGEN-RAY FEATURES

The roentgenologic and gross pictures of a malignant bone tumor depend upon the relative degree of osteolytic activity and, on the other hand, upon the extent of calcification and ossification. In the osteogenic sarcomas the processes of calcification and ossification may be both neoplastic and reactive, with one or the other predominant. The endotheliomas and myelomas form no neoplastic bone, but are generally characterized by small or extensive amounts of reactive bone. Osteolytic lesions are more common than bone and cartilage-forming lesions and ordinarily are more difficult to interpret roentgenographically.

CLASSIFICATION

The committee of the Registry of Bone Sarcoma, under the chairmanship of James Ewing, submitted a classification of malignant primary bone tumors in 1928, and a revised classification in 1939.

In the revised classification of 1939 the committee classified the chondrosarcomas as a special group of tumors separate from osteogenic sarcomas, recognized reticulum cell lymphosarcoma as a separate entity, and removed liposarcoma from the myeloma series.

The Registry committee's classification, while admittedly imperfect, has been an invaluable guide to pathologists, clinicians, and roentgenologists, as well as a stimulus to oncologists. As was anticipated there have been numerous disagreements and modifications. Considerable confusion has centered around the term osteogenic in that some have interpreted it to mean bone forming and others, to mean originating in bone. Ewing, in creating the term, emphasized that it means "originating in bone." While bone formation occurs frequently in the osteogenic sarcomas it is in no way an essential characteristic.

There is general agreement on the committee's designation of most bone tumors on the basis of their histogenesis. But considerable controversy has arisen from the use of the pathologic anatomy for naming the subvarieties under osteogenic sarcoma. There are no reliable gross pathologic or roentgenographic features that set the "periosteal" type of osteogenic sarcoma apart from the "subperiosteal and medullary" type. **Codman, Kolodny, Geschickter and Copeland, Budd and MacDonald**

REVISED CLASSIFICATION OF BONE TUMORS — 1939

(Registry of Bone Sarcoma)

	MALIGNANT	BENIGN

1. Osteogenic series
   Osteogenic sarcoma
	1. Medullary and subperiosteal
	2. Telangiectatic
	3. Sclerosing
	4. Periosteal
	5. Fibrosarcoma
	   (a) Medullary
	   (b) Periosteal
	6. Parosteal, capsular
		1. Exostosis
		2. Osteoma

2. Chondroma series	1. Chondrosarcoma 2. Myxosarcoma	1. Chondroma

3. Giant cell tumor series	1. Malignant	1. Benign
		2. Epiphyseal
		   giant cell
		   tumor

4. Angioma series	1. Angio-endothelioma	1. Cavernous
		   angioma
		2. Plexiform
		   angioma

5. Myeloma series	1. Plasma cell 2. Myelocytoma 3. Erythroblastoma 4. Lymphocytoma	
6. Reticulum cell lympho- sarcoma 7. Liposarcoma		

and others have preferred to forego the anatomic subdivision of osteogenic sarcoma.

Budd and MacDonald modified portions of the Registry classification. They retained chondrosarcoma with the osteogenic series and emphasized the importance of fibrosarcoma of bone. Osteoblastic osteogenic sarcoma, both sclerosing and osteolytic, was designated as osteosarcoma in order to match the terms used for the other two connective tissue sarcomas, chondrosarcoma and fibrosarcoma. This term, osteosarcoma, may be confusing to certain Europeans in that, as already mentioned, it was long used by them as a group term in referring to virtually all bone sarcomas.

Parosteal osteogenic sarcomas are not admitted to osteogenic status. Telangiectatic and sclerosing sarcomas are considered to be osteolytic and the sclerosing types of osteosarcoma in view of the fact that detailed studies have disclosed both sclerosing and osteolytic areas at some stage in the natural history of nearly all of these tumors. All degrees of vascularity exist from the relative avascularity of sclerosing areas to the rich vascularity of a pulstating, aneurysm-like telangiectatic area.

MODIFIED CLASSIFICATION OF BONE TUMORS (BUDD AND MACDONALD)

TYPE TISSUE	MALIGNANT	BENIGN
1. Connective	Osteosarcoma) osteogenic Chondrosarcoma) sarcoma Fibrosarcoma)	Osteoma Chondroma
2. Undetermined	Malignant giant cell tumor	Benign giant cell tumor Epyphyseal chondromatous giant cell tumor
3. Endothelial	(a) Angio-endothelioma (b) Diffuse endothelioma (Ewing sarcoma)	(a) Plexiform angioma (b) Cavernous angioma

4. Hematopoietic
    Erythropoietic
    Myeloid
    Lymphoid
	(a) Erythrocytoma
	(b) Myelocytoma; myeloma
	(c) Lymphocytoma
	(d) Reticulocytoma	

5. Adipose	Liposarcoma	

DIAGNOSIS

Christensen compiled a table of the distribution of 1000 bone tumors. In his series as well as in all other such studies the lower femur and upper tibia have proved to be the sites most frequently involved by practically all malignant bone tumors. Next in order is the upper humerus. In addition to favoring these sites, the giant-cell tumor also has a predelection for the distal radial epiphysis. As a generalization it can be stated that osteogenic sarcomas attack the tubular bone metaphyses, giant-cell tumors the epiphyses, endotheliomas the shafts, and myelomas the flat bones. Of course, the myelomas are the only malignant primary bone tumors in which multiple tumors are the rule. Age incidence may be generalized by stating that osteogenic sarcomas and endotheliomas are most frequently observed during the second decade, giant-cell tumors, the third decade; and myelomas the fourth and fifth decades.

The sex incidence is approximately equal except for a higher rate of occurrence in males in the instances of the osteogenic sarcoma series and Ewing's tumor.

BIOPSIES

Biopsies are indispensable to the proper management of the primary bone malignancies. Biopsies have been avoided in many instances because of a fear that the tumor would be disseminated. However, no convincing evidence has as yet been brought forth to indicate that the procedure of taking biopsies alters the incidence or time of occurrence of metastases. Under no circumstance should a multilating type of operation be performed without first having a microscopic study to corroborate clinical and roentgenographic diagnosis.

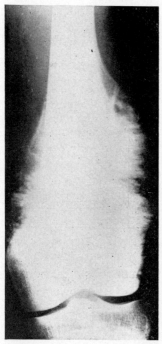

FIGURE 384. Sclerosing type of osteosarcoma of the lower femur showing a sun-ray pattern in the tumor bone and prominent Codman triangles of reactive bone.

Roentgenologists generally can make a diagnosis of osteogenic sarcoma with reasonable accuracy, but it is not possible to identify the subtype with regularity. The diagnosis of Ewing's tumor frequently has been based upon the response of the tumor to X-radiation, and a biopsy study considered unnecessary. This practice may have a defense in typical and advanced Ewing tumors, but to apply this method to other malignant tumors cannot be justified. MacDonald and Budd have stated the case well: "To employ intensive irradiation of bone lesions on roentgenographic evidence alone is an unwarranted intellectual obeisance to a fallible diagnostic measure."

An accurate microscopic diagnosis in osteogenic sarcoma is of value, not only as a guide to therapy, but as a basis for establishing the prognosis. MacDonald and Budd reviewed 118 of the Registry cases in which there was a five-year cure. Only 11.8 percent of the cases were osteosarcoma, thus emphasizing that this is the most highly malignant member of the osteogenic series. Chondrosarcoma accounted for 47.5 percent of the cases and fibrosarcoma, 31.4 percent. In a review of 47 fatal cases, 40 percent were osteosarcoma, 40 percent chondrosarcoma, and 15 percent fibrosarcoma.

Differential Diagnosis

This subject will be discussed in more detail when individual tumors are described. Bone tumors must be differentiated from syphilitic, tuberculous, and pyogenic osteomyelitic lesions. The Wasserman and tuberculin tests together with blood studies and generalized skeletal bone malignancies. Biopsies have been avoided in many instances because of a fear that the tumor would be disseminated. However, no convincing evidence has as yet been brought forth to indicate that the procedure of taking biopsies alters the incidence or time of occurrence of metastases. Under no circumstance should a multilating type of operation be performed without first having a microscopic study to corroborate clinical and roentgenographic diagnosis.

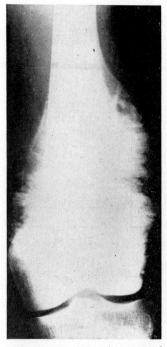

FIGURE 384. Sclerosing type of osteosarcoma of the lower femur showing a sun-ray pattern in the tumor bone and prominent Codman triangles of reactive bone.

Roentgenologists generally can make a diagnosis of osteogenic sarcoma with reasonable accuracy, but it is not possible to identify the subtype with regularity. The diagnosis of Ewing's tumor frequently has been based upon the response of the tumor to X-radiation, and a biopsy study considered unnecessary. This practice may have a defense in typical and advanced Ewing tumors, but to apply this method to other malignant tumors cannot be justified. MacDonald and Budd have stated the case well: "To employ intensive irradiation of bone lesions on roentgenographic evidence alone is an unwarranted intellectual obeisance to a fallible diagnostic measure."

An accurate microscopic diagnosis in osteogenic sarcoma is of value, not only as a guide to therapy, but as a basis for establishing the prognosis. MacDonald and Budd reviewed 118 of the Registry cases in which there was a five-year cure. Only 11.8 percent of the cases were osteosarcoma, thus emphasizing that this is the most highly malignant member of the osteogenic series. Chondrosarcoma accounted for 47.5 percent of the cases and fibrosarcoma, 31.4 percent. In a review of 47 fatal cases, 40 percent were osteosarcoma, 40 percent chondrosarcoma, and 15 percent fibrosarcoma.

DIFFERENTIAL DIAGNOSIS

This subject will be discussed in more detail when individual tumors are described. Bone tumors must be differentiated from syphilitic, tuberculous, and pyogenic osteomyelitic lesions. The Wasserman and tuberculin tests together with blood studies and generalized skeletal exist from the relative avascularity of sclerosing areas to the rich vascularity of a pulstating, aneurysm-like telangiectatic area.

MODIFIED CLASSIFICATION OF BONE TUMORS (BUDD AND MACDONALD)

TYPE TISSUE	MALIGNANT	BENIGN
1. Connective	Osteosarcoma) osteogenic Chondrosarcoma) sarcoma Fibrosarcoma)	Osteoma Chondroma
2. Undetermined	Malignant giant cell tumor	Benign giant cell tumor Epyphyseal chondromatous giant cell tumor
3. Endothelial	(a) Angio-endothelioma (b) Diffuse endothelioma (Ewing sarcoma)	(a) Plexiform angioma (b) Cavernous angioma
4. Hematopoietic Erythropoietic Myeloid Lymphoid	(a) Erythrocytoma (b) Myelocytoma; myeloma (c) Lymphocytoma (d) Reticulocytoma	
5. Adipose	Liposarcoma	

DIAGNOSIS

Christensen compiled a table of the distribution of 1000 bone tumors. In his series as well as in all other such studies the lower femur and upper tibia have proved to be the sites most frequently involved by practically all malignant bone tumors. Next in order is the upper humerus. In addition to favoring these sites, the giant-cell tumor also has a predelection for the distal radial epiphysis. As a generalization it can be stated that osteogenic sarcomas attack the tubular bone metaphyses, giant-cell tumors the epiphyses, endotheliomas the shafts, and myelomas the flat bones. Of course, the myelomas are the only malignant primary bone tumors in which multiple tumors are the rule. Age incidence may be generalized by stating that osteogenic sarcomas and endotheliomas are most frequently observed during the second decade, giant-cell tumors, the third decade; and myelomas the fourth and fifth decades.

The sex incidence is approximately equal except for a higher rate of occurrence in males in the instances of the osteogenic sarcoma series and Ewing's tumor.

BIOPSIES

Biopsies are indispensable to the proper management of the primary roentgenograms should be routine measures whenever a malignant bone tumor is suspected. Osteogenesis imperfecta, osteopetrosis, scurvy, and rickets have been responsible for lesions that were erroneously interpreted as malignant neoplasms. The reticulo-endothelial hyperplasias must also be kept in mind. Not infrequently the differentiation from a malignancy is made only after a study of biopsy material.

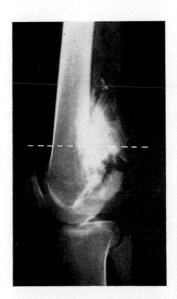
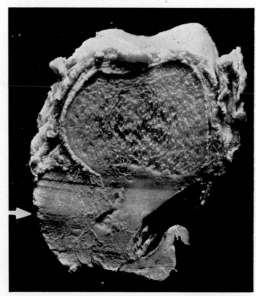

FIGURE 385. A. *(Left)* Lateral roentgenogram of a sclerosing osteosarcoma of the lower femur. B. *(Right)* Transverse section of the femur and tumor at the level of the broken line on Figure 385A.

OSTEOSARCOMA

SYNONYMS

When tumor bone formation is predominant osteosarcomas have been termed osteoblastic sarcoma, sclerosing osteogenic sarcoma, and osteoblastoma. When osteolysis is the dominant feature this tumor has been named osteolytic sarcoma, telangiectatic sarcoma, malignant bone aneurysm, osteoaneurysm and malignant bone cyst.

DEFINITION

The osteosarcomas are highly malignant primary bone tumors in which malignant osteoblasts are the principle cells. There is an intercellular deposition of osteoid and bone, the extent of which depends upon the degree of differentiation of the tumor osteoblasts. Just as the malignant osteoblast varies widely in its appearance so also does the

tumor bone. In fact, it can be said that no two osteosarcomas are pre-
cisely alike in their overall microscopic appearance.

PATHOGENESIS

By the time the tumor is diagnosed the exact site or origin is seldom
determinable. In an early stage the major portion of many osteosarcomas lies beneath the periosteum fused to the cortical surface. It is
thus tempting to conclude that these tumors have their origin in the
cambium of the periosteum. While there is evidence that this truly

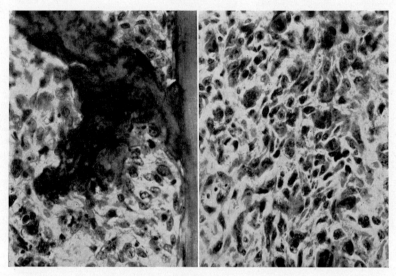

FIGURE 387. A. *(Left)* High power magnification of malignant osteoblasts and tumor
bone. B. *(Right)* High power magnification of the anaplastic tumor cells in an osteolytic
area of an osteosarcoma.

is the site or origin in a great many instances, there are numerous other
cases in which the origin may well have been either cortical or medullary. Regardless of the site of origin, all component parts of the bone
become invaded. In a late stage the scope of the tumor is obvious on
both gross and roentgenographic examinations. In an early stage the
cortical and marrow involvement may be identified only by the microscope.

When the tumor originates in the cambium layer of the periosteum,
a mass takes shape that elevates the periosteum. Growth of the tumor
tissue peripherally takes place beneath the fibrous layer of the pri-
osteum, for it is here that the youngest and most actively proliferating osteogenic cells are seen. Invasion of the cortex is by infiltration
of the tumor cells into the Volkmann and haversian canals. Consider-

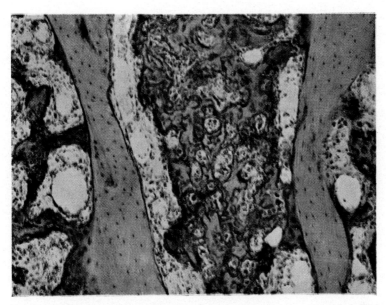

FIGURE 386. Osteosarcoma. The two orderly normal bone trabeculae are in striking contrast to the bizarre, purposeless arrangement of the tumor bone.

able time elapses before this infiltration creates sufficient destruction for its identification by gross and roentgenographic examinations. Ewing's tumor is characterized by a similar infiltration of the host bone. Conversely, most chondrosarcomas do not infiltrate, but perforate the cortex simply by pressure from the expanding tumor. Ultimately the cortex beneath an osteosarcoma becomes extensively destroyed and replaced by tumor tissue. Advance through the metaphyseal marrow spaces may take place rapidly, and tumor tissue may actively grow down

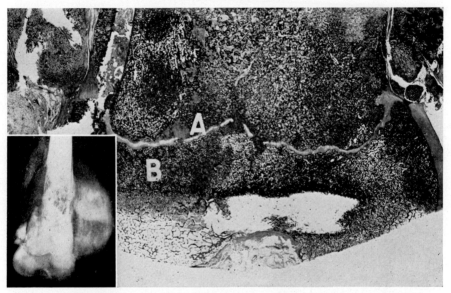

FIGURE 388. Histologic section of an osteosarcoma of the lower femur. Tumor cells have perforated the epiphyseal plate (A) and now the cells and tumor bone almost fill the epiphysis (B). The insert is a roentgenogram of the specimen.

the medullary canal of the diaphysis. The epiphyseal plate, particularly its zone of calcified cartilage, is a decided, although temporary, barrier to the advance of the tumor into the epiphysis. Ultimately there is a microscopic perforation of the cartilage plate and the tumor cells pour through it like water through a hole in a dyke. And like the hole in the dyke, the epiphyseal plate perforation steadily enlarges. Several such perforations may be seen in a single epiphyseal plate (Fig. 390). Cases have been reported in which the entire epiphysis became virtually filled with tumor tissue (Fig. 388). Another barrier is encountered when the tumor tissue reaches the articular cartilage; however, it is unusual for an osteosarcoma to advance so far. Generally, before this stage is attained, metastases and death overtake the patient, or a surgeon overtakes the tumor.

Bone formation in osteosarcomas is principally neoplastic and is the work of malignant osteoblasts (Fig. 358A). This bone forms for the most part just as it does in the ossification of membranous bones. Osseomucin is deposited in numerous slender rods which become surrounded by osteoblasts. In most instances the osteoid calcifies to form tumor bone, and through the activity of the tumor osteoblasts new tumor bone is apposed layer by layer to form a system of connected trabeculae. Bizarre masses of tumor bone may form by fusion of thick

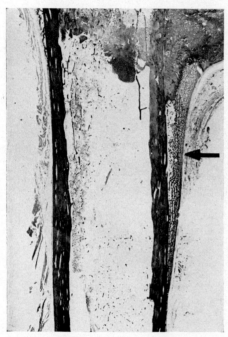

FIGURE 389. Codman triangle (arrow) of reactive, non-tumorus, bone.

trabeculae. Occasional areas of a primitive type of enchondral ossification are seen in osteosarcomas. Islands of tumor cartilage undergo matrical calcification at their periphery subsequent to which peripheral chondrocytes are released and tumor bone applied to projecting bars or buds of calcified matrix. This process may continue until the entire area of tumor cartilage is replaced by tumor bone. The transformation of tumor cartilage and fibroblastic tissue to bone by direct metaplasia is occasionally observed in scattered microscopic areas, but accounts for relatively little of the total mass of tumor bone.

It must be remembered that an osteosarcoma, as well as any other malignant bone tumor, may stimulate the formation of considerable quantities of **reactive bone**. There are times when the differentiation of reactive from tumor bone is difficult, but for the most part the reactive bone is at the periphery, is orderly, and its true character obvious. The most prominent example of reactive bone is the reactive triangle of Codman. This triangle of normal reactive bone is located on the diaphyseal side of the tumor where the periosteum leaves the tumor and rejoins the cortex of the host bone (Fig. 389). The base of the reactive triangle lies adjacent to the diaphyseal side of the tumor and the apex lies at the point where the periosteum reunites with the cortex. A Codman triangle certainly is not pathognomonic but roentgenographically it is one of the most important signs of a primary malignant bone tumor. In slow growing tumors a thin layer of reactive bone may overlie the entire extracortical mass.

MECHANISMS OF BONE RESORPTION

Bone destruction by an osteosarcoma is abetted by several factors. Osteoclastic action by the tumor cells themselves varies from pronounced

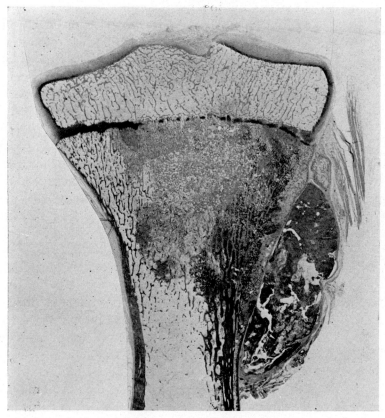

FIGURE 390. Histologic sections of advanced osteosarcomas of the upper tibia.
A. Minimal epiphyseal invasion.

activity as in certain osteolytic osteosarcomas, to no bone resorption whatever in fields in which tumor is being actively formed. Perhaps the most important source of osteoclasis in an osteosarcoma resides in the local proliferation of normal osteoclasts. Other factors stimulating osteoclasia are the ingrowth of new blood vessels, the hyperemia associated with the tumor, and the impingement of tumor masses against the host bone causing pressure atrophy. All osteosarcomas are destructive to the host bone regardless of the degree of tumor bone formation. Of course, the osteolytic or telangiectatic type is the most rapidly destructive and the most likely to lead to a pathologic fracture. Pathologic fractures generally are followed by an acceleration of tumor growth.

Perforation of the periosteum may occur early or late depending on the site of origin and the rate of growth of the tumor. A rapidly growing osteosarcoma originating in the cambium layer perforates the periosteum early. Perforation does not take place by a wide erosion or wholesale periosteal destruction. Rather there are columns or spearheads of tumor cells which create perforations of microscopic proportions. Tumor cells in great numbers proliferate through these perforations and consolidate into extra-periosteal masses. The major portion of the periosteum may long remain intact sandwiched between the subperiosteal and the extra-periosteal components of the tumor. It is an interesting phenomenon that once a barrier has been widely penetrated the remainder of the barrier may long persist unaltered.

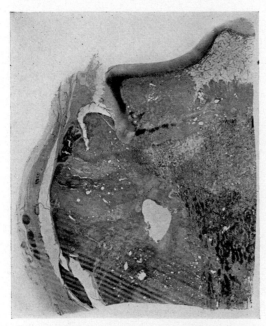

FIGURE 390. *(Continued)* B. Advanced epiphyseal invasion. (Courtesy, C. Howard Hatcher, M.D.)

After perforation of the periosteum a variable zone of fibrous tissue forms ahead of the advancing tumor margin. To say that this fibrous tissue represents a defensive response is open to question. The chances are that it is purely a reactive response since it offers little resistance to the spread of the tumor. In general the slower the tumor growth the better developed is this pseudocapsular wall of fibrosis. Spontaneous, surgical, and traumatic perforations of the periosteum in osteolytic osteosarcomas is often followed by a wild and rapid growth of the tumor into adjacent soft tissues, including the joint capsule. Cases have been reported where the tumor actually ulcerated the overlying skin (observed by Hertzler, denied by Kolodny).

Pathologic Anatomy

Gross

The gross examination of a series of osteosarcomas discloses the widest possible variation in appearance and density. At one end of the scale of densities lies the sclerosing osteosarcoma with its tumor bone of ivory-like density (Figs. 384 & 385) and at the opposite end of the scale the so-called telangiectatic or osteolytic osteosarcoma with its great vascularity, soft to firm consistency and a minimum of tumor bone (Figs. 394 & 395). Toward the middle of the scale might be said to lie the group of osteosarcomas in which neither sclerosis nor lysis predominate, both phenomena being well represented. The periosteal and medullary type in the Registry classification falls into this group. It is not unusual to see osteosclerosis in the medulla, and telangiectasis in the extracortical mass; and the reverse is also observed. Strictly speaking, the division into sclerosing and osteolytic types is a gross and roentgenologic division in that on a microscopic basis all sclerosing osteosarcomas possess fields of pronounced anaplasia and osteolysis.

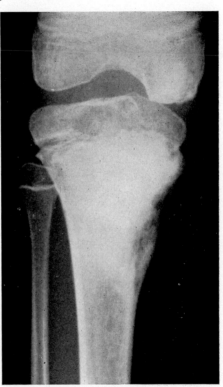

FIGURE 391. Osteosarcoma of the proximal tibial metaphysis.

As a rule the gross examination reveals a more extensive tumor involvement of the host bone than does the roentgenogram, and it can be added that the histologic study discloses more involvement than does the study of the gross specimen. At the operating table the vascularity of most osteosarcomas is an impressive feature, and in the osteolytic type the operative hemorrhage may, as Hertzler stated it, be dumbfounding to the surgeon. Older surgeons frequently described a bruit over the tumor mass, and it was the palpable pulsation of the mass that led to the term malignant bone aneurysm. It is extremely important, when possible, to employ a tourniquet, for it is mandatory that the surgeon have a clear unobstructed view of the tissue he visualizes with his scalpel. A biopsy of a sclerosing osteosarcoma may require a gouge or an osteotome for its removal. However, this is exceptional in that the extracortical mass, by growing at its periphery, is here the least mature and the least dense. An extracortical mass

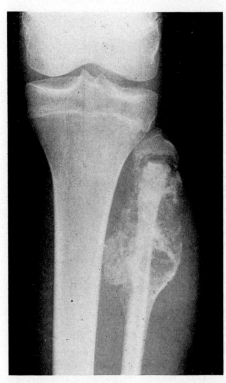

possessing minimal tumor bone is firm, flesh-like, vascular, and often gritty. As previously mentioned, a wall of fibrous tissue may over lie the tumor mass. Care must be taken not to limit the inspection and biopsy to this peripheral granulation and fibrous tissue.

Cortical involvement represents a permeation with honeycomb-like destruction leading to a great loss of strength in the host bone. On the cortical surface there is a distinct roughening. Digital pressure may reveal a crackling of the fragile bone and may actually perforate into the medulla. In instances of advanced osteolytic tumors it is not unusual to find one or more sizable sequestrated fragments of necrotic cortex isolated and enveloped by the tumor.

FIGURE 392. Osteosarcoma of the proximal fibular metaphysis.

Multiple large vascular sinuses may exist in both medullary and extracortical masses of the tumor. Some of these sinuses are engorged with blood, others are empty while still others are filled with tumor and blood thrombi. Aggressive tumors frequently destroy areas of their own blood supply leading to circumscribed mushy sites of necrosis having a purple, brown, or black color. In more advanced tumors it is the rule to find areas of necrosis that have undergone liquefaction to form pseudo-cysts filled with a dark brown fluid. Intense roentgentherapy often leads to large areas of tumor necrosis which may organize and become temporarily replaced by fibrogenic tissue.

Microscopic Features

Histologically osteosarcomas are among the most variable and most fascinating of all tumors. It is at once apparent that the degree of differentiation of the malignant osteoblasts dictates the extent and the density of the tumor bone. In the sclerosing areas of an osteosarcoma the osteoblasts attain a degree of differentiation capable of form-ing dense bone. However, there is no order to the internal or ex-ternal architecture of the bone, and, while masses of solid bone may form with complex irregular cementing lines, haversian sys-tems are not created. The struc-tural pattern could be referred to as pseudo-lamellar, but no true lamellar structure can be found. When solid sheets of tumor bone are seen there are numerous small vascular canals, but these are not haversian canals. In less dense areas a system of interconnected trabeculae and marrow spaces are seen, and the latter are packed with tumor osteoblasts. Many of the normal trabeculae of the host bone, particularly the longitudi-nal trabeculae, may survive un-altered by the tumor and, in fact, become enveloped by tumor trabeculae anchoring to their sur-faces. (Fig. 386, color plate).

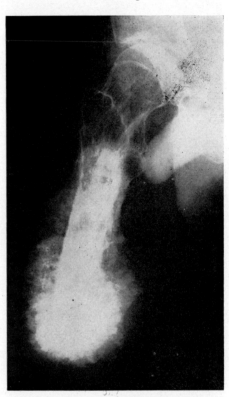

FIGURE 393. Osteosarcoma of the lower femur recurring in the femoral stump.

In osteolytic areas little or no tumor bone is laid down amongst the malignant osteoblasts. In such areas the trabeculae that do take shape frequently are isolated from each other and may not develop beyond the osteoid stage. Osteoblasts in these telangiectatic fields are poorly differentiated as indicated by their large and variable size, hyperchro-matic nuclei, and numerous mitotic figures. It is striking and not un-usual to find a field in which the osteoblasts are in a state of extreme anaplasia, lying near a field in which there is dense tumor bone and a higher differentiation of the tumor cells. The photomicrographs of figures 378A and 378B were from the same tumor. It has long been recognized that the sclerosing osteosarcoma has approximately as poor a prognosis as the osteolytic type. This is understandable when the entire tumor is examined histologically and numerous fields of anaplastic osteoblasts are noted. It is also well established that in the natural

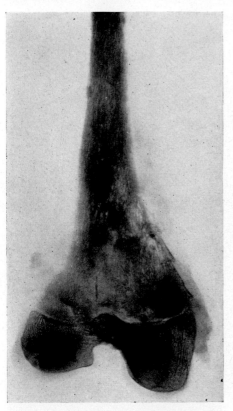

history of a given tumor the proportions between sclerosis and osteolysis are not fixed but undergo constant changes. After a long period of slow growth and an extensive formation of tumor bone, the tumor osteoblasts may become much more anaplastic, grow rapidly and assume the characteristics of an osteolytic osteosarcoma. The reverse is seen, particularly after a period of roentgentherapy; a rapidly growing osteosarcoma with little tumor bone will temporarily regress, then grow slowly, and form relatively large masses of tumor bone. This phenomenon forms an important link in the strong chain of evidence that links together the sclerosing and telangiectatic forms of osteosarcoma. There has been a rather widespread tendency to classify the predominately osteolytic form of osteosarcoma as a tumor having little or no relation to the pre-

FIGURE 394. Osteolytic osteosarcoma (Telangiectatic sarcoma) of the distal femoral metaphysis in a male age 11 years. Survived four months post-amputation. A. Roentgenogram of specimen.

dominately sclerosing form or even to the osteogenic group of sarcomas.

Blood vessels are numerous in all osteosarcomas, but are a great deal larger in telangiectatic areas where many of the blood vessels are lined by tumor cells. Ample explanation of the early pulmonary metastases can be viewed in the histologic sections of this tumor.

Small multinucleated giant cells with three to ten hyperchomatic nuclei are seen in some of the more anaplastic areas. Microscopic fields are occasionally seen that possess so many small multinucleated giant cells that, if viewed alone might be diagnosed as malignant giant cell tumor. A few foreign body giant cells may be seen around areas of hemorrhage and necrosis. Large spindle cells with large pale staining nuclei are mixed with pleomorphic rounded malignant osteoblasts which have hyperchomatic nuclei. Hyperchomatism of the nuclei is a reliable sign of malignancy when the histologic sections have been dependably stained.

The osteoblasts of osteosarcomas never attain a normal appearance, and the bone they form is similarly bizarre. In most normal physiologic process-es the osteoblasts and fibro-blasts are small, and are pur-posefully arranged; their in-terpretation seldom causes confusion. In the instance of bony callus formation in children, however, there are times when the histologic picture of fields of active cel-lular proliferation resemble those of sclerosing osteosar-coma. Of course, there is lit-tle excuse for an error in di-agnosis when the picture is studied in its entirety.

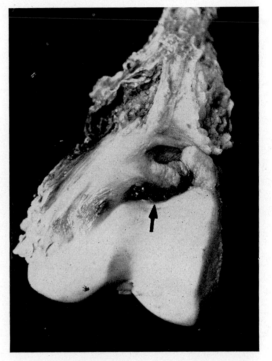

FIGURE 394. *(Continued)* B. Arrow points to perfo-ration of the tumor into the anterior aspect of the knee joint.

METASTASES

Virtually all metastases from osteosarcoma are pul-monary metastases and are carried to the lungs via the blood stream. In rare instances the metastatic tumor cells have passed through the lungs and have set up metastatic foci in the brain, abdom-inal viscera, and even in the skeletal system. Metastasis via the lymphat-ics also takes place, with involvement of neighboring lymph nodes.

Pulmonary metastases generally grow slowly and may exist for sev-eral months or years without detection clinically or roentgenologically. Slow growing metastases form tumor bone that may attain great density (Fig. 396). The amount of tumor bone formed by the primary tumor does not always dictate the amount of bone that will be formed in the metastases. Occasionally a primary tumor so anaplastic as to be difficult to diagnose as an osteosarcoma will form clear cut bone in the pulmonary metastases, thus removing all doubt regarding the diagnosis of the primary tumor.

Pathogenesis

The emboli of tumor cells are carried to the lung parenchyma by

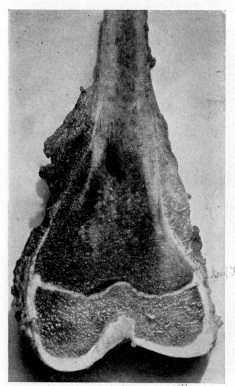

blood vessels, and while any portion of the lung can become the site of a metastatic focus the subpleural region is perhaps the most frequently involved. Hilar foci are also common and may become large. They must be differentiated from calcified hilar lymph nodes of tuberculosis. The metastases vary in consistency from soft to stoney hard, and are rounded in contour.

The capillaries of the involved pulmonary alveoli become engorged with tumor cells, after which the capillaries empty the tumor cells into the alveoli. Adjacent involved alveoli, filled with tumor cells, gradually fuse as the tumor cells proliferate and form tumor bone. Soon the alveolar markings disappear and the focus becomes a growing mass of tumor tissue. Alveoli adjoining the tu-

FIGURE 394. (Continued) C. Frontal section of specimen.

mor mass tend to become emphysematous.

Pulmonary Osteoblastic Bone Formation

Exponents of the osteoblastic theory of bone formation believe that the phenomenon of bone formation in pulmonary metastases is incontrovertible evidence that the osteoblast can possess a specific capacity to promote bone formation, regardless of its environment. The lung is not a favorable site for bone formation yet the metastatic tumor osteoblasts clearly demonstrate their predestined capacity to cause bone to form.

ROENTGENOLOGIC CORRELATION

"An essential safeguard for the pathologist in the diagnosis of bone tumors is the possession of full clinical and roentgenologic data. No breadth of experience can dispense with these aids in dealing with the variable structure of bone tumors" (Ewing).

Roentgenology plays an immensely important role in the diagnosis and understanding of the osteogenic neoplasms. The patient has distinctly benefited from the close cooperation of clinicians, roentgenologists, and pathologists. Roentgenologists no longer see mere shadows when they view their films; they visualize physiologic and pathologic processes; they see tissues and disease entities, living, growing, and unfolding their nature. This is dynamic diagnostic roentgenology.

Before viewing the roentgenologic picture as a whole, each individual structure should be studied; overlying soft tissues, periosteum, cortex, medullary canal, epiphyseal plate, epiphysis, and articular cortices may be examined in turn systematically. Destructive and proliferative lesions should be carefully analyzed to determine their pattern, extent, and if possible their origin.

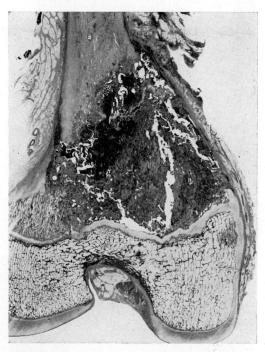

FIGURE 394. *(Continued)* D. Histologic section of specimen. Numerous blood sinuses were present throughout the tumor. Tumor cells were highly anaplastic and produced very little tumor bone.

Periosteum

Since the majority of osteosarcomas appear to originate in the cambium layer of the periosteum, this structure must be scrutinized for the early changes characteristic of this tumor. If tumor bone forms early in the subperiosteal mass the spicules tend to possess a fine caliber, radial alignment, and little calcium. A soft tissue exposure frequently gives the best portrayal of the early changes. A reactive triangle appears

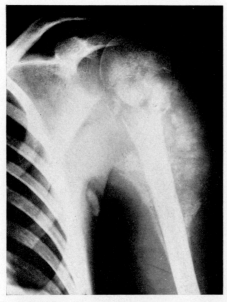

FIGURE 395. Osteolytic osteosarcoma of the humerus with a pathologic metaphyseal fracture.

early in some instances and may be the only indication of the presence of a periosteal mass. In a somewhat later stage, when tumor bone is a prominent feature, the typical shaggy sun-ray spicules may take shape. In a still later stage the extracortical mass may be so densely consolidated that the sun-ray structure entirely disappears.

The sun-ray structure is the best known of all the alterations observed in malignant bone tumors. It has been looked upon as virtually pathognomonic of osteogenic sarcoma. This is an error. The sun-ray pattern is far from pathognomonic; it is not only observed in other types of tumors, it has also been seen as a part of several non-tumorous lesions. Hasty conclusions are seldom warranted or safe when dealing with the complexities of malignant bone tumors.

Cortex

When the tumor originates either in the cambium cells of the periosteum or in the cortex proper there are relatively early localized changes in the cortex. These changes are represented by a surface area of cortical erosion and by localized osteoporosis. Both of these changes are due to the combination of the destructive action of the permeating tu-

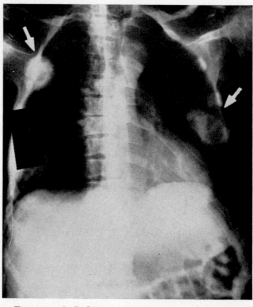

FIGURE 396. Pulmonary metastases of an osteosarcoma (arrows). Dense tumor bone has formed in the metastatic foci.

mor cells and the localized active hyperemia associated with the rich
blood supply that characterizes these tumors. Cortical changes are
limited to one aspect of the host bone, differing from the widespread
riddling of the cortex seen in many diffuse endotheliomas.

In sclerosing osteoblastic sarcomas the cortex may actually reveal
an increase in density at the site of the tumor. This is from the deposition of dense tumor bone following the resorption of the normal
cortical bone. Good roent-
genograms often disclose the
local interruption of the
normal pattern of the haversian systems. In other instances, a large dense extracortical mass of tumor bone
develops without there being any detectable roentgenographic changes in the cortex.

In osteolytic osteosarco-
mas a central destructive
lesion frequently destroys
the cortex from within. This
destructive process proceeds
so rapidly that no appreciable reactive periosteal bone
forms on the surface to give
rise to "expansion" of the
cortex. While the cortex
bounding such central le-
sions may be invaded

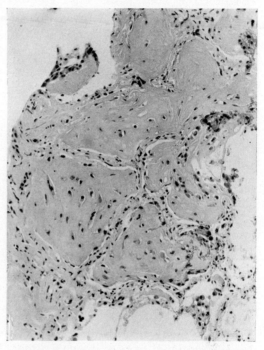

FIGURE 397. Tumor bone in a pulmonary metastasis of an osteosarcoma. (Courtesy, A. Purdy Stout,
M.D.)

throughout the circumference of the host bone, there is generally an
eccentric growth of the lesion to the extent that the cortex is perforated
in a circumscribed area. Pathologic fractures are not uncommon in this
type of osteosarcoma.

Subcortical Involvement

Metaphyseal cancellous bone and its marrow may be replaced extensively with tumor bone, thereby presenting increased density in the
roentgenogram. The process begins eccentrically and spreads across the
metaphysis, down the medullary canal and into the epiphysis. An accurate indication of the extent to which the tumor has advanced

down the medullary canal is seldom portrayed in the roentgenogram. Perforations of the epiphyseal plate cannot be detected until of considerable size. As with osteoporosis of cancellous bone from other causes, it is the transverse trabeculae that disappear first. This phenomenon is sometimes reflected in the roentgenogram by what appears to be an increased coarseness of the trabecular pattern.

Large central metaphyseal areas of destruction have been erroneously diagnosed as bone cysts. The resemblance to a solitary cyst is only superficial. Whereas a cyst has a sharply defined margin, the central lytic osteosarcoma has no clear definition at its periphery. A sharply

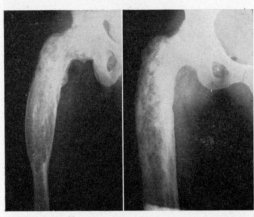

defined bone lesion is not likely to be malignant. A cyst expands the cortex, osteosarcoma does not. A cyst seldom perforates overlying cortex, whereas an osteosarcoma perforates the cortex early. Growth of a cyst is slow and relatively painless, growth of an osteosarcoma is generally rapid and often painful. Neighboring bone in a cyst posseses normal density, while the bone around an osteolytic osteosarcoma is porotic.

FIGURE 398. Osteosarcoma in a femur involved by osteitis deformans. (Roentgenogram on the right.) The roentgenogram on the left was taken prior to the appearance of the osteosarcoma.

Roentgenographically an osteolytic osteosarcoma cannot consistently be differentiated from a Ewing's tumor. Both of these tumors occur at the same age period, are profoundly destructive, develop in metphyses, and have peripheral soft tissue masses in association with their central destruction. One point is helpful: Many of Ewing's tumors are diaphyseal in origin and involve the metaphysis late whereas nearly all osteosarcomas are metaphyseal from the outset.

It cannot be overemphasized that bone lesions suspected of being malignant should be studied roentgenologically with films taken at several angles and with varied exposures. And the study should be repeated at close intervals until the diagnosis is established. A roentgenographic study of the entire skeleton is indicated whenever the diagnosis is in doubt. In not a small number of cases generalized processes such as hyperparathyroidism and syphilis have been erroneously diagnosed as bone sarcoma simply because the entire skeleton was not studied.

CLINICAL FEATURES

While osteosarcomas have been observed at all ages—infants to the aged—the peak incidence is seen between the ages of 12 and 25. Codman and Coley have emphasized the point that an osteosarcoma developing after the age of 50 is generally superimposed upon Paget's disease. Osteosarcomas, fibrosarcomas, and chondrosarcomas have all been observed as a complication of Paget's disease. The sex incidence gives males a slight edge.

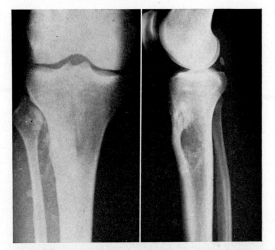

Distribution

Nearly all osteosarcomas develop in the metaphyses of long bones. Diaphyseal osteosarcomas are rare; capsular and paraosteal osteosarcomas have been reported but are decidedly rare. Approximately three-fourths of all osteosarcomas develop in the metaphysis of the lower femur and the upper tibia. Other sites at which this tumor has been observed include the upper femur, humerus, fibula, and ulna; the lower tibia and ulna; and the ilium, vertebral bodies, maxillae and the clavicle. No bone is immune.

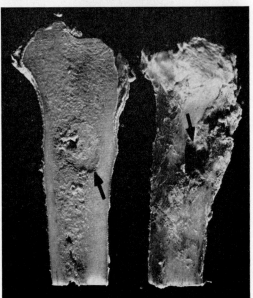

FIGURE 399. Chondrosarcoma of the upper tibia in a male age 52. A. *(Above)* Roentgenograms. B. *(Below)* Sagital section of amputation specimen. The extracortical tumor mass is not shown. Arrows point to the site of the intraosseous portion of the tumor.

Symptoms

Pain is generally the first symptom of an osteosarcoma. When growth of the tumor is slow the pain may be mild or moderate for several months. In rapidly growing tumors the pain may be severe from the outset. Intermittent pain is not nearly so characteristic as is a continuous dull boring pain that reaches its peak of severity during the night. Pain ordinarily precedes a palpable tumor by several months and usually is unexplained during this period. In 72 of 100 cases of bone sarcoma reviewed by Ewing, the first physician consulted by the patient failed to recognize the significance of the pain. Pain gradually becomes intractable. Perforation of the periosteum may give temporary partial relief, but an accelerated growth of the tumor takes place. The pain may be greatly aggravated by weight bearing or even by movements of the adjacent joint. This accounts for pronounced muscle atrophy of late stages. A pathologic fracture generally increases the pain, but such fractures are uncommon when osteolysis predominates and are rare in the sclerosing type.

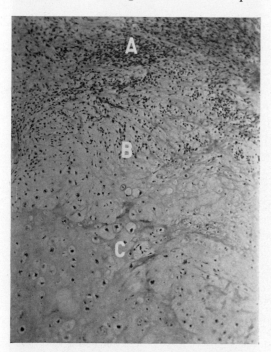

FIGURE 399. *(Continued)* C. Photomicrograph showing evolution of the tumor cartilage. *A*. Fibroblastic tissue. *B*. Myxomatous tissue. *C*. Cartilage.

Objective Findings

The palpable tumor varies widely in size, is firm to hard, moderately tender and partially fixed to overlying soft tissues. In a late stage the overlying soft tissues become solidly fixed to the tumor, at which stage the skin becomes a brown or copper color and the superficial veins distended. Telangiectatic extracortical masses may pulsate. In palpating malignant tumors, gentleness is in order. It must be kept in mind that a firm squeeze of a malignant tumor is capable of sending tumor emboli on their road to the lungs and the patient on the road to his grave. These deadly tumors must not be aided and abetted.

A low grade fever and leucocytosis are the rule in later stages but do not reach the high levels seen in the endotheliomas and myelomas.

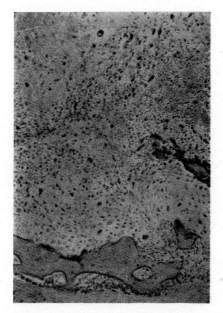

Figure 400. Photomicrograph of malignant cartilage.

Woodward and Higginbotham have shown that the alkaline serum phosphatase is elevated in osteosarcoma and is highest in the presence of metastases. A persistent elevation of the serum phosphatase after total removal of the primary tumor is said to be evidence of the presence of meta- stases.

Diagnosis

Biopsies are indicated in nearly all cases, and, as has been previously stated, should be routine proce- dure prior to a mutilating operation. It sounds trite to say that a biopsy must in- clude tumor tissue, but all too frequently the peripher- al reactive tissue is all that the surgeon has to show for his efforts. On theoretical grounds, at least, the inci- sion into the tumor proper should be repaired. When frozen sections are inconclu- sive, time should be taken to prepare a permanent sec- tion with the necessary stain- ing for a comprehensive study. A single biopsy does

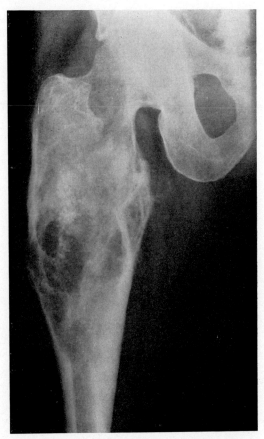

FIGURE 401. Chondrosarcoma of the upper femur in a male age 60.

not always establish the diagnosis. A second biopsy should be taken if the first proves inadequate.

Lesions most frequently diagnosed erroneously (pre-biopsy) as osteo- sarcoma include traumatic periostitis, pyogenic, leutic, and tuberculous osteomyelitis, myocitis ossificans, solitary bone cysts, metastatic carci- noma, Ewing's tumor, myeloma, eosinophilic granuloma, the benign bone tumors, gout, and rheumatoid arthritis. With so much at stake when the lesion is an osteosarcoma, it is reasonable and proper to view every suspicious lesion in its worst light until its benignity is es- tablished.

Prognosis

There is no such thing as a good prognosis when the lesion is an osteosarcoma. It deserves to be stated again that of all osteogenic sarcomas the prognosis in osteosarcoma is the worst.

A particularly poor prognosis can be made when the tumor is growing rapidly, is predominately osteolytic, highly vascular, soft consistency, has no appreciable reactive margin of fibrosis, highly anaplastic with little intercellular substance, severely painful, and located in the proximal aspect of an extremity or in the torso.

At the time of amputation more favorable prognosis, but by no means good prognosis, is indicated when the tumor is slow growing, the cells better differentiated and more uniform in size with less hyperchomatism of the nuclei, dense tumor bone, intact periosteum, well formed zone of marginal reactive fibrosis, lymphocytic infiltration (Kolodny), and location of the tumor in the distal aspect of an extremity. To this can be added a low alkaline phosphatase, and a near-normal erythrocyte and leukocyte study, and of course, a negative chest roentgenogram.

CHONDROSARCOMA

Chondrosarcomas are malignant connective tissue tumors, nearly all of which are found in the bones. In this treatise the chondrosarcomas will be classified with the osteogenic series of sarcomas. As previously stated, the term osteogenic is defined as originating in bone, but not necessarily forming bone. As the name implies, chondrosarcomas are composed principally of cartilage in various states of differentiation and calcification. Myxomatous tissue forms a part of these tumors and may be negligible or be so extensive as to constitute most of the tumor volume. As is true with tumors of the osteogenic series, all of the osteogenic tissues (bone, cartilage, and fibrous tissue) are represented in nearly every tumor. However, when the entire tumor is examined the cartilage element is found to far exceed the quantity of bone and fibrous tissue.

While the degree of malignancy varies through as wide a range as it does in osteosarcoma, the chondrosarcomas as a group are said to be less deadly than the osteosarcomas. The incidence of chondrosarcoma is approximately that of osteosarcoma, particularly so when osteolytic (telangiectatic) sarcoma is included, as it should be, with the osteosarcomas.

PATHOGENESIS

While a chondrosarcoma is most likely to originate in the periosteum at the metaphyseal level, it may take its origin in any portion of the bone. An extremely important group of these tumors originates in the perichondrium of a chondroma or an osteochondroma. Thus, a

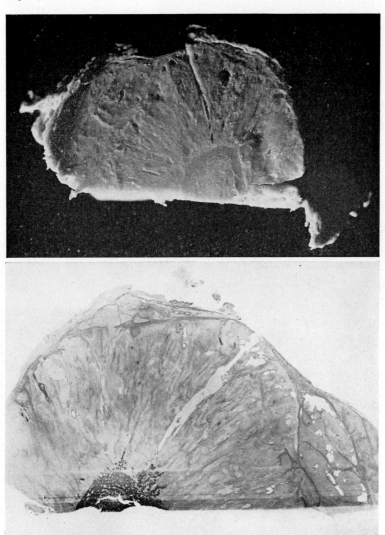

FIGURE 402. Chondrosarcoma. A. *(Above)* Cross section of specimen. B. *(Below)* Histologic section.

chondrosarcoma may be primarily malignant, or represent a secondary malignant degeneration of a benign cartilage tumor.

A chondrosarcoma originating in the periosteum forms a firm, often rubbery, dome-shaped mass. Growth of the tumor is principally by expansion, rather than by infiltration. The underlying cortex is steadily eroded until it perforates and admits the tumor to the cancellous bone of the metaphysis or to the medullary canal of the diaphysis. As the intraosseous portion of the tumor enlarges it assumes a rounded contour.

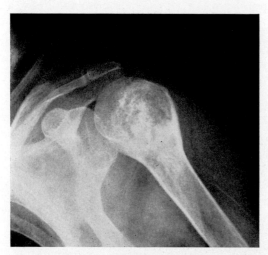

FIGURE 403. Chondrosarcoma of the humeral head in a female age 65.

When a chondrosarcoma is superimposed upon a chondroma or an osteochondroma it evolves from the perichondrial tissue, for herein resides the mother tissue of the benign tumor. A chondroma is so completely enveloped and replaced by the chondrosarcoma that it is usually impossible to identify remains of the original tumor tissue. In fact, it is very often impossible to learn whether or not a given chondrosarcoma originated in a chondroma. In general, primary chondrosarcomas are more common before the third decade, and secondary chondrosarcomas after the third decade.

An osteochondroma (cartilaginous exostosis), when involved by a chondrosarcoma, undergoes changes in the region of the cartilaginous cap. Following displacement of the tumor cap there may be invasion of the osseous portion beneath the cap. But even in advanced stages the base of the osteochondroma may be preserved (Fig. 405).

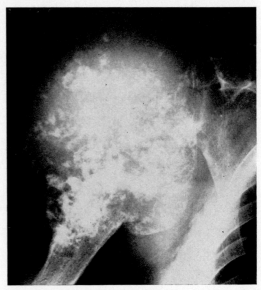

FIGURE 404. Far advanced chondrosarcoma of the upper humerus.

Growth of cartilaginous sarcomas varies from extremely slow to rapid. After a protracted period of virtual quiescence the tumor may suddenly start to grow rapidly. Trauma appears capable, in some instances, of accelerating the rate of growth of these tumors.

Phemister and others have reported instances in which a chondrosarcoma has grown into and along the lumen of the femoral vein.

Pathologic Anatomy

Gross Examination

Gross examination of a chondrosarcoma generally reveals a white or gray, glistening, opalescent, rounded tumor mass fixed to both the

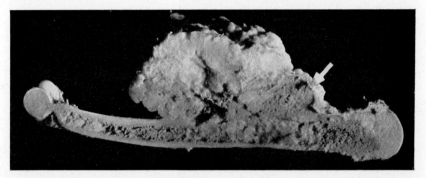

FIGURE 405. Chondrosarcoma secondary to an osteochondroma. The arrow points to the base of the osteochondroma.

underlying cortex of the host bone and the overlying soft tissues. The mass tends to be lobulated and may contain both cystic areas of necrosis and multiple scattered white areas in which the cartilage is densely calcified. Soft myxomatous areas are composed of neoplastic and degenerative myxomatous tissue. In some instances radially arranged cords of tumor tissue, some of which are calcified, extend out from the cortex in a sun-ray pattern through the extraosseous mass. The tumor may overlie much of the circumference of the bone but the cortex is seldom perforated at more than one site. At this site, the intraosseous tumor mass is continuous with the extraosseous portion of the tumor. If the chondrosarcoma is superimposed upon an osteochondroma there may be no intraosseous involvement, even in chondrosarcomas.

Pathologic fractures are uncommon in chondrosarcomas.

Microscopic Features

The histologic picture of chondrosarcoma is characterized by purposeless masses of hyalin and chondral matricial substances in which are imbedded anaplastic chondrocytes and myxomatous cells. Chondrocytes, varying as they do from small to large, at no time assume a column or other orderly alignment (Fig. 400). Mitoses vary in number from few to many and it is common for some of the chondrocytes to possess two or more nuclei. It is in the more cellular areas that the best opportunity is found for identifying the malignant character of the tumor. Large, plump, chondrocytes with or without dual nuclei and mitotic figures are evidence of maligancy. Areas of foetal cartilage are packed with chondrocytes, show a high degree of anaplasia, and generally possess very little intercellular substance.

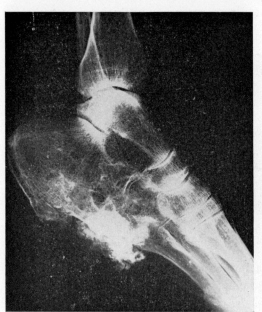

FIGURE 406. Chondrosarcoma of the os calcis.

Extremely anaplastic areas, viewed alone, frequently prove to be inadequately differentiated to serve as a basis for making the diagnosis of chondrosarcoma. In general it can be said that more chondrosarcomas have few mitotic figures than have many mitotic figures. The most ominous-appearing fields in the sections must be searched out and the final diagnosis based upon these, rather than upon the better differentiated, less cellular areas. Differentiation from a chondroma can be difficult—even impossible. In no tumor is it more necessary to weigh the roentgenologic and clinical pictures along with the pathologic appearance. Histologically the phalangeal chondromas may appear malignant, but be entirely benign. Malignant changes in phalangeal cartilage tumors are extremely rare. The chondrocytes in chondromas tend to be considerably smaller than they do in chondrosarcomas, and this is true even when they possess dual nuclei.

Myxomatous connective tissue generally constitutes an important part of chondrosarcomas, and it develops on the basis of both degeneration and neoplasia, the latter being predominant (Fig. 399C). Myxomatous tissue may exist within the tumor as scattered patches blending with cartilage areas or, in exceptional cases, represent the bulk of the tumor tissue. Fields of cartilage can always be identified in the so-called pure myxomas of bone.

The cells in chondrosarcoma do not engage in the direct formation of tumor bone. Bone, seldom a prominent feature of this tumor, forms either by direct metaplasia of tumor cartilage or by the action of disorderly enchondral lines encircling areas of cartilage. At these enchon-

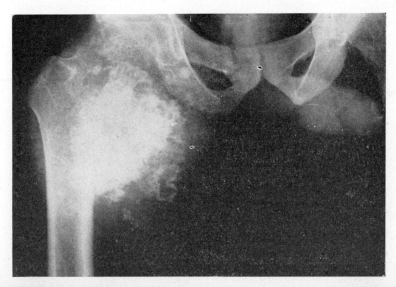

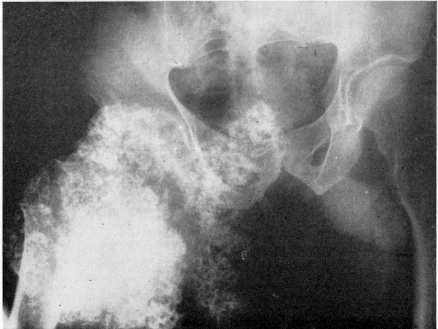

FIGURE 407. Chondrosarcoma secondary to an osteochondroma of the lesser trochanter. A *(Above)* taken approximately one year prior to B.

dral lines a zone of calcified cartilage can be seen, but an orderly zone of columns is not found. Reactive, non-tumorous bone, frequently takes shape at the periphery of the extracortical mass and may form typical Codman triangles.

Areas of necrosis are common, particularly among fields of calcified cartilage.

There are no essential differences in the microscopic pictures of primary and secondary chondrosarcomas.

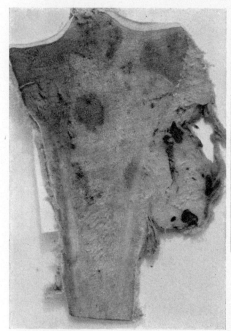

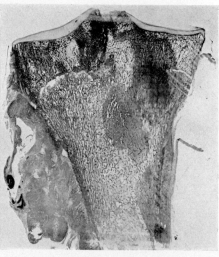

FIGURE 408. Fibrosarcoma of the upper tibia of a male, age 16 years. The tumor had infiltrated throughout the metaphysis and epiphysis. A. *(Left)* Photograph of the specimen. B. (Right) Histologic section of specimen.

ROENTGENOLOGIC FEATURES

The tumor mass of a chondrosarcoma may be totally radiolucent, possess scattered rounded or elongated areas of calcification and ossification, or present a nearly solid mass made up of multiple foci of dense calcified cartilage. There are exceptions, but as a rule the calcified areas of the tumor are limited to the extraosseous portion of the tumor. Chondrosarcomas superimposed upon chondromas and osteochondromas tend to become large and to possess massive calcified areas.

Sun-ray patterns of the areas of calcification and ossification are seldom seen. To visualize the base of an osteochondroma when it lies beneath a secondary chondrosarcoma may require roentgenograms taken at several angles.

Since a chondrosarcoma is frequently difficult to diagnose, it may be necessary to repeat the roentgenograms several times. Differentiation from myocitis ossificans is often clarified after the roentgenograms are repeated a time or two. Chondrosarcomas grow more rapidly and progressively lose their definition. Myocitis ossificans tends to gain in its definition during a series of examinations.

CLINICAL FEATURES

Age incidence

Primary chondrosarcoma ordinarily occurs in adolescents and young adults, whereas a chondrosarcoma superimposed upon a chondroma or an osteochondroma generally develops at an age period beyond the third decade.

Distribution

The metaphyseal level of the lower femur and the upper tibia are the sites most frequently involved; approximately fifty percent of

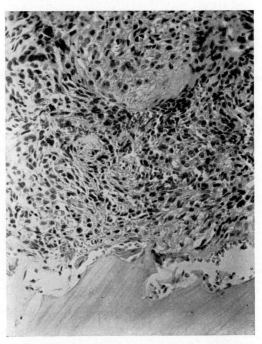

FIGURE 408. *(Continued)* C. Photomicrograph of tissue from the tumor.

all chondrosarcomas develop near the knee. Other sites at which these tumors are seen include the upper femur, upper humerus, pelvis, os calcis, costochondral junctions, and the lower tibia.

Symptoms

Like other osteogenic sarcomas, the pain is intermittent in early stages and constant in advanced stages; and is most severe at night. Pathologic fractures are uncommon. Leukocytosis, fever, and secondary anemia characterize the terminal stage.

Chondrosarcoma, like any other member of the osteogenic series, can develop as a complication of Paget's disease.

Therapy

Roentgen therapy has little or no influence on the growth and outcome of a chondrosarcoma.

Secondary chondrosarcoma is frequently treated by local excision, on the basis of an erroneous diagnosis of chondroma. A high incidence of local recurrence follows this type of surgical therapy. With the advent of a recurrent growth, amputation is still successful in effecting a cure in a great many instances. Most secondary chondrosarcomas grow slowly and metastasize late. No other osteogenic sarcoma responds so well to proper surgical therapy.

FIBROSARCOMA

Fibrosarcomas, essentially similar to those occurring in the soft tissues of the body, develop in both the periosteum and in the medullary canal of the bones. Whether or not these tumors should be assigned to the osteogenic series is an unsettled question. In view of the fact that fibrosarcoma of bone, from the standpoint of pathologic anatomy, is a clear-cut entity, this tumor will be included with the other connective tissue tumors of bones, namely, the osteosarcoma and chondrosarcoma. It will not be contended that the tumor fibroblasts of the skeletal fibrosarcoma definitely originated in cells that were predestined to form bone and cartilage. Proof of this theory is not substantial. An occasional skeletal fibrosarcoma forms a small amount of tumor bone, but so also do the fibrosarcomas of the soft tissues.

Two types of osseous fibrosarcoma are seen, periosteal or peripheral and medullary or central. The two types have approximately the same rate of occurrence and a similar distribution.

Fibrosarcoma is the least common and the least malignant of the connective tissue tumors of the bones. Batts reviewed 200 malignant primary bone tumors at the University of Michigan and found 27 or 13.5 percent to be fibrosarcoma. In the MacDonald and Budd series of 47 uncured cases seven, or 15 percent, were fibrosarcoma. In their series of 118 cases of cured osteogenic sarcoma, 37 (31.4 percent) were fibrosarcoma.

PATHOGENESIS

Periosteal fibrosarcoma originates in the fibrous layer of the periosteum and grows by expansion, crowding adjacent soft tissues and in the instances of more aggressive tumors, the periosteum is perforated and the overlying soft tissues are invaded. While the majority of fibrosarcomas grow by expansion there are a few of the more anaplastic and rapidly growing type that grow by infiltration. The underlying bone is eroded, and a shallow or deep concave defect is created. Eventually the cortex may be perforated and a portion of the medullary canal occupied. In rapidly growing fibrosarcomas large areas of bone are demolished and very little reactive bone is deposited. In the slow growing type, which is much the more common, reactive bone appears beneath the periosteum at each pole of the tumor in the form of a Codman reactive triangle.

Medullary fibrosarcomas originate centrally in the host bone and expand to create a round or oval defect devoid of bone elements. Fibrosar-

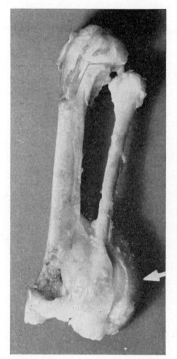
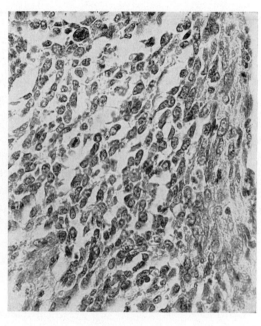

FIGURE 409. Fibrosarcoma of the lower tibia of infant age two months. The tumor was rapidly fatal. A. *(Left)* Specimen (arrow points to tumor). B. *(Right)* Photomicrograph of tissue from the tumor.

comas are purely osteolytic. As the tumor enlarges and reaches the cortex there is no so-called expansion of the cortex as seen in bone cysts, rather there is slow but progressive destruction of the cortex. In the more anaplastic fibrosarcomas large areas of the host bone may be destroyed leading to collapse of the bone. When the overlying cortex and periosteum are perforated, the tumor moves into adjacent soft tissues.

As the tumor grows, some of its blood vessels are obliterated, frequently leading to areas of necrosis. Necrotic tumor tissue may liquify, undergo calcification, or be replaced by an ingrowth of either normal fibrous tissue (scar tissue), or tumor tissue.

Factors responsible for the formation of this tumor are not known. However, fibrosarcomas have been produced experimentally in the soft tissues in numerous instances and by many of the more familiar carcinogenic agents. But a definitely osteogenic fibrosarcoma has thus far resisted experimental reproduction. Franceen, Aub, and Simpson implanted carcinogenic agents into the upper tibia of rats and mice. They succeeded in producing 17 tumors, all of which were fibrosarcoma. None of the tumors disclosed more than faint traces of alkaline phosphatase, so, on this basis, the authors concluded that the fibrosarcomas were extraosseous in their origin.

PATHOLOGIC ANATOMY

Gross Pathology

Fibrosarcomas develop in and around metaphyses and diaphyses. In the Batts series the incidence of involvement of metaphyses was greater than that of diaphyses in the ratio of five to three. Epiphyses are rarely involved. The long bones are the principle sites of predelection, but the skull, mandible, and vertebrae are not infrequently involved. The primary tumor is solitary. A multicentric origin apparently occurred in the Steiner case. In that remarkable and unique case a male age 43 developed medullary fibrosarcomas in nearly all of the bones of the entire skeletal system. Metastases were found in most of the viscera.

Fibrosarcoma of the mandible originates at one of three sites: (1) Periosteum, (2) Mandibular canal, or (3) The peridental membrane of the alveolar processes.

Goldman and Adams reported a fibrosarcoma of the sphenoid bone. The tumor invaded the sphenoid and encroached upon the cavernous sinus.

Several cases of fibrosarcoma of the skull have been reported and generally have been associated with Paget's disease. Kirshbaum recommended that every case of fibrosarcoma of the skull be investigated for Paget's disease. Fibrosarcoma of a long bone is not an unusual complication of Paget's disease.

In a fibrosarcoma of the upper tibia reported by Morley, Ghormley, and MacDonald there was an associated generalized neurofibromatosis. No proof could be offered that the fibrosarcoma originated from a neurofibroma.

Diaphyseal periosteal fibrosarcoma of a tubular bone may slowly grow around the shaft and eventually accomplish a complete encirclement without seriously eroding the bone. Or a periosteal fibrosarcoma may remain spherical and gradually destroy a circumscribed area of the underlying cortex.

Cross section of a fibrosarcoma reveals a solid, fibrous, firm, white, glistening tissue. Areas of necrosis and calcification are relatively common, particularly in the highly malignant type. In the majority of instances a capsule-like structure envelops the tumor mass. The more slowly the tumor grows the better formed is this pseudo-capsule. Mac-Donald and Budd found that the presence of some degree of encapsulation of the tumor was "a most favorable prognostic indication." In 73 percent of the 5 year cures of fibrosarcoma in their series the tumor possessed encapsulating tissue.

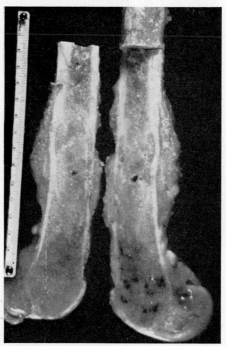

FIGURE 410. Fibrosarcoma of the distal one-half of the femur of a female, age 26 years. A. Photograph of the specimen.

Histopathology

Microscopically the fibrosarcoma presents a wide variety of spindle cells in a similarly varied matricial substance. The cells may closely resemble fibroblasts except for their larger size. When the degree of malignancy is minimal it is often difficult to differentiate a fibrosarcoma from a fibroma. When the degree of anaplasia is more pronounced spindle cells of proportions several times the size of fibroblasts are seen and their cell wall and cytoplasm are almost invisible. In such instances mitotic figures are numerous and multinucleated cells frequent. Round and stellate cells may be scattered through many fields giving the cell pattern a polymorphous character. There is more cell uniformity from one portion of a fibrosarcoma to another than is generally found in osteosarcoma and chondrosarcoma.

Matricial substance varies from scanty to abundant and from homogeneous deposits to well formed collagenous bundles. Collagenous bundles, both straight and wavy, assume a variety of patterns; they run parallel, become intertwined and crisscrossed, or lie in whorls. The proportion of the tissue area occupied by cells compared to that occu-

pied by matricial substance varies through an extremely wide range.
In general the greater the malignancy the greater is the proportion

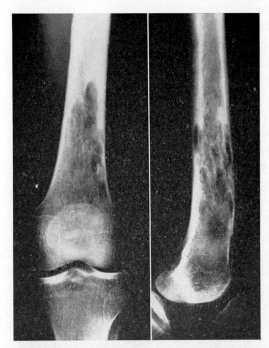

of cells to matricial substance. Highly malignant
fibrosarcomas may be so
cellular that matricial substance is virtually non-exist-
ent. In a state of extreme
anaplasia it is impossible in
many instances to identify
the type of connective tissue
the cells were destined to
form.

A slow growing, well dif-
ferentiated fibrosarcoma has
well formed matricial substance which is generally in
the form of clearly visible
collagenous bundles. It has
been widely stated that the
proportion of cells to matricial substance is an accurate
criterion of the degree of
malignancy—the more cel-
lular, the more malignant.
However, there are so many
exceptions to this rule that
it cannot be stated that
abundant matricial sub-
stance is an indication of benignancy. MacDonald and
Budd reviewed histologic
sections of cured and un-
cured fibrosarcomas with an

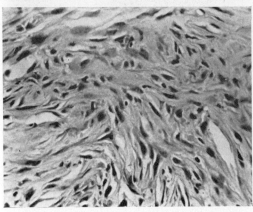

FIGURE 410. *(Continued)* B. *(Above)* Roentgenograms. C. *(Below)* Photomicrograph showing the
anaplastic character of the tumor.

eye toward identifying prognostic indications and concluded that the amount of
matricial substance is not a reliable basis for the prognosis. The character of the cells themselves is the most accurate single prognostic
criterion.

Retrograde changes in some degree are the rule. These changes are manifest by hyalinization, mucoid degeneration, necrosis and calcification. Reactive bone in small amounts may appear within the tumor as well as at the margins and tends to develop in areas of calcification.

Tumor bone is never a prominent feature as compared with that formed in osteosarcoma. Cases of so-called ossifying fibrosarcoma have been reported but when an extensive amount of tumor bone is present the tumor is more likely to be an osteosarcoma. The stroma of an osteosarcoma frequently is fibrosarcomatous in character. Occasions have arisen where the differentiation between fibrosarcoma and osteosarcoma was not made until the autopsy gave an opportunity to study the pulmonary metastases. Metastases sometimes reflect the true character of the primary tumor more clearly than does the primary tumor itself.

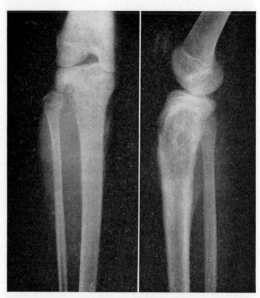

FIGURE 411. Ewing's tumor of the upper tibia in a female, age 12 years. A. Roentgenograms of the tibia.

ROENTGENOGRAPHIC FEATURES

Fibrosarcoma is a radiolucent tumor. Occasionally the diffuse radiolucency is interrupted by scattered small patches of calcium.

A central or medullary fibrosarcoma destroys and displaces one or more areas of cancellous bone giving a cyst-like radiographic appearance (Fig. 410). Unlike a cyst no periosteal new bone develops to give rise to the so-called cortical expansion so frequently associated with a bone-cyst. The margin of a central fibrosarcoma is less well defined than is the wall of a bone cyst. As the central fibrosarcoma grows it erodes the inner aspect of the cortex, ultimately destroying a small or large area of cortex. Cortical destruction occurs within a localized area by erosion or becomes riddled (motheaten) in a wide area by tumor-cell infiltration. At an even later stage a large segment of cortex may be completely demolished, continuity being maintained only by the radiolucent tumor mass. Spicules of bone at the periphery of such an aggressive tumor represents feeble attempts at reactive bone formation by the periosteum.

A periosteal fibrosarcoma appears in the roentgenogram as a radio-lucent mass overlying the cortex of the host bone. Soft tissue roentgeno-grams are helpful in visualizing the tumor mass. The first radiographic evidence of the presence of a periosteal non-ossifying tumor may be

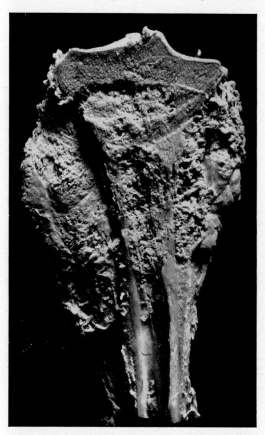

a smooth, shallow defect in the outer aspect of the bony cortex. Roentgenograms taken at several angles are sometimes needed to visualize the defect. A small Codman triangle of reactive bone may appear at the proximal and distal poles of the tumor mass and of course is the periosteal response to being elevated by the tumor. In a later stage the reactive triangles are lost. Invasion of the medullary canal occurs when the tumor perforates the cortex. Cancellous bone disappears at the site of tumor tissue. But tumor tissue can advance down the medullary canal of a tubular host bone and offer the roentgenologist no clue to its presence.

FIGURE 411. *(Continued)* Ewing's tumor. B. Frontal section of amputation specimen of tibia.

The distribution and size of pulmonary metastases are similar to those from osteo-sarcoma and chondrosarcoma but being radiolucent are somewhat less prominent in the roentgenograms.

CLINICAL FEATURES

Fibrosarcoma is slightly more common in males and the age incidence reaches its peak during the second and third decades. In the Batts series the youngest patient was one year, the oldest was 76, and the average age was 32. The author has observed a highly anaplastic periosteal fibrosarcoma of the lower tibia in an infant age four months. Three weeks following an amputation at the knee the infant died of pulmonary metastases.

Symptoms are similar to those caused by the other types of osteogenic sarcoma. A slow growing fibrosarcoma may cause little disability for months. The duration of symptoms prior to treatment is usually longer than with osteosarcoma and chondrosarcoma. Pathologic fractures are not uncommon, particularly in association with the medullary type of fibrosarcoma.

Therapy

Treatment of a fibrosarcoma is primarily surgical. In the more anaplastic forms an immediate amputation well above the tumor is indicated whenever the tumor resides in an extremity. In instances of a minimal degree of malignancy as indicated by a reliable microscopic study a radical local excision can be considered. However, if the tumor then recurs, as it will in a great many cases, the degree of malignancy has increased, thereby calling for an amputation. Fibrosarcoma in the pelvis, vertebra, thorax and skull can only be treated by wide excision of the tumor.

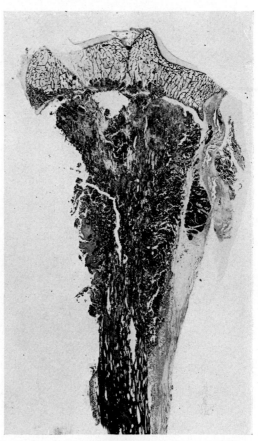

FIGURE 411. (*Continued*) Ewing's tumor. C. Histologic section of the specimen.

Roentgentherapy is not considered to be of great value in fibrosarcoma, but is usually recommended after local excisions and as palliative therapy in hopeless cases.

Prognosis

As poor as the prognosis is in fibrosarcoma it is better than in osteosarcoma and chondrosarcoma. When there is pronounced anaplasia and rapid growth, the chances of a recovery, even with relatively early amputation, are nil. A review of the "cured" cases of fibrosarcoma indicates that in nearly all instances the tumor was fairly well differentiated and slow growing. As has been mentioned, the presence of an encapsulating margin is a favorable sign.

BONE SARCOMA IN PAGET'S DISEASE

Paget's disease may be complicated by the formation in Paget bone of a fibrosarcoma, chondrosarcoma, or osteosarcoma. This is the most

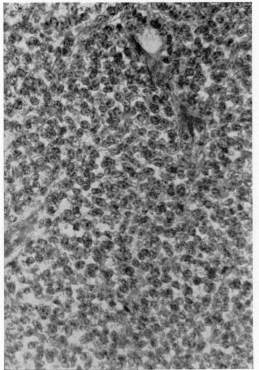

serious complication that can befall a patient with Paget's disease. The incidence of sarcomas of the osteogenic series in Paget's disease is given variously from 5 to 14 percent.

Platt (1947) reported a review of 180 primary sarcomas of bone among which there were ten cases in which the sarcoma was superimposed upon Paget's disease. Coley and Sharp (1931) reviewed 72 cases of osteogenic sarcoma in patients over 50 years of age. Paget's disease was an underlying factor in 28 percent.

When a sarcoma develops in the skeleton of a patient with Paget's disease, the tumor invariably appears in bone involved by the osteitis

FIGURE 411. *(Continued)* Ewing's tumor. D. Photomicrograph of the tumor cells.

deformans. Multiple bone sarcomas are far more common in association with Paget's disease than in skeletal systems uninvolved by Paget's disease. Summey and Pressly (1946) found 76 cases in the literature of sarcoma in Paget's disease; they added three new cases of their own. They listed the sites of the tumors in the following order: femur, humerus, skull, tibia, scapula, vertebrae, and ilium.

Periodic roentgenograms of the skeleton have been recommended, particularly in polyostotic osteitis deformans. Detection of an osteogenic sarcoma in an early stage is the only hope of improving an otherwise grave prognosis. An early amputation is indicated when the complicating sarcoma is located in an extremity. Roentgentherapy has only palliative benefit. The average life expectancy in the Coley-Sharp series proved to be an average of ten months shorter than would have been expected with osteogenic sarcomas unassociated with Paget's disease.

EWING'S TUMOR
(Diffuse endothelioma of bone)

Ewing described the entity which now bears his name in 1921, and called it endothelial myeloma. A far reaching polemic was touched off by Ewing's contentions but it is now generally conceded that what he described represents a clearcut pathologic and clinical entity that needed to be extracted from the "endothelioma" group. The term endothelioma was introduced by Golgi in 1889. He applied the term to a large group of poorly understood tumors whose cellular composition appeared to be endothelial in character.

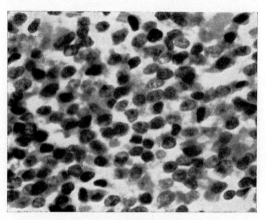

FIGURE 412. Ewing's tumor. Photomicrograph of the tumor cells.

Two great groups of tumors stem from the bone marrow. From the marrow blood cells and their progenitors stems the myeloma series (multiple myeloma), and from the supporting structure of the marrow (the reticulo-endothelial tissues), stem three tumors: Ewing's tumor, reticulum cell sarcoma, and hemangioendothelioma. Lipomatous tumors may also have a place in the latter group. Conner in 1926 classified the reticulo-endothelial marrow tumors into three types: (1) Angioendothelia, (2) Reticulum cell, and (3) Diffuse endothelioma (Ewing's). Ewing did not believe that the reticulum cell sarcoma was related to the endotheliomas.

Oberling Theory

Oberling (1928) contends that Ewing's tumor and the reticulum cell sarcoma are variants of the same tumor and that both tumors originate from reticulum cells. Stout, Jaffe, Lichtenstein, Weinmann, and Sicher share this view. It is Oberling's further belief that the reticulum cell is also the ancestral cell for lymphocytes, plasma cells, myelocytes, and erythroblasts. The present trend is toward Oberling's concept of the disease and away from Ewing's. But a vast realm of the histogenesis remains unfathomed. Stout has given words to the feeling shared by all who have earnestly studied this disease: "The histopathological picture is difficult to record because in my experience it is the most complex and poorest defined in all oncology."

ETIOLOGY

The cause or causes of Ewing's tumor are unknown. Attempts have been made to credit trauma and several of the infectious diseases as etiologic factors but thus far the evidence brought forward is not convincing.

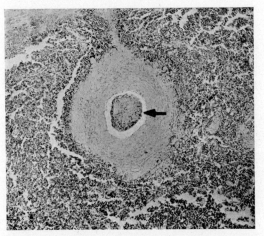

FIGURE 413. Ewing's tumor cell thrombus (arrow).

PATHOGENESIS

As has been stated the precise cell from which Ewing's tumor originates is not known. Geschickter and Copeland, and others, denying that the cells are endothelial in origin, see evidence of a lymphogenous origin and consider Ewing's tumor to be a lymphoma.

Once the primary tumor is well established it is impossible to accurately identify the site of origin. The evidence at hand indicates that the tumor begins in either the cortex or in very close proximity to the cortex, and then spreads in all directions by infiltration. Following perforation of the cortex a subperiosteal mass takes shape and ultimately the periosteum is perforated. In the majority of cases the tumor originates in the diaphysis of a long tubular bone, then soon spreads to the nearest metaphysis. The epiphyseal plate presents a substantial barrier, so there is a long delay before the plate is perforated and the epiphysis invaded. There is no tendency for Ewing's tumor to invade joints.

Reactive Bone

While no tumor bone forms in any of the marrow tumors, there is formed a variable amount of reactive (non-tumorous) bone. Multiple myeloma stimulates the formation of very little reactive bone whereas Ewing's tumor frequently is associated with considerable reactive bone, particularly in early stages. Reactive bone is both central and periosteal. Examples of *central reactive bone* have been seen in Ewing's tumor of the os calcis and the tibial diaphysis. The entire tumor area presents the picture of osteosclerosis. In a late state the reactive bone together with a segment of the host bone may be utterly demolished as the aggressive tumor cells destroy all bone with which they come in contact (Figs. 411 & 416).

PERIOSTEAL REACTIVE BONE around a diaphyseal Ewing's tumor in an early stage frequently forms two to several thin layers of periosteal bone. When the tumor cells penetrate the cortex of the host bone and a thin layer of the cells lie beneath the periosteum the periosteum reacts by forming a thin sheet of fibrous bone parallel to the shaft. The tumor cells then penetrate the layer of periosteal bone and thereby prompt the formation of a second layer of fibrous bone. Several such layers of bone may form in succession, the most mature being adjacent to the cortex. The layers of periosteal bone and the layers of tumor cells sandwiched between them are of approximately equal thickness and seldom exceed one

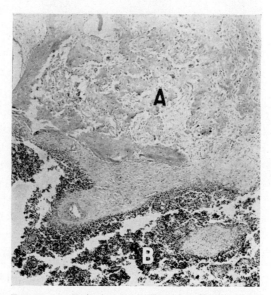

FIGURE 414. Ewing's tumor. Reactive fibrous bone, *A*, adjacent to tumor tissue, *B*.

or two millimeters. In a late stage all evidence of this so-called "onion skin" structure is generally lost. Layering of periosteal bone in this manner is by no means pathognomonic of Ewing's tumor. It is observed occasionally in low grade pyogenic osteomyelitis, and rarely in chronic granulomatous infections of bone (e.g., tuberculosis, syphilis). Once the extracortical portion of Ewing's tumor forms a dome-shaped mass there is generally a Codman triangle of reactive bone to be found at the upper and lower blending of the tumor with the host bone periosteum, particularly on the diaphyseal side. The protruding portion of the extracortical mass develops around it a zone of reactive fibrous tissue. As the tumor mass grows the tumor cells infiltrate and destroy portions of the fibrous tissue. More fibrous tissue is then laid down to preserve the confining margin. Unfortunately, this reactive margin has no capacity to halt the growth of the tumor.

METASTASES

Pulmonary metastases are an ultimate development in nearly all cases of Ewing's tumor. The lung metastases from a Ewing's tumor are similar to those from an osteogenic sarcoma except in the character of the component cells. Unlike an osteogenic sarcoma, Ewing's tumor

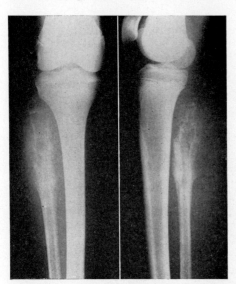

frequently metastasizes to regional lymph nodes and to other bones. Lymph node and skeletal metastases may even precede the pulmonary metastases. So frequently have metastases developed in various parts of the skeletal system that several investigators have believed the disease to be of multicentric osseous origin. Far more skeletal metastases have been observed in the skull, vertebrae, ribs and pelvis than in the long tubular bones.

PATHOLOGIC ANATOMY

FIGURE 415. Ewing's tumor of the upper fibula. A. Preoperative roentgenograms.

Distribution

The primary Ewing's tumor may occur in any bone but the incidence is highest in the long tubular bones of the lower extremities. The following sites are listed according to the frequency with which they are involved by Ewing's tumor: proximal one-half of the tibia, lower and upper femoral metaphyses and an adjacent segment of diaphysis, proximal humeral metaphysis and the proximal one-half of the diaphysis, the fibula, ilium, lower radius, clavicle and ribs, and the os calcis and other tarsals.

Gross Pathology

The tumor mass is firm to soft and is light gray in color. Reddish gray and dark brown areas represent sites of hemorrhage and necrosis. Small pseudo-cysts are not infrequently seen where necrotic tissue has liquefied. Multiple fibrous bands criss-cross through the tumor mass. In a great many cases, except those where the tumor is of brief duration, the extracortical mass represents the largest portion of tumor. Forty-one percent of Stout's cases had an extraosseous mass greater than the intraosseous involvement. The zone of reactive fibrous tissue overlying the tumor mass is usually clearly visible on gross examination.

In late stages a large segment of the host bone may become so riddled by the infiltrating tumor tissue that it possesses no strength or

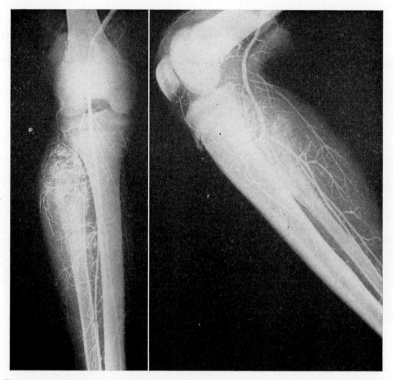

FIGURE 415. *(Continued)* Ewing's tumor. B. Arteriograms of amputation specimen.

rigidity. Continuity is often maintained by tumor tissue, not bone (Fig. 417C).

The vascularity of Ewing's tumor varies rather widely but is generally pronounced.

Histopathology

The cells that make up Ewing's tumor are as monotonously uniform as the cells in the osteogenic sarcoma are varied. Masses of closely packed round or oval cells measuring approximately ten microns in diameter characterize the tumor (Figs. 411D & 412). When individual cells are closely examined in the less crowed areas it is found that the hyperchromatic, sharply outlined nucleus rarely has a nucleolus. Only a poorly defined narrow rim of cytoplasm surrounds the nucleus and can be identified in but few of the cells. Crowded areas give the cells a polyhedral appearance. Not a few of the numerous blood vessels of this tumor are lined by tumor cells, and thrombi formed of tumor cells are not at all unusual (Fig. 413).

A few mitotic figures are seen. Campbell and Hamilton used the total number of mitotic figures ("chromatin knots") per high power field as a basis for establishing the prognosis. Cases were graded from one to four. Five or less mitotic figures per field was classified as Grade I; Grade II had six to ten mitotic figures; Grade III, 11 to 15; and Grade IV, more than 15. Thirty cases were analyzed. Patients in Grade I had a 31 percent chance of living five years and a 23 percent chance of living ten years. Patients in Grades III and IV would probably not survive longer than a little over one year.

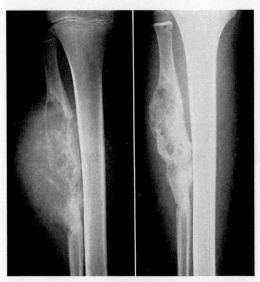

FIGURE 416. Ewing's tumor of the fibula. A. *(Left)* Roentgenogram prior to roentgentherapy. B. *(Right)* Roentgenogram three months after roentgentherapy showing a reduced tumor mass and increased reactive ossification.

One of the outstanding histological characteristics of many cases of Ewing's tumor is the perithelial arrangement of the cells. Pseudo-rosettes are formed and are similar to those in a neuroblastoma. A neuroblastoma may resemble Ewing's tumor both histologically and clinically (Willis).

Areas of necrosis are the rule. In these areas it is common to find numerous islands of living tumor cells, and the center of many of the islands is marked by a blood vessel.

The osteolytic capacity of the tumor cells varies widely. In some instances, particularly in the early stages the cells infiltrate marrow spaces and very often appear to cause little change in the bony trabeculae. In the majority of instances, however, the cells are actively osteolytic. Bone in the path of the tumor is destroyed both by tumor cells and by giant cell osteoclasts.

Whereas a reticuum cell sarcoma regularly presents a delicate reticulum network, seldom does Ewing's tumor. Oberling and Stout found reticulum cells in Ewing's tumor; Ewing denied that his tumor possesses any reticulum cells.

The strands of fibrous tissue in Ewing's tumor represent remains of reactive fibroblastic tissue formed within the tumor and at the periphery. Areas of tumor necrosis may fill in with fibro-cellular tissue, and it is not unusual for trabeculae of fibrous bone to appear in such

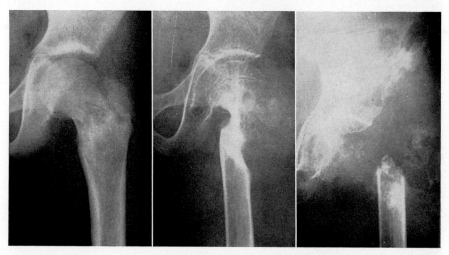

FIGURE 417. Ewing's tumor of the upper femur. (Childrens Hospital, Los Angeles.) A. *(Left)* 1-3-1929. B. *(Center)* 2-6-1930. C. *(Right)* 4-19-1930. Rapid destruction of the upper femur occurred in spite of roentgentherapy.

fields. Neutrophils and lymphocytes frequently infiltrate the fibrous pseudo-capsule enveloping the extracortical mass.

Growth of Ewing's tumor is principally by infiltration. An extracortical mass, in addition to extending its boundaries by infiltration, also grows by expanson.

ROENTGENOGRAPHIC FEATURES

Early evidences of Ewing's tumor are reflected in roentgenograms by a Codman triangle (unassociated with tumor bone and calcium), localized widening of the medullary canal, localized cortical mottling, and in some sites such as the os calcis, with considerable reactive bone. In a few cases, a pathological fracture may be the cue for the initial roentgenographic study.

Periosteal bone may take several forms of which the "onion peel" structure and Codman triangles have been the most discussed. A short segment of fusiform dense thickening of long bone diaphyseal cortex is not a rare observation and represents reactive periosteal bone. Heavier exposure of such a sclerotic segment generally discloses localized cortical mottling. In rare instances reactive bone in an extracortical tumor mass takes the form of radially arranged spicules resembling the sun-ray structure of an osteosarcoma. Reactive bone may become conspicuous for a few weeks or months following roentgen therapy. As the tumor becomes immune to the roentgen rays the reactive bone is demolished.

The extensive destruction of bone in advanced stages, so dramatically portrayed by the roentgenogram, needs no further elucidation.

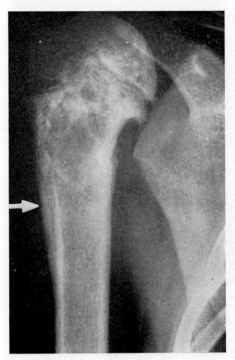

FIGURE 418. Ewing's tumor of the upper humerus. Arrow points to the "onion peel" pattern of periosteal bone.

CLINICAL FEATURES

Ewing's tumor is a catastrophic disease of childhood and adolescence. While the incidence during the first decade is higher than it is for the osteogenic sarcoma series, the majority of cases occur during the second and third decades. A few cases have been observed during middle and old age. The incidence of the disease is approximately twice as high in males as in females. In 79 percent of Stout's series of 42 cases the known duration of the disease at the time of diagnosis was less than one year.

Symptoms

Pain is the most frequent single symptom and exists in nearly all cases. During the early stage the pain tends to be intermittent in character and moderate in degree. Long remissions are not unusual. Just as with most malignant bone tumors the pain in the advanced stage is generally constant and severe, and is more distressing at night than during the day.

A palpable mass is present in virtually all cases, particularly when the tumor is located in an extremity. The overlying soft tissues are trequently tender, and excessively warm, and the skin somewhat red-dened. It is little wonder that so many of Ewing's tumors are explored under the diagnosis of pyogenic osteomyelitis.

FEVER is a part of the clinical picture. In the early stage the fever is low grade, seldom rising above 100 degrees. In the advanced stage temperatures of 103 and 104 degrees are not at all excep-tional.

THE BLOOD PICTURE re-veals a moderate secondary anemia and generally a leu-cocytosis. White blood cell counts as high as twenty to forty thousand have been observed.

Pulmonary symptoms (from metastases), and pro-gressive loss of weight char-acterize the late stage.

Differential Diagnosis

Ewing's tumor often re-quires detailed study to con-clusively differentiate it from the many diseases with which it has been confused. Pyogenic osteomyelitis heads the list but tubercu-losis and syphilitic osteomye-litis must also be included. The other tumors that enter into the differential diagno-sis include neuroblastoma,

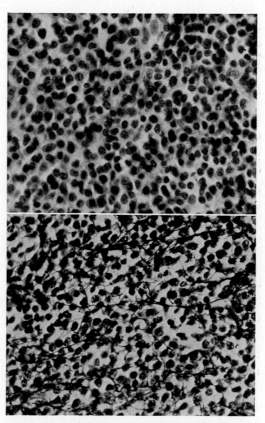

FIGURE 419. Reticulum cell sarcoma (x 560). A. *(Above)* Photomicrograph of a typical field of tumor cells. B. *(Below)* Silver reticulin stain to show the network of reticulin fibrils.

osteosarcoma, chondrosarcoma, fibrosarcoma, myeloma, and metastatic carcinoma. Hand-Christian's disease and the other reticulo-endo-thelioses must also be ruled out.

Treatment

Amputation is still recommended by most surgeons whenever the tumor involves an extremity. A few surgeons view the disease with such a deep sense of futility that they do not recommend surgery, particularly when the patient is a child. In some instances local resection of the tumor has proved feasible and beneficial. Roentgen therapy is widely used in the treatment of Ewing's tumor, both in conjunction with surgery and without surgery. At the outset the tumor is decidedly radiosensitive and rapidly melts away under the action of the roentgen rays. But, unfortunately, the tumor recurs and each time it recurs after roentgentherapy it is more resistant to the rays. Few proved cases have been cured by roentgentherapy alone. The best results have been with an amputation followed by roentgen radiation.

Prognosis

In Bradley Coley's words, "Ewing's tumor is truly a catastrophic disease." In general the younger the patient the more grave the prognosis. Early and well-directed treatment in an adolescent or adult offers a small chance for recovery. The reliable evidence available appears to indicate that *less* than ten percent of the patients with Ewing's tumor recover from the disease.

RETICULUM CELL SARCOMA OF BONE

Primary reticulum cell sarcoma of bone appears well-established as a solitary malignant primary bone tumor. It must, of course, be differentiated from the generalized form of reticulo-sarcoma (Craver and Copeland).

According to Ewing, reticulum cell sarcoma was first recognized by Kaufmann. Important contributions to this subject have since been made by Oberling and others.

Parker and Jackson (1939), in a clinico-pathological study, reviewed 17 cases. Their cases had the following skeletal distribution: femur, five cases; clavicle, four cases; tibia, three cases; humerus, three cases; scapula, one case; and mandible, one case.

Sherman and Snyder (1947) described the roentgenographic characteristics of the tumor in 17 cases. The ages of the patients varied from 13 to 76, and the distribution of the tumors was as follows: femur, four; tibia, five; humerus, two; scapula, two; vertebrae, two; fibula, one; and rib, one.

In seven instances in each of the two series of 17 cases (41 percent) the tumor was located in the knee region. Of the 12 cases of the Sherman-Snyder series in which the tumor was located in a tubular bone, five were diaphyseal, and seven were either metaphyseal or epiphyseal.

GROSS PATHOLOGY

A medullary origin is the rule, and from the central origin the tumor mass either extends along the medullary canal or perforates the over-

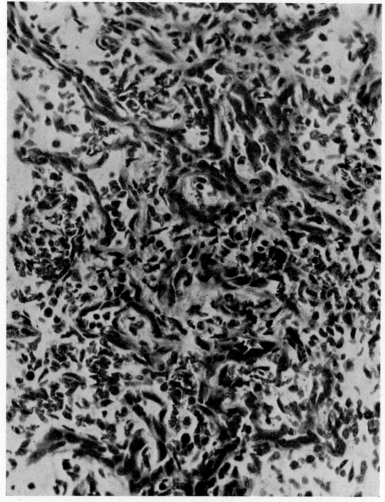

FIGURE 420. Hemangio-endothelioma. The tumor cells form numerous vascular channels which contain circulating blood cells. (Courtesy, A. Purdy Stout, M.D.)

lying cortex to form an extracortical mass. Cases representing these two patterns of extension are approximately equally divided. In those instances where an extracortical mass develops, the mass is rarely of large dimensions. The incidence of a metaphyseal origin is higher than in Ewing's tumor.

While it is not unusual to observe considerable reactive bone in and around the tumor, no tumor bone is ever seen. The tumor grows, and destroys the bone in its path, both by infiltration and by the erosion incident to expansion. Codman triangles may form but extensive periosteal bone formation leading to cortical expansion is not seen. Because of the infiltrating cells at the periphery of the tumor, the tumor margin is poorly defined both grossly and in roentgenograms.

Pathologic fractures are not uncommon, as indicated by the presence of four instances in the Sherman-Snyder series.

HISTOPATHOLOGY

The cells of reticulum cell sarcoma somewhat resemble those of Ewing's tumor except for a wider variation in size and the presence of numerous cells that are considerably larger than those of Ewing's tumor (Fig. 419A). Except for the association with bone the histology is similar to that of reticulum cell sarcoma of lymph nodes.

A reticulin fiber network (Fig. 419B) is a consistent part of the picture, whereas in Ewing's tumor there is seldom a well-formed reticulum framework. Reticulin stains should be routine in these tumors.

The reactive bone is fibrous in type. Specimens secured following a period of roentgen therapy show a considerable increase in reactive bone.

CLINICAL FEATURES

Diagnosis

It may be impossible to differentiate a reticulum cell sarcoma from Ewing's tumor except by biopsy. Both tumors respond to radiation therapy and later recover their aggressiveness. As a rule reticulum cell sarcoma forms less periosteal bone and a smaller extracortical mass than does Ewing's tumor. The average age of the patient is higher in reticulum cell sarcoma than in Ewing's tumor. Osteolytic osteosarcoma must occasionally be differentiated from reticulum cell sarcoma, as must also osteolytic carcinoma metastases. Reticulum cell sarcoma is more radiosensitive and grows more slowly than either osteosarcoma or carcinoma metastases. It must be remembered that the generalized form of reticulum cell sarcoma (Craver and Copeland's lymphosarcoma in bone) can be associated with one or more skeletal foci and thus present a problem in differential diagnosis.

Therapy

Parker and Jackson recommended amputation for reticulum cell sarcoma of an extremity. Sherman and Snyder, on the other hand, advised radiation therapy. There appears to be a place for both of these forms of therapy.

Prognosis

The prognosis in reticulum cell sarcoma is decidedly better than in Ewing's tumor. In the 17 cases of the Sherman-Snyder series there were five, five-year cures, and five, three-year cures. Three of the patients were dead and four were still under treatment.

HEMANGIO-ENDOTHELIOMA

Hemangio-endothelioma, or angio-endothelioma as it is also termed, has been observed in a few instances as a primary bone tumor. Stout reported a series of 18 cases of hemangio-endothelioma, and in two of his series the tumor was primary in bone. Other primary sites of these tumors include the breast, uterus, liver, spleen, pleura, and skin.

Ewing observed three cases in which the lower humerus was the site of the tumor. Ewing described these tumors as bulky, cystic, and characterized by pulsations and a bruit.

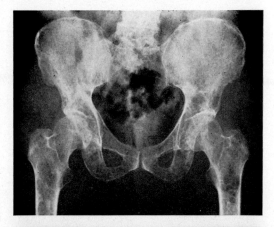

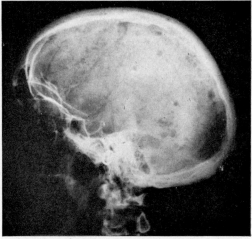

FIGURE 421. Multiple myeloma in a male, age 56. A. *(Above)* The femora and the pelvis are riddled by the tumor tissue. B. *(Below)* Multiple characteristic punched out osteolytic skull lesions.

Thomas (1942) reported similar cases. Pulmonary metastases are said to be common. Nearly all of the reported cases have involved adults. The sex incidence is approximately equal.

Hemangio-endothelioma, a malignant vascular tumor, is characterized by a mass of anastomosing vascular channels. The vascular tubes are neoplastic but serve to carry the circulating blood throughout the tumor, thus making this an extremely vascular tumor (Fig. 420). Whereas in the benign vascular tumors the vessels are generally lined by a single layer of normal endothelium, the vessels of a hemangio-endothelioma are characterized by multiple layers of atypical endothelial cells. A complex pattern of anastomosis is seen and between the vessels there is a delicate reticulin framework. As would be anticipated, extensive hemorrhages are liable to occur within and around the tumor.

Both Ewing and Stout emphasize that metastic carcinoma, particularly of the kidney, adrenal and thyroid, must be ruled out before making a diagnosis of primary osseous hemangio-endothelioma. The resemblance between hypernephroid carcinoma metastases and hemangio-endothelioma is striking. It is Stout's opinion that the illustrative cases used by both Thomas and Ewing more closely resemble metastatic hypernephroid carcinoma than true hemangio-endothelioma. When the cells lining the vascular channels are large, possess clear cytoplasm, are cylindrical in shape, and have small nuclei the lesion is more likely the metastasis of a hypernephroma.

MULTIPLE MYELOMA
(Myelomatosis)

Multiple myeloma is a fatal malignant neoplastic disease of middle and old age in which the primary lesions are in the hematopoietic marrow of the skeletal system.

The first reported case was described in two historic articles, the first by William McIntyre in 1848 and the second by McIntyre, Bence-Jones and Dalrymple in 1850. In the past one-hundred years scores of articles have been written about this interesting disease. It is now acknowledged by most investigators that multiple myeloma is a well-defined clinical and pathologic entity.

In the bone tumor classification of the Bone Sarcoma Registry multiple myeloma is divided into four types: (1) Plasma cell, (2) Myelocytoma, (3) Erythroblastoma, and (4) Lymphocytoma. This classification is based upon the assumption that the individual types arise from specific and different marrow cells. The exact origin of the cells that make up multiple myelomas has not been established. In view of this fact plus the fact that all types have approximately similar clinical manifestations has led Wallgren, Gaschickter and Copeland, Lichtenstein and Jaffe, and others to abandon the histologic subdivisions.

Virtually nothing is known of the etiology. Infection has not been a factor, neither has trauma, and the heredity factor has not proved to be significant. No race has been spared.

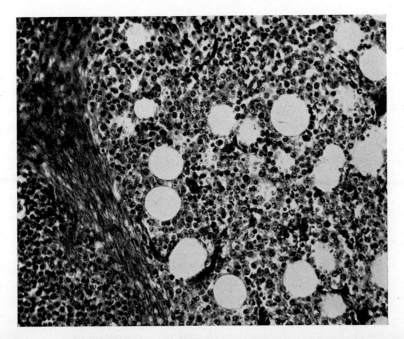

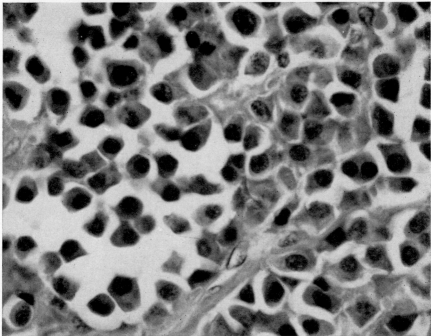

FIGURE 422. Multiple myeloma. A. *(Above)* Photomicrograph, low power, of the tumor tissue showing a preponderance of plasma cells. B. *(Below)* Photomicrograph, high power (x 900).

Pathologic Anatomy
Distribution

In most instances the bone lesions are multiple when they are first observed. However, a number of cases are now on record in which the lesion was solitary (in a single bone) for several months to several years prior to dissemination (myelomatosis). Solitary lesions have been observed most frequently in the ilium (Fig. 423). In virtually all instances the dissemination through the skeleton has followed the solitary lesion regardless of the type of treatment employed. However there is the outstanding case reported by Stewart and Taylor in which a large solitary myeloma of the proximal one-third of the humerus was removed by a forequarter amputation, and the patient was alive and well 8 years later.

The classical picture of multiple myeloma is one in which the spine, skull, pelvis, femora and humeri are riddled with a multitude of rounded osteolytic lesions (Fig. 421). Contrary to popular opinion there are many cases in which the skeleton does not present this striking alteration. Instead there is generalized osteoporosis and scattered central areas of cortical erosion.

Myelomas have occurred in the greatest numbers in the vertebrae, ribs, sternum, skull, and pelvis. Involvement of the femora and humeri is generally limited to a late stage; involvement of the bones distal to the knee and elbow seldom occurs.

Extra-skeletal myelomas, also known as extramedullary plasma cell tumors are much less common than skeletal myelomas but do occur more frequently than is generally realized. Hellwig, in 1943, reviewed 127 published cases. Sixty-three of this number originated in the air passages (antrum, larynx, pharynx, tongue and beneath tongue, tonsils, uvula, turbinates, and septum). Thirty-nine of these plasmacytomas were benign and remained localized; thirty were invasive. Nine of the thirty metastasized to lymph nodes, and nine to the bones, all of which were fatal. Extra skeletal myelomas have also been observed in the spleen, liver, lungs, and heart. Several years may elapse between the appearance of a primary malignant extraskeletal myeloma and the metastases. Jackson, Parker and Bethea removed a plasmacytoma of the tonsil eight years prior to generalized bone involvement.

Gross Pathology

Myelomas tend to be spherical, solid, though friable and moderately firm. Their color is a dark red, dark gray or a mixture of these colors.

The moderate to considerable vascularity of these tumors is indicated by the active bleeding that takes place when they are incised. Areas of old hemorrhage and necrosis are a frequent observation. A wall of reactive bone overlying a tumor mass is exceptional but when present it assumes a parchment-like character. Pathologic compression fractures and collapse of host bones is the rule. Such fractures occur in large numbers in ribs, in vertebral bodies and even in the sternum. Vertebral body collapse frequently leads to the formation of a kyphosis, a gibbus, or a scoliosis. Pathologic fractures heal in approximately one half of the cases.

Histopathology

Microscopically there are masses of closely packed round or oval cells averaging about 10 microns in diameter (Fig. 422). No supporting stroma is seen; in fact, there is no visible intercellular substance. The majority of the cells resemble plasma cells in that the nucleus is eccentrically

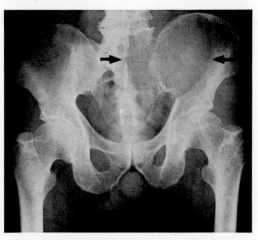

FIGURE 423. Solitary myeloma of the ilium and sacrum in a male, age 72.

placed, frequently possesses a spoke-like chromatin pattern, and a sharply defined nuclear wall. The cytoplasm takes an eosinophilic stain and the cell has a fairly clear outline, particularly in fields where the cells are not crowded. There is an occasional mitotic figure and a few of the cells have double nuclei. Red blood cells and scattered leucocytes are the result of hemorrhage. Granulation and fibrous tissues are found around areas of necrosis and at pathologic fractures.

The cell from which myelomas originate has not yet been identified. It is presumably a fixed, (non-circulating) marrow cell. Lichtenstein and Jaffe, and Wallgren emphasize "the unity of myelomas." There is considerable evidence that the variations in the component cells of multiple myeloma represent variations in cell maturity rather than variations in the character of the ancestral cell. Lichtenstein and Jaffe divide the myelomas on a histologic basis into two types. The first is the classical and more common plasma cell type with its uniform small size; the second type is characterized by cells most of which are considerably larger than the "plasma cell." In the second type the majority of cells, even though larger, have an eccentric nucleus and eosinophilic cytoplasm, just as in the first type.

Microscopically, the myeloma picture must be differentiated from Ewing's tumor, neuroblastoma, carcinoma metastases, and Hand-Christian's disease.

Amyloidosis is not an infrequent associated finding in myelomatosis. The amyloid deposits appear in microscopic proportions in the myelomas and in medullary canals. Larger accumulations of amyloid have been found in a few instances.

The histologic diagnosis of myeloma is most reliable when made from tissue taken directly from a myeloma. However, in establishing the diagnosis in the living, it is not always feasible or possible to remove tissue from a tumor mass. *Sternal* punctures have been employed in recent years with considerable diagnostic success. Myeloma cells, scattered or numerous, tell of the presence of myelomatosis.

Kidney Lesions

Kidney damage, principally from a nephrosis, is the rule in myelomatosis; 70 per cent of the Geschickter and Copeland series disclosed renal changes. An atypical nephritis frequently represents one of the earlier changes. Foord has advised that the finding of an atypical nephritis should arouse the clinician to suspect multiple myeloma. Albuminuria is present in a large proportion of cases of myelomatosis.

BENCE-JONES PROTEINURIA

In the first reported case Bence-Jones noted an albuminoid substance in the urine. The Bence-Jones bodies appear as a cloudy white precipitate when the urine is heated to a temperature of 45° to 60° C. Near the boiling point (100° C.) the white precipitate goes back into solution.

It was formerly believed that virtually all patients with myelomatosis had Bence-Jones bodies in their urine. It is now well established that less than three-fourths of the patients have positive tests. In the early stages of the disease Bence-Jones proteinuria may be present only at irregular intervals. It is only in an advanced stage that the urine is likely to be consistently positive. Obviously, one or several negative tests do not rule out myelomatosis.

It deserves to be emphasized that Bence-Jones proteinuria is not pathognomonic of myelomatosis. Carcinomatosis with skeletal metastases, some of the chronic leukemias, sarcomatosis, and senile osteomalacia have been known to be associated with Bence-Jones proteinuria.

Blood Changes

The principle abnormal findings in the blood consist of hyperproteinemia, hypercalcemia, secondary anemia, and rarely, pseudoleukemia.

HYPERPROTEINEMIA: Hyperglobulinemia is found in half or more of all cases. When serum globulins are high there is frequently an associated lowering of the serum albumin.

HYPERCALCEMIA: An increase in serum calcium is said to occur in approximately 50 per cent of cases. In the Lichtenstein-Jaffe series levels up to 18 mg. percent were recorded. There is rapid mobilization of calcium when skeletal myelomas are actively growing. A secondary parathyroid gland hyperplasia is said to be a factor in some instances. Metastatic calcium deposits are not unusual in the kidneys, and lungs. Hypercalcemia associated with hyperproteinemia or Bence-Jones proteinuria is strong diagnostic evidence of multiple myeloma.

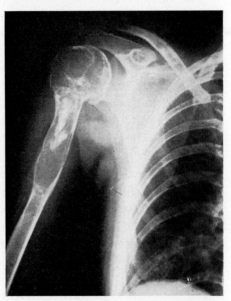

FIGURE 424. Myeloma of the upper humerus in a female, age 48. The tumor began in the right humerus and later became disseminated. A pathologic fracture is present at the surgical neck of the humerus (Los Angeles County Hospital).

SECONDARY ANEMIA: Displacement of hemopoietic marrow by tumor tissue plus kidney deterioration are among the factors responsible for the high incidence of secondary anemia in myelomatosis. A leucopoenia may also be observed together with a substantial increase in immature leucocytes. The Schilling blood differential count may disclose a pronounced shift to the left. Plasma cells, and normoblasts may also be seen.

PSEUDO-LEUKEMIA: In far advanced cases it is not rare for large numbers of myeloma cells (principally "plasma cells") to enter the blood stream. This phenomenon, termed "plasma cell leukemia" is not in reality a leukemia, but merely an uncommon phase of late myelomatosis. The total leucocyte count may undergo pronounced elevation.

ROENTGENOGRAPHIC FEATURES

The roentgenogram is often of immeasurable help in establishing the diagnosis of myelomas. While it is admitted that many cases are not associated with spectacular roentgenographic changes, it must be conceded that in the majority of instances the skeletal tumors are portrayed in a most striking manner. The pure osteolytic character, the rounded contour, and their central location give the lesions sharp definition. Of course, in advanced cases when the areas of the skeleton are "riddled" with myelomas the individual tumors are not discernible.

The bony defects created by myelomas possess a "punched out" appearance. An overlying periosteal reaction, when present, is seldom associated with the formation of new bone, except at sites of pathologic fractures. Reactive osteosclerosis adjacent to the lesions does not occur.

Solitary myelomas occasionally grow to large proportions. An entire ilium, upper humerus, or a vertebral body may be destroyed before dissemination takes place. A large area of bone may utterly disappear, leaving a radiolucent area uninterrupted by either visible flakes of calcium or spicules of bone.

The skull defects are most numerous in the frontal and parietal regions. Vertebral involvement takes place principally in vertebral bodies and is generally most extensive in the lower dorsal and upper lumbar vertebra. Intervertebral discs become narrowed and may even disappear whenever adjacent vertebral bodies are invaded. Collapse of vertebrae is reflected by kyphotic and scoliotic curvatures.

Pulmonary metastases are conscpicuous for their absence. This fact serves as a useful differential diagnostic point, not seldom needed. On occasion the multiple osteolytic rib lesions offer a superficial resemblance to pulmonary lesions.

CLINICAL FEATURES

Myelomatosis generally makes its appearance between the ages of forty and sixty. A few cases in young adults are on record but are exceptional. Children do not acquire this disease. In all of the series reported there have been more males than females. It was formerly taught that the proportion was two males to one female. More recent statistics give the males only a "slight edge."

Symptoms

Pain is a prominent symptom in myelomatosis and it often begins in the spine. In early stages the pain is intermittent and tolerable, in late stages it is often excruciating and constant. Compression of spinal nerve roots and the spinal cord are relatively common observations. In fact, it is not unusual for a paraplegia to usher in the clinical phase of the disease. Radiating pain in the lower extremities is usually bilateral. This is one of the few instances where organic lower extremity radiations are bilateral.

A chronic bronchitis and an emphysema may follow the collapse of one or more dorsal vertebrae.

Tumors occasionally protrude through the host bone and extend into the overlying soft tissues sufficiently to be identified by palpating fingers. Widespread bone tenderness may be a prominent finding and does not depend upon cortical perforation for its existence. Exquisite tenderness is generally localized to a site directly over a myeloma.

Malaise and loss of weight, progressive in late stages, are subject to remissions in early stages.

Treatment

The treatment is symptomatic and palliative. Blood transfusions offer a temporary diminution of the secondary anemia; a laminectomy is indicated when the spinal cord is compressed; and a period of immobilization must be employed for many of the pathologic fractures. In a small number of cases an amputation has been performed for the treatment of a solitary myeloma in an extremity. This has rarely altered the ultimate fatal outcome but offers the patient his only chance for recovery.

Roentgen therapy has proved temporarily beneficial in many cases in that pain was lessened. Radioactive phosphorus (P_{32}) has been employed in some quarters but the results thus far have been disappointing.

Snapper has reported temporary relief from bone pain following the use of preparations called "stilbamidine" (4, 4'-diamidinostilbene) and "pentamidine" (4, 4' [pentamethylenedioxy] dibenzamidine) administered in conjunction with a low protein diet. Fifteen patients were so treated, all of which appeared to experience a remission of the disease. This form of therapy is in the experimental stage and cannot yet be evaluated.

Prognosis

All cases of myelomatosis have a fatal termination. The average duration of life after the onset of symptoms is approximately two years, but varies from a few months to 16 years (Davison and Balser).

LIPOSARCOMA

Primary osseous liposarcoma is not universally accepted as an established entity. The existence of liposarcoma as a primary bone tumor is said to rest entirely upon circumstantial data. However, new case reports continue to appear in the literature.

Attention was first called to liposarcoma of bone by Ewing in 1928. In 1931 Stewart reported a detailed description of three cases. Rehbock and Hauser added two cases in 1936 and reviewed the five cases previously reported. Four of the seven patients were males, and all were adults, the ages varying from 23 to 60 years. The following bones were sites of the primary tumor: phalanx 3rd finger, left fibula, right fibula, right ilium, left scapula, and right femur. Growth of the tumor is generally slow. Skeletal and pulmonary metastases have been common. Five of the seven patients said to have had liposarcoma of bone were dead at the time of the Rehbock-Hauser report. While the tumor is generally radiosensitive the treatment of choice is radical surgery whenever it is feasible.

HISTOPATHOLOGY

Microscopically, a liposarcoma consists of masses of adult or foetal lipoblasts. While there is wide variation in the size of the cells, the large granular cell is the more common. Cells are characterized by abundant acidophilic cytoplasm and a small, often eccentrically placed, nucleus. Occasional mitotic figures and multinucleated giant cells are seen. A fine reticulin network is also characteristic.

Fat stains (Sharlach R.) should be employed whenever a liposarcoma is suspected. Fat stains identify numerous fat droplets in the cytoplasm.

REFERENCES

Sarcomas of the Osteogenic Series

Badgley, C. E. and Batts, M.: Osteogenic sarcoma. *Arch. Surg., 43*:4, 1941.

Batts, M.: Periosteal fibrosarcoma. *Arch. Surg., 42*:566, 1941.

Coley, B. L. and Sharp, G. S.: Paget's disease; predisposing factor to osteogenic sarcoma. *Arch. Surg., 23*:918, 1931.

Coley, B. L. and Stewart, F. W.: Bone sarcoma in fibrous dysplasia. *Ann. Surg., 121*:872, 1945.

Davie, T. B. and Cooke, W. E.: The supervention of osteogenic sarcoma in Paget's disease. *Brit. J. Surg., 25*:299, 1937.

Desjardins, A. U.: Radiosensitiveness of tumors derived from cartilage. *Am. J. Cancer, 1*:15, 1933.

Fennel, E. A.: Osteogenic sarcoma from exostoses. *Am. J. Surg., 39*:121, 1938.

Franceen, C. C., Aub, J. C., and Simpson, C. L.: Experimental production of fibrosarcoma of bone. *Cancer Research, 1*:393, 1941.

Fry, H. J. B. and Shattock, C. E.: Chondrosarcomatous permeation of the inferior vena cava and right side of heart. *Brit. J. Surg., 14*:337, 1926.

Geschickter, C. F.: Fibrocartilaginous tumors of bone. *Arch. Surg., 23*:215, 1931.

Geschickter, C. F. and Copeland, M. M.: Tumors of bone. *Am. J. Cancer,* 1936.

Goldman, M. and Adams, R. D.: Fibrosarcoma of the sphenoid bone. A case report. *J. Neuropath. & Exper. Neurol., 5*:155, 1946.

GUTMAN, A. B.: Tumors of the skeletal system; medical aspects. *Bull. New York Acad. Med., 23*:512, 1947.

HALDEMANN, K. O.: Development of bone in relation to the formation of neoplasms. *Radiology, 40*:247, 1943.

HERTZLER, A. E.: *Surgical Pathology of the Diseases of Bones.* J. B. Lippincott Co., Philadelphia, 1931.

HODGES, P. C., PHEMISTER, D. B., and BRUNSCHWIG, R.: *The Roentgen-Ray Diagnosis of the Diseases of Bones and Joints.* Thomas Nelson and Sons, New York, 1938.

KIRSHBAUM, J. D.: Fibrosarcoma of the skull in Paget's disease. *Arch. Path., 36*:74, 1943.

KNAGGS, R. L. and GRUNER, O. C.: A contribution to the study of ossification in sarcomata of bone. *Brit. J. Surg., 2*:366, 1914-15.

KOLODNY, A.: Bone sarcoma. *Surg., Gynec. & Obst., 44*:126, 1927.

LICHTENSTEIN, L. and JAFFE, H. L.: Chondrosarcoma of bone. *Am. J. Path., 19*:533, 1943.

LUCK, J. V.: Correlation of roentgenogram and pathologic changes in ossifying and chondrifying primary osteogenic neoplasms. *Radiology, 40*:253, 1943.

MACDONALD, I. and BUDD, J. W.: Osteogenic sarcoma I. *Surg., Gynec. & Obst., 77*:413, 1943.

MACDONALD, I. and BUDD, J. W.: Osteogenic sarcoma II. Roentgenographic interpretation of growth patterns in bone sarcoma. *Surg., Gynec. & Obst., 82*:81, 1946.

MACDONALD, I. and BUDD, J.: Osteogenic sarcoma. 1. A modified nomenclature and a review of 188 five-year cures. *Surg., Gynec. & Obst., 77*:413, 1943.

McREYNOLDS, I. S.: Osteolytic osteogenic sarcoma with a report of eight five-year survivals. *Surg., Gynec. & Obst., 67*:163, 1938.

MEYERDING, H. W., BRODERS, A. C., and HARGRAVE, R. L.: Clinical aspects of fibrosarcoma of the soft tissues of the extremities. *Surg., Gynec. & Obst., 62*:1010, 1936.

MEYERDING, H. W. and VALLS, J. E.: Primary malignant tumors of bone. *J. A. M. A., 117*:237, 1941.

MORLEY, T., GHORMLEY, R. K., and McDONALD, J. R.: Neurofibromatosis with sarcoma of the leg. Report of case. *Proc. Staff Meet., Mayo Clin., 20*:478, 1945.

PHEMISTER, D. B.: Chondrosarcoma of bone. *Surg., Gynec. & Obst., 50*:216, 1930.

PIKE, M. M.: Paget's disease with associated osteogenic sarcoma. *Arch. Surg., 46*:750, 1943.

PLATT, H.: Sarcoma in abnormal bones. *Brit. J. Surg., 34*:233, 1947.

PUTTI, V.: Malignant bone tumors. *Surg., Gynec. & Obst., 48*:324, 1929.

STEINER, P. E.: Multiple diffuse fibrosarcoma of bone. *Am. J. Path., 20*:877, 1944.

SUMMEY, T. J. and PRESSLY, C. L.: Sarcoma complicating Paget's disease of bone. *Ann. Surg., 123*:135, 1946.

EWING'S TUMOR

BLOODGOOD, J. C.: Differential diagnosis of periosteal lesions. *Radiology, 3*:432, 1924; *8*:727, 1926.

CALLENDAR, G. R.: Tumors and tumor-like conditions of the lymphocyte, the myelocyte, the erythrocyte and the reticulum cell. *Am. J. Path., 10*:443, 1934.

CAMPBELL, W. C.: An analysis of the living patients with primary malignant bone tumors. *J. A. M. A., 105*:1496, 1935.

CAMPBELL, W. C. and HAMILTON, J. F.: Gradation of Ewing's tumor (endothelial myeloma). *J. Bone & Joint Surg., 23*:869, 1941.

COLEY, W. B.: The differential diagnosis of sarcoma of the long bones. *J. Bone & Joint Surg., 10*:420, 1928.

CONNER, C. L.: Endothelial myeloma. *Arch. Surg., 12*:789, 1926.

EWING, J.: Endothelial myeloma of bone. *Proc. N. Y. Path. Soc., 21*:17, 1921; *24*:93, 1924.

EWING, J.: *Neoplastic Diseases,* 4th Ed. W. B. Saunders Co., Philadelphia, 1940.

GESCHICKTER, C. F. and COPELAND, M.: Tumors of bone. *Am. J. Cancer,* 1936.

GESCHICKTER, C. F. and MASERITZ, I. H.: Ewing's sarcoma. *J. Bone & Joint Surg., 21*:26, 1939.

HOWARD, W. T., JR. and CRILE, G. W.: Contribution to knowledge of endothelioma and perithelioma of bone. *Ann. Surg., 42*:358, 1905.

KOLODNY, A.: Bone sarcoma. *Surg., Gynec., & Obst., 44*:126, 1927.
MARCKWALD: A case of multiple intravascular endothelioma in all of the bones of the skeleton. *Virchows Arch. f. path. Anat., 141*:128, 1895.
MELNICK, P. T.: Histogenesis of Ewing's sarcoma of bone. *Am. J. Cancer, 19*:353, 1933.
OBERLING, C.: Les reticulosarcomes et les reticulo—endothéleosarcomes de le moelle osseuse. *Bull. Assoc. franç p. l'étude du cancer, 17*:259, 1928.
STOUT, A. P.: Discussion of pathology and histogenesis of Ewing's tumor of bone marrow. *Am. J. Roentgenol., 50*:334, 1943.
WELLS, H. G.: Relation of multiple vascular tumors of bone to myeloma. *Arch. Surg., 2*:435, 1921.
WILLIS, R. A.: Metastatic neuroblastoma in bone presenting the Ewing syndrome, with a discussion of Ewing's sarcoma. *Am. J. Path., 16*:317, 1940.

RETICULUM CELL SARCOMA

CALLENDER, G. R.: Tumors and tumor-like conditions of the lymphocyte, the myelocyte, the erythrocyte, and the reticulum cell. *Am. J. Path., 10*:443, 1934.
CRAVER, L. F. and COPELAND, M. M.: Lymphosarcoma in bone. *Arch. Surg., 28*:809, 1934.
DOUB, H. P. and HARTMAN, F. W.: Lymphocytic, myelocytic, and monocytic neoplasms. Roentgen diagnosis and treatment. *J. A. M. A., 105*:942, 1935.
KAUFMANN: Cited by Ewing, J. A review of the classification of bone tumors. *Surg., Gynec. & Obst., 68*:971, 1939.
OBERLING, C.: Les réticulosarcomes et les réticulo-endotheliosarcomes. de la Moelle ossense. *Bull. Assoc. franç u. l'étude du cancer, 17*:259, 1928.
PARKER, F., JR. and JACKSON, H., JR.: Primary reticulum cell sarcoma of bone. *Surg., Gynec. & Obst., 68*:45, 1939.
SHERMAN, R. S. and SNYDER, R. E.: The roentgen appearance of reticulum cell sarcoma. *Am. J. Roentgenol., 58*:291, 1947.

HEMANGIO-ENDOTHELIOMA

EWING, J.: Neoplastic Diseases, 4th Ed. Pages 361 and 362. W. B. Saunders Co., Philadelphia, 1940.
HAUSER, H.: Angiosarcoma of bone. *Am. J. Roentgenol., 42*:656, 1939.
MURRAY, M. R. and STOUT, A. P.: Cultural characteristics of hemangio-endothelioma. *Am. J. Path., 20*:277, 1944.
STOUT, A. P.: Hemangio-endothelioma; tumor of blood vessels featuring vascular endothelial cells. *Ann. Surg., 118*:445, 1943.
THOMAS, A.: Vascular tumors of bone: Pathologic and clinical study of 27 cases. *Surg., Gynec. & Obst., 74*:777, 1942.

MULTIPLE MYELOMA

AEGERTER, E. and ROBBINS, R.: The changing concept of myeloma of bone. *Am. J. M. Sc., 213*:282, 1947.
BENCE-JONES: *Philosoph. Tr. Roy. Soc., London, 1*:55, 1848.
CARLTON, T. J.: Multiple myeloma. *Arch. Int. Med., 40*:98, 1927.
COLEY, W. B.: Multiple myeloma. *Ann. Surg., 93*:77, 1931.
DALRYMPLE, ..: *Dublin Quart. J., 2*:85, 1848.
DAVISON, C. and BALSER, B. H.: Myeloma and its neural complications. *Arch. Surg., 35*:913, 1937.
FOORD, A. G.: Hyperproteinemia, autohemagglutination, renal insufficiency and abnormal bleeding in multiple myeloma. *Ann. Int. Med., 8*:1071, 1935.
FREUND, E.: *Frankfurt. Ztschr. f. Path., 40*:400, 1930.
GESCHICKTER, C. F. and COPELAND, M. M.: Multiple myeloma. *Arch. Surg., 16*:807, 1928.
GUNN, F. D. and MAHLE, A. E.: Megakaryoblastic myeloma with crystalline protein in the renal tubes. Report of a case. *Arch. Path., 26*:377, 1938.
GUTMAN, A. B.: Tumors of the skeletal system; medical aspects. *Bull. New York Acad. Med., 23*:512, 1947.

HELLWIG, C. A.: Extramedullary plasma cell tumors as observed in various locations. *Arch. Path., 36*:95, 1943.

JACKSON, H., PARKER, F., and BETHEA, J. M.: Studies of disease of the lymphoid and myeloid tissues. II. Plasmatocytomata and their relation to multiple myeloma. *A. J. M. Sc., 181*:169, 1931.

JACOX, H. W., and KAHN, E. A.: Multiple myeloma with spinal cord involvement. *Am. J. Roentgenol., 30*:201, 1933.

KAHLER, O.: *Prog. Med. Wchnschr., 14*:33, 1889.

LICHTENSTEIN, L., and JAFFE, H.: Multiple myeloma. *Arch. Path., 44*:207, 1947.

LOW-BEER, B. V. A., LAWRENCE, J. H., and STONE, R. S.: The therapeutic use of artificially produced radioactive substances. *Radiology, 39*:573, 1942.

McINTYRE, W.: A case of mollities and fragilitas ossium. *Med.-Chir. Tr., 33*:211, 1850.

SNAPPER, I.: *Medical Clinics on Bone Diseases.* Interscience Publishers, Inc., New York, 1945.

SNAPPER, I.: Stilbamidine and pentamidine in multiple myeloma. *J. A. M. A., 133*: 157, 1947.

TAYLOR, A. L. and STEWART, M. J.: Observations on solitary plasmocytoma. *J. Path. & Bact., 35*:541, 1932.

WALLGREN, A.: *Untersuchungen über die myelomkrankheit.* Upsal, Almquist, and Wiksell, 1920. William Wood & Co., Baltimore, 1920.

WARREN, S.: Generalized amyloidosis of the muscular systems. *Am. J. Path., 6*:161, 1930.

WARREN, S.: The therapeutic use of radioactive phosphorus. *Am. J. M. Sc., 209*:701, 1945.

WOOD, A. C. and LUCKE, B.: Multiple myeloma of the plasma cell type. *Ann. Surg., 78*:14, 1923.

LIPOSARCOMA

BARNARD, L.: Primary liposarcoma of bone. *Arch. Surg., 29*:560, 1934.

EWING, J.: The classification and treatment of bone sarcoma. *Rep. Internat. Conf. Cancer.* Page 365. London, 1928.

FENDER, F. A.: Liposarcoma; report of case with intracranial metastases. *Am. J. Path., 9*:909, 1933.

KHANOLKAR, V. R.: Liposarcoma of bone. *Indian Physician, 4*:19, 1945.

REHBOCK, D. J. and HAUSER, H.: Liposarcoma of bone. *Am. J. Cancer, 27*:37, 1936.

STEWART, F. W.: Primary liposarcoma of bone. *Am. J. Path., 7*:87, 1931.

WILLIFORD, H. B. and FATHERREE, T. J.: Primary sarcoma of bone. Report of a case. *U. S. Nav. M. Bull., 46*:1750, 1946.

CHAPTER XX

Secondary Involvement of the Bones by Malignant Diseases

Contents

Secondary involvement of the skeletal system takes place by one or more of the following three methods: (1) through the formation of metastases, (2) the direct extension of a neighboring soft tissue malignancy, and (3) by the action of blood cells in malignant diseases of the blood. Whereas primary bone tumors are almost always solitary, the secondary bone lesions of malignancies are generally multiple. By far the most frequent secondary lesions of bones are the carcinoma metastases. Secondary malignant lesions are decidedly more frequent than are the primary bone malignancies. Whereas most primary bone tumors occur prior to the third decade, the secondary malignant lesions ordinarily appear during and after the third decade.

METASTASES TO BONES
CARCINOMA

Carcinoma metastases residing in bones are of two types, osteolytic and osteoplastic. *The osteolytic type,* as the name implies, is purely de-

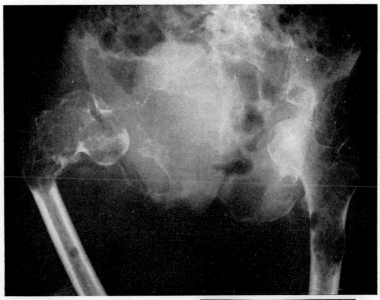

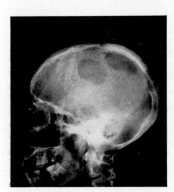

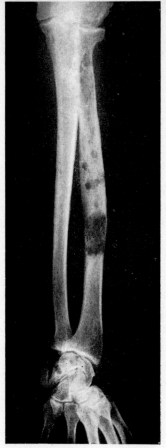

FIGURE 425. Osteolytic adenocarcinoma metastases as portrayed by roentgenograms. A.
(Above) Pelvis and upper femora. B. *(Left)* Skull. C. *(Right)*
Radius and ulna.

structive. Bone within the mass of metastatic tumor tissue is destroyed. At the periphery there is neither reactive osteosclerosis nor periosteal new bone. *Osteoplastic metastases,* on the other hand, are associated with a striking increase in bone trabeculae at each of the sites at which the tumor cells are deposited. Virtually all osteoplastic metastases have their origin in carcinoma of the prostate. Rarely, a carcinoma of the breast gives rise to this type of metastasis.

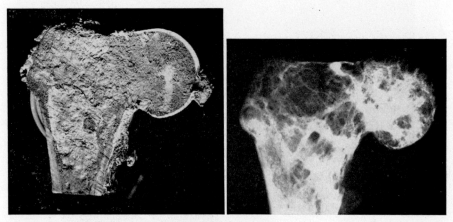

FIGURE 426. Osteolytic adenocarcinoma metastases to the upper femur. A. *(Left)* Frontal section of specimen. B. *(Right)* Roentgenogram of specimen.

Distribution of Metastases

All bones are susceptible, but only rarely are metastatic foci found in the bones distal to the knees and the elbows. The most frequent sites at which skeletal metastases are observed are the vertebral bodies, pelvis, skull, femora, humeri, ribs, and the sternum. Neal and Robnett concluded that: "The nearer a bone is to the site of a primary cancer the greater is its liability to secondary involvement."

Incidence of Skeletal Metastases

Certain of the carcinomas possess a high incidence of skeletal metastasis, whereas other carcinomas only rarely metastasize to the skeleton. There appears to be no type of carcinoma incapable of metastasizing to bones. In Kaufmann's series of cases, 52 percent of the breast carcinomas and 66 percent of the prostatic carcinomas metastasized to one or more bones. Hypernephromas are the third most frequent source of skeletal metastases. Of 63 cases reviewed by Geschickter and Copeland, 22 or 34.9 percent metastasized to bone. Carcinoma of the thyroid also has a relatively high incidence of bone metastases. In the Ehrhardt series of 238 cases there were 66 instances of skeletal system metastasis.

Carcinoma of the lung is said to metastasize to the skeleton in approximately 25 percent of cases. Carcinomas of the gastro-intestinal tract, uterus, ovaries, testicles and bladder metastasize to bones in from 1 to 10 percent of cases.

Routes of Dissemination

Adequate proof exists to warrant the conclusion that carcinomas may metastasize via both the lymphatic system and the blood stream. Recklinghausen and Piney were among the first to emphasize the spread of carcinoma by tumor cell emboli carried in the circulating blood. Handley, Carnett, and Howell, on the other hand contended that carcinoma spreads principally through lymphatics. These investigators produced evidence of retrograde extension of the tumor through lymphatics; the spread of tumor cells along lymphatics

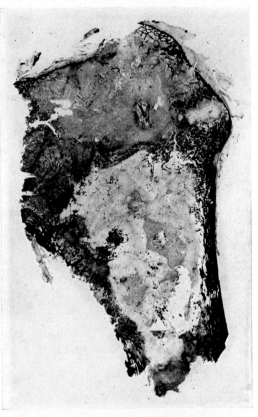

FIGURE 426. *(Continued)* C. Histologic section of the trochanteric region showing the massive metastases.

of fascial planes was also demonstrated. Neal and Robnett observed conclusive evidence of hematogenous metastases. In patients with widespread skeletal carcinomatosis it is difficult to explain the pattern of the dissemination on any other than a hematogenous basis. In most instances a combination of the methods of metastasis probably takes place.

Invasion of bone by direct extension is not uncommon, particularly in pelvic carcinomas. Breast carcinomas may extend directly into the ribs. Epitheliomas of the skin and mucous membranes occasionally spread directly into underlying bone.

Gross Pathology

Most secondary bone tumors are located centrally and either expand in a circumscribed manner or extend proximally and distally along the medullary canal. At one or many levels the tumor tissue destroys small or large areas of the bony cortex (Figs. 425-430). While entire bones may become riddled in late stages of the disease, it is the proximal one-

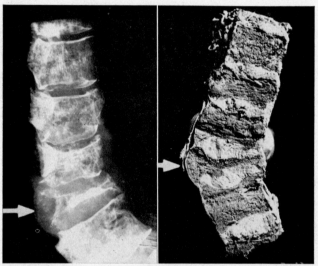

FIGURE 427. Carcinoma metastases to vertebral bodies at the dorso-lumbar junction. A. *(Left)* Sagital section of the specimen. The vertebral body at the arrow has collapsed pathologic compression fracture). B. *(Right)* Roentgenogram of the specimen.

third of the long bones that is more likely to be invaded in early stages.

The masses of tumor tissue are light to dark gray, and rather frequently have a yellowish cast. The tissue is friable and may be either highly vascular or virtually avascular.

Osteoplastic metastases are seen grossly as rounded masses of dense cancellous bone lying in the medullary canal or metaphysis, in the cortex, or even subperiosteally. In late stages as large areas of the involved bones become invaded, the many small masses coalesce to form large nodular masses. Extensive areas of cortex may thus become replaced by the tumor tissue and the associated reactive cancellous bone. A diffuse replacement of one or many vertebral bodies is not unusual.

Histopathology

An osteolytic metastasis is seen as a solid mass of tumor cells. Reactive fibrous tissue in small or extensive amounts is seen in and around the mass of tumor tissue. Normal bone at the site of the tumor is

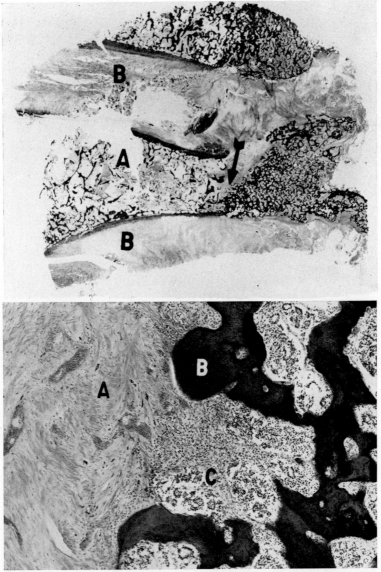

FIGURE 427. *(Continued)* C. *(Above)* Histologic section of the collapsed vertebra. Arrow points to site of photomicrograph shown in D. *A.* Vertebral body. *B.* Intervertebral discs. D. *(Below)* Photomicrograph from the field opposite the point of the arrow in C. *A.* Herniated disc and scar tissue. *B.* Bone trabeculae. *C.* Adenocarcinoma.

destroyed by the tumor cells themselves and apparently also by giant cell osteoclasts. With the exception of carcinoma of the kidney (hypernephroma) and of the prostate, the site of the primary tumor cannot

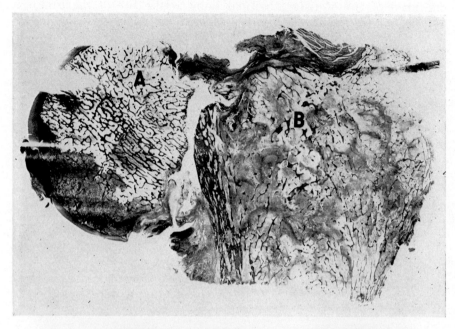

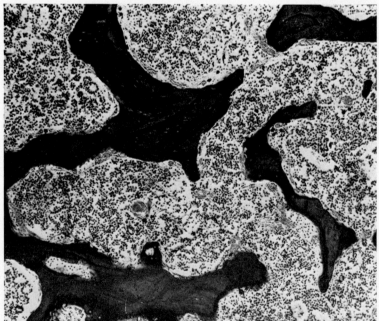

FIGURE 428. Adenocarcinoma metastases to the upper femur with a pathologic fracture and resorption of the entire femoral neck. A. *(Above)* Frontal section of the specimen. The dark areas are metastatic foci. *A.* Femoral head. *B.* Trochanteric region. B. *(Below)* Photomicrograph from the histologic section in Figure 428A. Numerous acini are seen.

often be identified by the microscopic appearance of the metastatic lesions. In metastases from hypernephroma the cells are relatively large, the cytoplasm clear, and the nuclei small and hyperchromatic. No stroma is present.

OSTEOPLASTIC METASTASES do not present the abundant masses of tumor cells of the osteolytic lesions; rather, they are characterized by small bits and clusters of tumor cells crowded into narrow intertrabecular spaces undergoing progressive stenosis from the formation of new bone layer upon layer. The spongy bone identified with the tumor cells may be either fibrous or lamellar in type, but is always reactive in character and never the creation of the tumor cells. Tumor cells may form clearly recognizable acini when the cells are well or moderately well differentiated (Fig. 431). In less well differentiated tumors, the acini may be few or even absent.

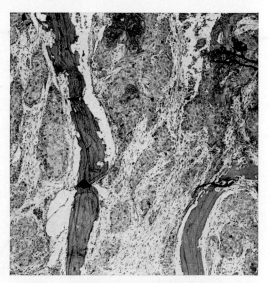

FIGURE 429. Osteolysis in carcinoma metastases. A. Lacunar resorption of bone trabeculae by osteoclasts in an epithelioma metastasis.

Growth of the osteoplastic prostatic carcinoma metastasis is slow and is under the influence of the male hormone, testosterone. It is now clearly established that this hormone must be present for uninhibited growth of the tumor. Orchiectomy, or roentgen radiation of the testicles inhibits the growth of the metastases through a reduction of the secretion of testosterone.

ACID PHOSPHATASE is increased, often to a profound degree, by metastases from a carcinoma of the prostate. Hovenanian, et al have shown that the enzyme acid phosphatase is a product of cellular metabolism (tumor cells) and is produced by both the nucleus and the cytoplasm.

Roentgenographic Features

Solitary metastatic foci are less commonly observed when extensive and careful roentgenographic studies are made. Osteolytic metastases are much more common than are the osteoplastic type, and of course this is decidedly so in the female. Osteolytic foci give a punched out

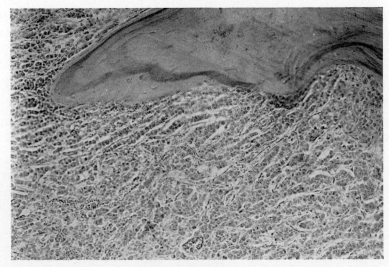

FIGURE 429. *(Continued)* B. Smooth resorption of a bone trabeculum by adenocarcinoma cells.

appearance whenever the cortex is involved. As with myelomatosis, a large tumor mass may lie in the medullary canal of a long bone and give the roentgenologist little evidence of its presence.

Periosteal bone formation is exceptional, except at sites of pathologic

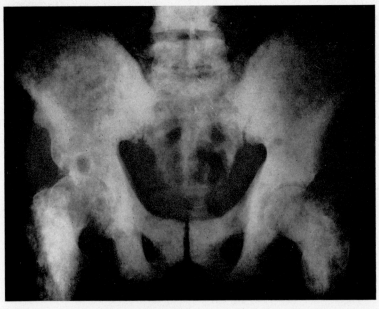

FIGURE 430. Osteoplastic metastases from a carcinoma of the prostate. Roentgenogram of the pelvis.

fractures. Overlying periosteum may be destroyed as the tumor tissue infiltrates through the cortex and into adjacent soft tissues.

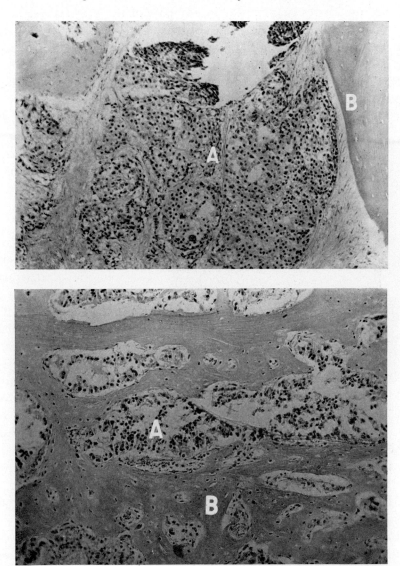

FIGURE 431. Photomicrographs, carcinoma prostate. *A*. Adenocarcinoma. *B*. Bone trabeculae.

Pathologic fractures are commonplace, particularly in relation to osteolytic metastases. In the Geschickter and Copeland series of hypernephromas with skeletal metastases, 45.5 percent developed pathologic fractures.

Clinical Features

Since metastases may appear in any part of the skeletal system, any bone may become the site of disabling symptoms. Skeletal metastases may cause only mild and fleeting pain at the outset but in late stages the pain is generally excruciating. There is a wide variation in the reaction of the patient to the metastatic foci. Some patients deteriorate rapidly, others slowly.

Pathologic fractures, if properly immobilized, occasionally heal. Part of the tumor tissue at the site of a fracture is destroyed and replaced by fibrous tissue or callus.

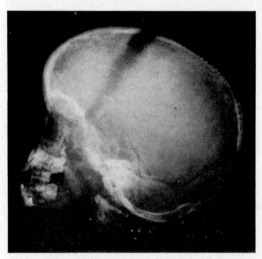

FIGURE 432. Neuroblastoma. Roentgenograms disclosed generalized metastases. A. Skull, showing the characteristic diastasis of the suture lines.

NEUROBLASTOMA

The neuroblastomas originate from primitive neuroblasts in the adrenal gland medulla. Two types are seen: I. Pepper type. This type only rarely associated with bone metastases, is characterized by massive involvement of the mesenteric lymph nodes and the liver. II. Hutchinson's type. This form of the disease is associated with a high incidence of early metastasis to the bones. Sites at which the metastases tend to concentrate are the skull, femora, vertebrae, pelvis, ribs, and sternum.

Metastases are osteolytic, giving a punched out appearance in roentgenograms (Figs. 432 B & C).

In the skull the invasion of the orbits may be associated with exophthalmus and with ecchymosis of the lids. The increased intracranial pressure often produces a striking spread of the suture lines (Fig. 432A). In a long bone a solitary metastatic lesion may resemble a Ewing's tumor both radiographically and pathologically. Willis reported the case of a 17 year old female with a large tumor of the distal two-thirds of the femur. On the basis of the clinical findings, the roentgenograms, and a biopsy, the tumor was diagnosed a Ewing's tumor. At autopsy the correct diagnosis of neuroblastoma became evident. This diagnostic error is probably not rare.

Histopathology

Microscopically there are masses of cells resembling lymphocytes. A narrow rim of cytoplasm surrounds a hyperchromatic nucleus. Rosettes are seen and generally appear as a well formed circle of nuclei surrounding a rounded microscopic mass of cytoplasm.

Prognosis

The prognosis is hopeless after metastases are identified.

THE OSTEOGENIC SARCOMAS

In rare instances sarcomas of the osteogenic series have metastasized to other parts of the skeletal system (Fig. 433). In Paget's disease complicated by an osteogenic sarcoma, the question has occasionally arisen regarding whether the multiple skeletal foci of the sarcoma represented multicentric primary foci or metastases from a solitary primary focus. Several skeletal foci may be discovered simultaneously.

EWING'S TUMOR

As mentioned under the description of Ewing's tumor (Chapter XIX), metastases to the skeletal system is an ultimate de-

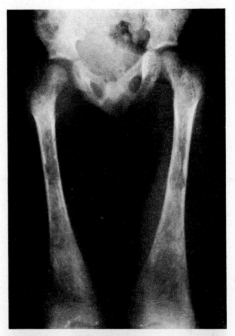

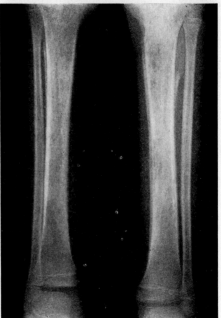

FIGURE 432. *(Continued)* B. *(Above)* Femora showing multiple osteolytic metastases. C. *(below)* Tibiae and fibulae. Tibiae show osteolytic lesions and periosteal bone.

velopment in nearly all cases of Ewing's tumor, and may precede the pulmonary metastases. The skull, vertebrae, ribs, and pelvis are much more frequently the site of the metastatic foci than are the long bones (Fig. 434).

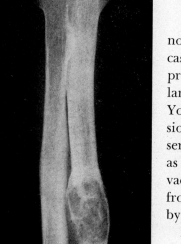

FIGURE 433. A skeletal metastasis to the ulna from an osteosarcoma of the upper tibia. Such a metastasis is rare indeed.

LYMPHOSARCOMA

Skeletal system involvement has been noted in approximately ten percent of the cases of lymphosarcoma. In a series of 164 proved cases studied by Craver and Copeland at the Memorial Hospital in New York, 17 cases (10.4 percent) disclosed lesions of the bones. The patients in this series were from 9 to 65 years of age. Just as in Hodgkin's disease, the disease may invade the bones either by direct extension from involved neighboring lymph nodes or by hematogenous metastases.

In the distribution of the bone lesions there is no predelection for hematogenous marrow. Principle sites of involvement are the spine, skull, pelvis, femur, tibia, fibula, and ribs.

PATHOLOGIC ANATOMY

Areas of cortex of an invaded bone may be destroyed from without by a process of direct extension from overlying soft tissues, or be destroyed centrally from medullary canal metastatic foci (Fig. 435). The process does not tend to remain limited to any certain area of the bone, the tendency being to gradually spread throughout the bone.

Reactive bone may form to a moderate degree in the periosteum, and within the bone.

Microscopically the picture of the bone lesions is one of masses of osteolytic lymphoid cells actively advancing by infiltrating through the marrow spaces and the haversian canals. Reticulin stains reveal a well formed reticular network.

Lymphosarcoma of bone must be differentiated from Hodgkin's disease, carcinoma metastases, the leukemias, the chronic osteomyelitides, and Ewing's tumor.

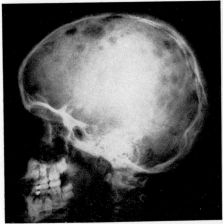

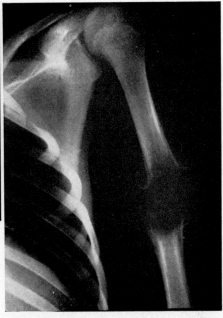

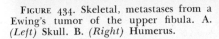

FIGURE 434. Skeletal, metastases from a Ewing's tumor of the upper fibula. A. *(Left)* Skull. B. *(Right)* Humerus.

Irradiation therapy is a useful palliative measure. The disease is generally fatal within three years from the onset of symptoms.

HODGKIN'S DISEASE

The incidence of bone involvement in Hodgkin's disease is considerably higher than formerly believed. Symmers goes so far as to contend

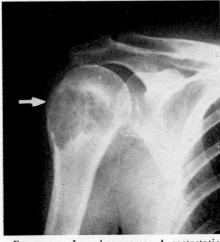

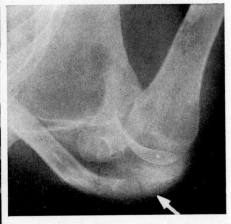

FIGURE 436. Hodgkin's disease. A metastatic skeletal focus in the acromion process of the scapula (arrow).

FIGURE 435. Lymphosarcoma. A metastatic focus in the head and neck of the humerus.

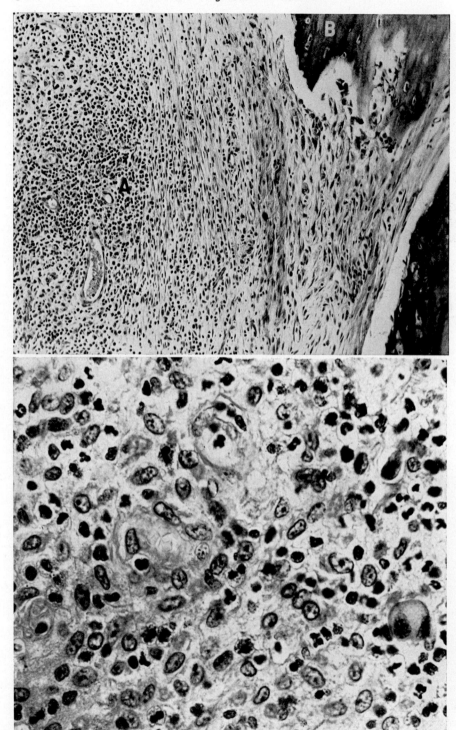

that there is involvement of the bone marrow in all cases of Hodgkin's disease. Craver and Copeland reviewed 172 proved cases and found bone changes in 27 instances. Ages varied from 17 to 40, and there were two males to one female. In Vieta's series of 257 cases, bone lesions were found in 14.8 percent.

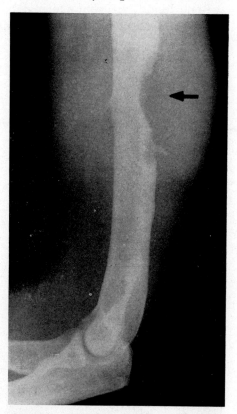

Distribution

The bone lesions are found at sites of hematopoietic marrow. Sites of involvement according to frequency are as follows: Vertebrae, sternum, pelvis, femur, ribs, skull, humerus, scapula, and clavicle. Lesions in the long bones are generally localized to the proximal one-third of the bone.

Etiology

None of the numerous theories of the etiology of Hodgkin's disease appears near to being established. Twenty percent of the patients in Parker's series had pulmonary tuberculosis. However, there is no incontrovertible proof that the tubercle bacillus causes Hodgkin's disease. It may be that

FIGURE 438. Extra osseous fibrosarcoma eroding the cortex of the humerus. The arrow sets in the center of the large soft tissue mass and points to the concave humeral defect.

Hodgkin's disease tends to activate tuberculosis.

While Hodgkin's disease is a clear-cut and well-established entity, it is not settled whether the pathologic changes represent a neoplasm or a granuloma.

Gross Pathology

In the majority of cases the process is first noted in the lymph nodes. The involved lymph nodes lose their internal architecture and often

FIGURE 437. Hodgkin's disease. A. (Above) Photomicrograph of a granulomatous focus, A, in bone, B. B. (Below) Photomicrograph, high power, of a typical field.

enlarge to such large dimensions that they impinge nerve trunks, great vessels, and respiratory tubes. Epidural masses have been known to compress the spinal cord (Weil).

Bone lesions are characterized by accumulations of granulomatous tissue or sarcoma-like tissue of Hodgkin's disease in the form of focal collections or confluent masses located in the medullary canal or beneath the periosteum. As the disease advances, large areas of the bone marrow may be displaced by the tissues of Hodgkin's disease.

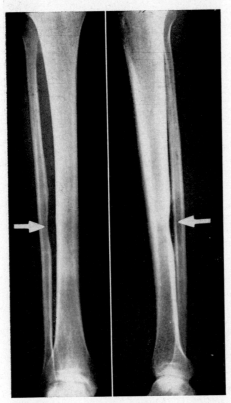

FIGURE 439. Extraosseous fibrosarcoma eroding the tibia and fibula (arrows) by direct extension.

Most of the periosteal lesions and superficial cortical erosions represent direct extensions from neighboring diseased lymph nodes. Medullary lesions generally represent hematogenous metastases. The metastatic lesions often destroy areas of overlying cortex (Fig. 436). Reactive osteosclerosis around the osteolytic areas is not uncommon.

Histopathology

The tissues created by the disease vary considerably in make-up. The following three patterns are seen: (1) granulomatous tissue, (2) highly cellular sarcoma-like tissue, and (3) fibrotic tissue.

A preponderance of endothelial cells and endothelial giant cells characterize the early stages. Other cells seen in varying proportions in the reticulum network include lymphocytes, plasma cells and eosinophils (Fig. 437). The Dorothy Reed giant cells seen in typical cases are large (40 microns) cells with multilobed nuclei.

In a substantial percentage of cases the granulomatous character undergoes a transformation to terminate as a sarcoma-like process. The cells become much more uniform and generally take the form of large round cells. A malignant transformation and the appearance of numerous areas of fibrosis are developments of an advanced stage of the disease. Areas of necrosis, rare in early stages, are quite common in advanced stages.

Roentgenographic Features

Bone changes visible in roentgenograms are not ordinarily an early finding in Hodgkin's disease. However, Blount reported a case (1929) in which bone lesions were noted two years prior to the appearance of the lymphadenopathy.

As already mentioned, the superficial cortical erosions represent direct extentions of the disease from adjacent soft tissue, whereas the central osteolytic lesions generally represent metastatic foci. Periosteal bone, reactive in type, forms only in a limited manner. Reactive zones of osteosclerosis form at the periphery of the osteolytic lesions whenever expansion of the central lesion is slow.

Pathologic fractures are rare except for

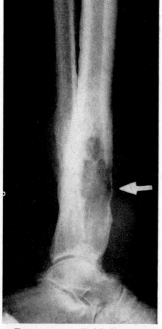

FIGURE 440. Epithelioma involving the lower tibia. The tumor represented a complication of chronic pyogenic osteomyelitic sinuses of many years duration.

a moderately high incidence of compression fractures of vertebral bodies.

Clinical Features

The most outstanding symptom is the painless generalized lymphadenopathy starting usually in the cervical region. Other regions that may serve as a starting point for the lymphadenopathy include the supraclavicular, axillary, inguinal, retroperitoneal, and mediastinal. An enlarged liver and spleen is the rule.

A diagnosis can be clearly established by the histologic study of a lymph node. An easily accessible node that can be removed intact is preferable.

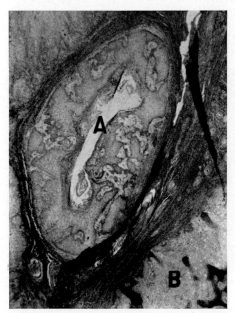

FIGURE 441. Epitheliomatous sinus, A, in bone, B, Malignant epithelium lines the sinus tract.

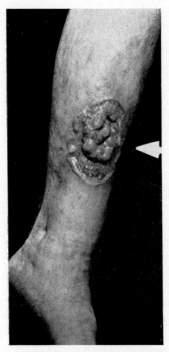

FIGURE 442. Epitheliomatous ulcer associated with chronic pyogenic osteomyelitis.

According to Woodard the alkaline phosphatase is increased with the advent of bone involvement.

The three diseases that are the most often necessary to differentiate from Hodgkin's disease are carcinomatosis, lymphatic leukemia, and lymphosarcoma.

Hodgkin's disease is invariably fatal. Roentgentherapy is employed as a palliative measure.

DIRECT EXTENSION OF A SOFT TISSUE MALIGNANCY

SARCOMAS OF THE SOFT TISSUES

It is not rare for a sarcoma of one of the soft tissues in the vicinity of a bone to erode the bone. While any of the soft tissue sarcomas may invade a neighboring bone, the two that most frequently involve bone by direct extension are fibrosarcoma and neurogenic sarcoma.

Most of the soft tissue sarcomas that invade bone are seen in adults. While no part of the skeleton is immune from this form of neoplastic invasion the two sites with the highest incidence of involvement are the lower femur and the upper tibia. Involvement of the fibula is also relatively common. When the tumor has resided near the end of a long bone, invasion of the adjacent joint has not been rare.

The *fibrosarcomas* constitute the great majority of the bone-invading tumors. As a rule the tumor is rounded, sharply circumscribed, and grossly encapsulated. At the outset the periosteum is perforated, usually without precipitat-

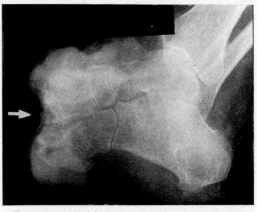

FIGURE 443. Epithelioma, in crater opposite arrow, originated in a protracted stump skin ulcer. The underlying bone was involved by the epithelioma.

ing the formation of periosteal bone, and the cortex eroded to create a smooth, shallow, concave defect (Figs 438 and 439). Ultimately the cortex may be perforated. When a long bone is entered the tumor tends to advance along the medullary canal. In an advanced stage of an aggressive tumor it may be difficult to identify the paraosseous origin of the tumor. Ordinarily the paraosseous mass is large and the size of the bone defect relatively small.

Reactive bone is seen when growth of the tumor is slow, whereas rapidly growing tumors are purely osteolytic. No tumor bone ever forms in conjunction with the tumors that involve the bones by direct extension. Growth of these tumors is generally by expansion; however, the highly malignant types may grow principally by infiltration.

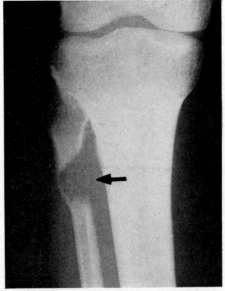

FIGURE 444. Epitheliomatous extension to the upper fibula (arrow). The epithelioma originated in the overlying skin scar of a burn.

Pulmonary metastases are relatively common.

CARCINOMA

There are numerous instances of the direct extension of a primary carcinoma to a neighboring bone. A carcinoma of the breast may extend to underlying ribs, a carcinoma of the prostate or bladder to bones of the pelvis, and a carcinoma of the kidney to vertebrae. This is a manifestation of an advanced stage.

Epitheliomas of the skin and mucous membranes occasionally invade the underlying bone. The most important instance of this in bone pathology is seen in the appearance of an epithelioma in long standing

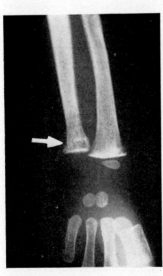

FIGURE 445. Aleukemic leukemia. The infiltration of the distal ulnar metaphysis resembles an osteomyelitic focus (Los Angeles Childrens Hospital).

skin sinuses of chronic osteomyelitis (Figs. 440-444). This type of epithelioma gradually grows down the sinus tract to enter the bone. In Chapter III under the subject of *Chronic Pyogenic Osteomyelitis* will be found a description of this entity.

MALIGNANT DISEASES OF THE BLOOD

LYMPHATIC AND MYELOGENOUS LEUKEMIA

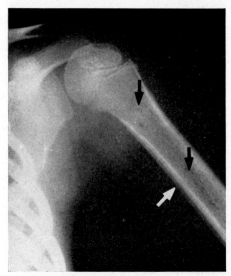

FIGURE 446. Lymphatic leukemia with involvement of the humerus. White arrow points to periosteal bone, and the black arrows to the numerous punctate osteolytic cortical lesions (Los Angeles Childrens Hospital).

The leukemias seldom cause bone changes visible in roentgenograms. Craver and Copeland reviewed the Memorial Hospital cases and found among 86 patients with lymphatic leukemia only 6 (7 percent) that presented roentgenographic evidence of bone involvement. Four of these six patients were females. A similar review of 82 cases of myelogenous leukemia disclosed only one patient, a 59 year old female, that had bone changes. Involvement in this one patient was seen as a mottling and multiple central punched out lesions in the upper one-third of the femur. The incidence of bone involvement is unquestionably higher than is indicated by the statistics in medical literature. Many of the cases that have been reviewed were of patients treated prior to the time of roentgenographic studies of the complete skeleton.

Just as in Hodgkin's disease, the leukemic bone lesions have a predelection for bones containing hematogenous marrow. The principle sites of the bone changes are the vertebrae, ribs, skull, femur, and humerus.

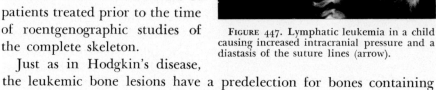

FIGURE 447. Lymphatic leukemia in a child causing increased intracranial pressure and a diastasis of the suture lines (arrow).

Pathologic changes in the bones are medullary in origin and make their appearance in an advanced stage of the leukemia. Multiple central cortical erosions may extend throughout the length of the bone, appearing as circumscribed lesions (Figs. 445 & 446). A coalescence

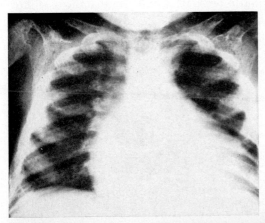

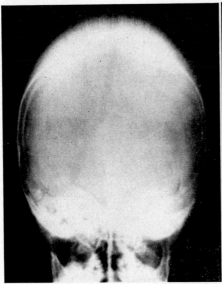
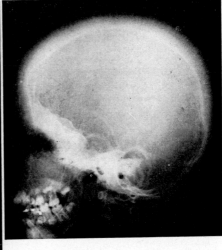

FIGURE 448. Cooley's erythroblastic anemia. This entity together with familial jaundice, and sickle cell anemia may produce punctate osteolytic lesions *(Above)* similar to those of the leukemias. These anemias of infancy and childhood often widen medullary canals and cause a peculiar ossification pattern on the outer table of the skull resembling the hair standing on end *(Below)*. Rapid hyperplasia of the hemopoietic marrow to keep pace with the rapid destruction of erythrocytes by the reticuloendothelial system is responsible for the skeletal changes.

of the numerous foci ultimately takes place. Perforation of the cortex and the formation of slight amounts of periosteal bone occasionally occurs (Fig. 446).

Clinical Features

In addition to symptoms of the disease there may be localized pain and tenderness at the sites of bone changes.

The diagnosis is usually established by blood counts, blood smears, a lymph node biopsy, or a bone puncture. In the six cases of the Craver-Copeland series of lymphatic leukemia with bone changes the lymphocytes in the blood stream were only slightly or moderately increased in numbers. These authors concluded that bone changes may occur more frequently in low grade lymphatic leukemia than in instances where the total leucocyte count is high.

The bone changes of the leukemias must be differentiated from Hodgkin's disease, lymphosarcoma, Cooley's anemia, carcinoma metastases, multiple myeloma, and the chronic osteomyelitides.

REFERENCES

CARCINOMA

CARNETT, J. B. and HOWELL, J. C.: Bone metastases in cancer of the breast. *Ann. Surg., 91*:811, 1930.

EHRHARDT, O.: *Bruns' Veitr. z. klin. Chir., 35*:343, 1902.

EWING, J.: *Neoplastic Diseases,* 4th ed. W. B. Saunders Co., Philadelphia, 1940.

GESCHICKTER, C. F. and COPELAND, M. M.: Tumors of bone. *Am. J. Cancer.,* 1936.

HANDLEY, W. S.: *Cancer of the Breast and Its Operative Treatment.* John Murray, London, 1906.

HOVENANIAN, M. S. and DEMING, C. L.: The heterologous growth of cancer of the human prostate. *Surg., Gynec. & Obst., 86*:29, 1948.

JENKINSON, E. L.: Primary carcinoma of the gastrointestinal tract accompanied by bone metastases. *Am. J. Roentgenol., 11*:411, 1924.

KAUFMANN, E.: Sekundare Geschwülste der Knocken. *Spez. Path. Anat., 1*:954, 1922.

MOON, V. H.: Primary carcinoma of the liver with metastases to bone. *Arch. Path., 8*:938, 1919.

NEAL, M. P. and ROBNETT, D. A.: Generalized osseous metastases secondary to atrophic scirrhus carcinoma of left breast. *Arch. Surg., 14*:529, 1927.

PAGET, J.: The distribution of secondary growths in cancer of the breast. *Lancet, 1*:571, 1889.

PINEY, A.: Carcinoma of the bone marrow. *Brit. J. Surg., 10*:235, 1922-1923.

SIMPSON, W. M.: Three cases of thyroid metastasis to bone. *Surg., Gynec. & Obst., 42*:489, 1926.

VON RECKLINGHAUSEN, F.: *Festschrift der Assistenen für Virchow.* 1891.

NEUROBLASTOMA

DOUB, H. P.: The roentgen aspect of sympathetic neuroblastoma. *J. A. M. A., 109*:1188, 1937.

FREW, R. S.: On carcinoma originating in the suprarenal medulla in children. *Quart. J. Med., 4*:123, 1910.

HUTCHINSON, R.: On suprarenal sarcoma in children with metastasis in the skull. *Quart. J. Med., 1*:33, 1908.

PEPPER, W.: A study of congenital sarcoma of the liver and suprarenal. *Am. J. M. Sc., 121*:287, 1901.

WILLIS, R. A.: Metastatic neuroblastoma in bone presenting Ewing's syndrome; with discussion of "Ewing's sarcoma." *Am. J. Path., 16*:317, 1940.

LYMPHOSARCOMA

BALDRIDGE, C. W. and AWE, C. D.: Lymphoma: A study of 150 cases. *Arch. Int. Med., 45*:161, 93c.

CRAVER, L. F. and COPELAND, M. M.: Lymphosarcoma in bone. *Arch. Surg., 28*:809, 1934.

DESJARDINS, A. U. and FORD, F. A.: Hodgkin's disease and lymphosarcoma. *J. A. M. A., 81*:925, 1923.

POHLE, E. A. and RITCHIE, G.: Lymphosarcoma of the femur. *Radiology, 18*:635, 1932.

SCHREINER, B. F. and HERGER, C. C.: Radium and x-rays in the treatment of round cell sarcoma. *Radiology, 5*:399, 1925.

STOUT, A. P.: Is lymphosarcoma curable? *J. A. M. A., 118*:968, 1942.

HODGKIN'S DISEASE

ALLEN, I. M. and MERCER, J. O.: Spinal symptoms with lymphadenoma. *J. Neurol. & Psychopath., 17*:1, 1936.

ARNELL, S.: Two cases of Hodgkin's disease with bone destruction. *Acta radiol., 8*:259, 1927.

ASKANAZY, M.: Lymphogranuloma of the bone marrow. *Centralbl. f. allg. Path. u. path. Anat., 31*:557, 1920-21.

BELOT, J., NAHAN, L. and KIMPEL, J.: Involvement of bones in the course of malignant granulomatosis. *J. de radiol. et d' électrol., 12*:257, 1928.

BLOUNT, W. P.: Hodgkin's disease; orthopedic problem. *J. Bone & Joint Surg., 11*:761, 1929.

BRUNSCHWIG, A. and KANDEL, E.: Correlation of the histologic changes and clinical symptoms in irradiated Hodgkin's disease and lymphoblastoma lymph nodes. *Radiology, 23*:315, 1934.

CONE, S. M.: Bone in Hodgkin's disease. *J. Bone & Joint Surg., 25*:458, 1927.

CRAVER, L. F.: Local and general irradiation in Hodgkin's disease. *Radiology, 31*:42, 1938.

CRAVER, L. F. and COPELAND, M. M.: Changes in the bone in Hodgkin's disease. *Arch. Surg., 28*:1062, 1934.

DESJARDINS, A. U.: Salient features in the treatment of Hodgkin's disease and lymphosarcoma with roentgen rays. *Am. J. Roentgenol., 54*:707, 1945.

DRESSER, R.: Lymphogranuloma of bones. *Strahlentherapie, 41*:401. 1931.

DRESSER, R. and SPENCER, J.: Hodgkin's disease and allied conditions of bone. *Am. J. Roentgenol., 36*:809, 1936.

FRIEDRICH, H.: Lymphogranulomatosis (Hodgkin's disease) of the bones. *Fortschr. a. d. Geb. d. Röntgenstrahlen, 41*:206, 1930.

JOBY, M.: Bone lesions in lymphogranulomatosis. *Bull. et mém Soc. de radiol. med. de France, 19*:45, 1931.

JOHNSON, J. M.: Hodgkin's disease with invasion of spinal column. *Pennsylvania M. J., 34*:877, 1930-31.

KREMSER, K.: On bone changes in Hodgkin's disease. *Röntgenpraxis, 2*:998, 1930.

LOCKWOOD, I. H., JOHNSON, E. T., and UARR, F. C.: Hodgkin's disease with bone and skeletal muscle involvement. *Radiology, 14*:445, 1930.

MONTGOMERY, A. H.: Hodgkin's disease of bones. *Ann. Surg., 87*:755, 1928.

SYMMERS, D.: The clinical significance of the pathological changes in Hodgkin's disease. *Am. J. M. Sc., 167*:157 and 313, 1924.

TETZNER, E.: Lymphogranulomatosis in the spinal column. *Frankfurt Ztschr. f. Path., 42*:545, 1931-32.

UEHLINGER, E.: On bone granulomatosis. *Virchows Arch. f. path. Anat., 288*:36, 1933.

UEHLINGER, E.: Ueber Knochen-lymphogranulomatose. *Virchows Arch. f. path. Anat., 288*:36, 1933.

VIETA, J. O., FRIEDELL, H. L. and CRAVER, L. F.: A survey of Hodgkin's disease and lymphosarcoma in bone. *Radiology, 39*:1, 1942.

WALLHAUSER, A.: Hodgkin's disease. *Arch. Path., 16*:522 and 672, 1933.

WOODARD, H. Q. and CRAVER, L. F.: Serum phosphatase in lymphomatoid diseases. *J. Clin. Investigation, 19*:1, 1940.

ZIEGLER, K.: *Ueber die Hodgkinsche Krankheit; das maligne lymphogranulom.* Fischer, Jena, 1911.

Sarcomas of the Soft Tissues

Bick, E. M.: End results in cases of fibrosarcoma of the extremities. *Arch. Surg.,* *37*:973, 1938.

Stout, A. P.: Sarcomas of the soft parts. *J. Missouri M. A., 44*:329, 1947.

Warren, S. and Sommer, G. N. J.: Fibrosarcoma of soft parts. *Arch. Surg., 33*:425, 1936.

The Leukemias

Apitz, K.: Ueber Knochenveranderungen Bei Leukämia. *Virchows Arch. f. path. Anat., 302*:301, 1938.

Baty, J. M. and Vogt, E. C.: Bone changes in leukemia in children. *Am. J. Roentgenol., 34*:310, 1935.

Craver, L. F.: Tenderness of the sternum in leukemia. *Am. J. Med. Sc., 174*:799, 1927.

Craver, L. F. and Copeland, M. M.: Changes in the bones in the leukemias. *Arch. Surg., 30*:639, 1935.

Hoffman, W. J. and Craver, L. F.: Chronic myelogenous leukemia. *J. A. M. A., 97*:836, 1931.

Melchior, E.: Spondylopathia leucaemia. *Zentralbl. f. Chir., 49*:1737, 1922.

Mettier, S. R.: Hematologic aspects of space consuming lesions of bone marrow (myelophthisie anemia). *Ann. Int. Med., 14*:436, 1940.

Rolleston, H. D. and Frankan, C. H. S.: Acute leukemia simulating caries of the spine. *Lancet, 1*:173, 1914.

Taylor, H. K.: Periosteal changes in a case of lymphatic leukemia. *Radiology, 6*:523, 1926.

CHAPTER XXI

Tumors of Joints

Contents

The great and growing literature and attention centered around bone tumors had not been associated with a similar interest in joint tumors. Joint tumors do not deserve this relative neglect.

BENIGN TUMORS OF JOINTS

XANTHOMATOUS GIANT CELL TUMOR

Virtually all so-called giant cell tumors of the synovial membrane are said by DeSanto and Wilson (1939) to be xanthomas. These investigators reported 9 cases of xanthomatous joint tumors and reviewed 32 cases in medical literature. Of the total of 41 patients, 24 (59 percent) were males. The majority of the patients in this series were between the ages of 20 and 40.

The predelection for the knee joint is strikingly indicated by the fact that in 36 of the 41 cases the knee was the site of the tumor.

Gross Pathology

Three anatomical types are described:

1. *Pedunculated.*—This is the commonest type. The tumor mass

varies from one to several centimeters in diameter, is spherical and is attached to the synovial membrane by an adequate pedicle. A yellowish color derives from blood pigment and the xanthoma cells of the tumor.

2. *Multiple.*—Generally represented by several small tumor masses fixed to the synovial membrane.

3. *Diffuse.*—This is a rare type in which much or all of the synovial membrane becomes covered by numerous small nodular masses.

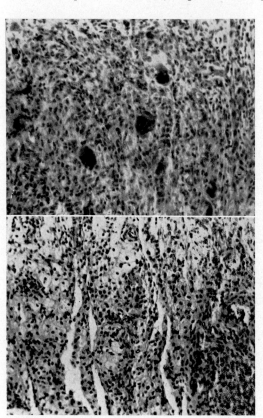

FIGURE 449. Xanthomatous giant cell tumor. A. *(Above)* Photomicrograph of a field in which there is a preponderance of stroma cells and multinucleated giant cells. B. *(Below)* A field with a preponderance of Xanthoma cells (foam cells).

Histopathology

The microscopic picture is characterized by foam cells and multinucleated giant cells in a fibrocellular stroma (Fig. 449). Xanthoma or foam cells are large rounded cells with a clear, colorless cytoplasm and a small nucleus; these cells exist as diffuse masses or simply scattered through the stroma. A fat stain clearly reveals the fat content of these cells.

Considerable variation exists in the cellularity and collagen content of the stroma. Scattered blood pigment is a feature of most xanthomas.

After a comprehensive study of this subject, Jaffe, Lichtenstein, and Sutro (*Arch. Path. 31*:731, 1941) concluded that these lesions are neither giant cell tumors nor xanthomas, and recommended the term *pigmented villinodular synovitis.*

Clinical Features

Pain is a symptom in most cases, as is also some degree of distention of the joint. A tumor mass is not often palpable. None of the DeSanto-Wilson cases were diagnosed preoperatively. A history of trauma was present in 23 of the 41 cases, and an internal derangement of the knee in seven cases. Hemarthrosis is common.

The treatment is complete excision of the tumor. In seven of the 41 cases the tumor recurred; however, malignant transformation did not occur in a single instance.

HEMANGIOMA

Bennett and Cobey (1939) reviewed 24 cases reported in medical literature and added five cases of their own. In 1943 Cobey added 4 more cases. The tumors were divided into two types:

1. Localized
    a. Pedunculated
    b. Flat
2. Diffuse

These tumors, most of which were in the knee joint, were only rarely diagnosed preoperatively. A history of intermittent swelling over a long period was the rule; it was seldom possible to palpate the tumor mass. A family history was not unusual. In several instances hemangiomas were located elsewhere on the patient's body.

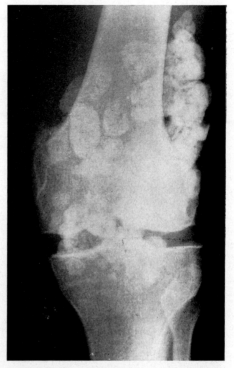

FIGURE 450. Osteochondromatosis of the knee joint. A. Antero-posterior roentgenogram.

The histopathology is similar to that of hemangiomas elsewhere.

Surgical excision proved to be the treatment of choice for the pedunculated type, but was not feasible for the diffuse type. Radiation therapy was recommended for the diffuse type.

FIBROMA

True fibromas are rarely found within joints. Histologically the picture is similar to fibromas elsewhere. Surgical excision is usually simple and curative.

LIPOMA

Most so-called lipomas of joints are fatty hyperplasias and not neoplasms. On the basis of their anatomical location two types of true lipomas are recognized: (1) intracapsular and, (2) extracapsular.

Intracapsular lipomas are moderately large and solitary or else small and multiple. Multiple small lipomas have been termed lipoma arborescens. The inflammatory type must be differentiated from the neoplastic type. An extraarticular lipoma, in rare instances, has protruded into a joint; the hip and the knee have been the usual sites.

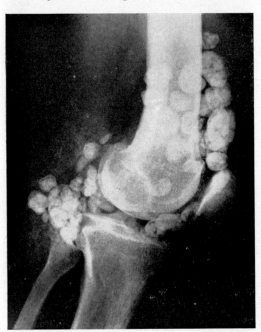

All lipomas are composed of fatty tissue plus a variable fibrotic element.

Surgical excision is the treatment if the tumor causes disabling symptoms. Malignant transformation does not occur.

OSTEOCHONDROMATOSIS
(Chondromatosis)

The term osteochondromatosis refers to multiple benign osseocartilaginous tumors having their origin in the synovial membrane and subsynovia. Except for reactive changes the articular cartilage and the articular cortex are not involved.

FIGURE 450. *(Continued)* B. Lateral roentgenogram.

Lannec is said by Halstead to have described the first case in 1813. Brodie reported this entity in 1836 and classified it as a neoplasm. Reichel's report in 1900 and Hugh Jones' article of 1924 are landmarks in our understanding of this disease.

Most investigators writing on this subject have agreed with Sir Benjamin Brodie and Lexer that the disease is a blastomatous growth arising from numerous cell rests in the synovial membrane. Freund, on the other hand, contended that the process is simply one of synovial hyperplasia associated with a metaplastic change of islands of the synovialis to cartilage and bone. The process was compared to myocitis ossificans. Spontaneous disappearance of some or all of the joint bodies has not been a rare observation and this phenomenon was viewed by Freund as evidence that the osseocartilaginous bodies are not blastomatous.

The etiology is unknown.

Pathogenesis

The joint capsule originates embyrologically from the same primi-

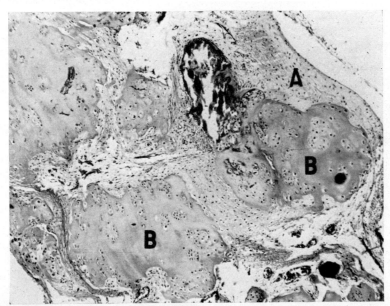

FIGURE 451. Chondromas forming in the synovial membrane showing origin of synovial osteochondromatosis. *A*. Synovial membrane. *B*. Islands of hyalin cartilage.

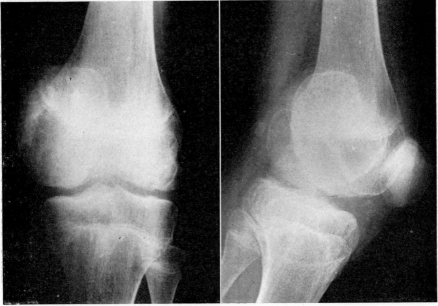

FIGURE 452. Epiarticular osteochondromas of the left distal femoral articular surface and the left ankle joint in a female age 16 years. All other joints were normal. There was no history of trauma or infection. A. Roentgenogram of the left knee.

tive tissue that creates periosteum and perichondrium. Microscopic islands of hyaline cartilage, believed by many to arise from mesenchymal

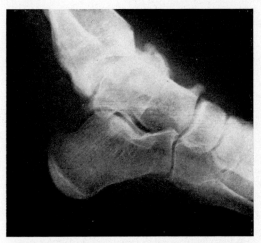

cells rests, are found in the synovialis (Fig. 451). These nests of chondrocytes grow into cartilaginous capsular bodies. Ultimately, many of these synovial chondromas hang from the synovial membrane by a narrow vascular pedicle. Through the friction and pressure incident to joint motion numerous of the chrondromas are separated from the membrane and become free joint bodies (Fig. 450).

FIGURE 452. *(Continued)* B. Roentgenogram of the left ankle.

The core of those chondromatous joint bodies attached to the synovial membrane may or may

not calcify. In several reported cases none of the cartilage bodies became calcified or ossified. Thus the joint bodies gave no notice of their presence in roentgenograms. These were cases of articular chondromatosis. In most instances the cartilage masses undergo central calcification. Blood vessels then make their way to the site of the calcified cartilage and through the cellular activity that ensues the cartilage is absorbed and replaced by primitive bone. The process is one of primitive enchondral ossification. Ossification by metaplasia of cartilage may also be observed. Part or all of the individual chondroma is replaced by bone, transforming

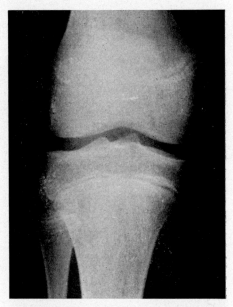

FIGURE 452. *(Continued)* C. Roentgenogram of the normal right knee.

the joint body to an osteochondroma. Once the ossified joint body is separated from its vascular pedicle the bone element promptly undergoes avascular necrosis. Subsequently if the osteochondroma again attaches itself to the synovial lining and acquires a blood supply the necrotic bone may be revitalized by the process of creeping replacement.

While bone dies if separated from a blood supply, cartilage is able to survive on the nourishment derived from the synovial fluid. Free chondromatous joint bodies are capable of acquiring a perichondrium and through its proliferative activity, layer upon layer of chondrocytes

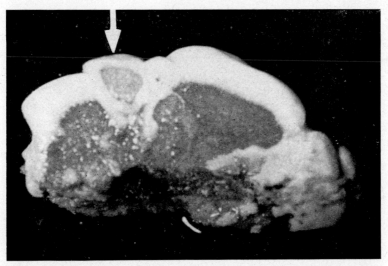

FIGURE 452. *(Continued)* D. Specimen removed from left knee shows how osteochondromas are crowded out to become loose joint bodies (arrow).

are added to the periphery of the joint body. This phenomenon, once doubted, is now well established.

Clinical Features

Chondromatosis and osteochondromatosis is a disease of young and middle aged adults.

In one of Jones' cases a chondrosarcoma developed in a knee joint that was the site of an osteochondromatosis. However, there is little basis for expecting an articular osteochondromatosis to undergo malignant transformation.

The treatment is surgical and consists of removing the synovial membrane and all accessible joint bodies.

EPIARTICULAR OSTEOCHONDROMAS
(Articular osteomatosis)

Whereas the osteochondromas in articular osteochondromatosis originate in the synovial membrane, the osteochondromas of articular osteo-

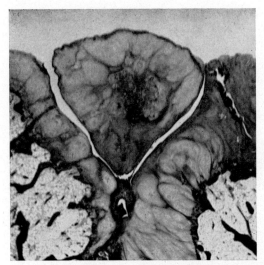

FIGURE 452. *(Continued)* E. Photomicrograph of the site of the arrow in D.

matosis originate on the joint surfaces. The term "osteomatosis" was employed by Lexer (1907) and by Lieberman (1936). It is the writer's opinion that the term epiarticular osteochondromas is more descriptive, and therefore preferable.

A review of English medical literature disclosed only one case report of this entity, and this was reported by Freund in an article dealing with unusual cartilaginous tumors. In a review of foreign literature six cases were found in German literature, two in Italian journals, and one in Russian literature.

This interesting entity is not as rare as is indicated by the small number of cases reported in medical literature. The writer has collected seven new cases which will be reported.

Pathogenesis

At one or many small areas along the enchondral line lying beneath the articular cartilage, the process of enchondral ossification is sharply accelerated. Through this localized accelerated growth, tumor-like bodies are formed which grossly and histologically resemble osteochondromas (Figs. 452 & 453).

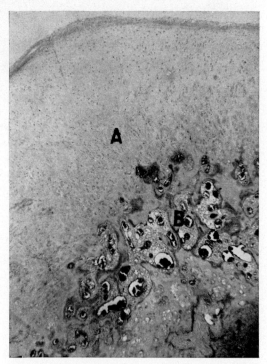

FIGURE 452. *(Continued)* F. Photomicrograph showing the cartilaginous cap, *A,* and the enchondral line, *B,* of a growing epiarticular osteochondroma.

These epiarticular osteochondromas, having a cartilaginous cap and a bony core, vary widely in shape, and size. They grow largest at the periphery where they are less subjected to pressure and friction. Since there is often extreme crowding, some of the tumors are crowded out or broken off to become free bodies in the joint (Figs. 452 D & E).

Most of the epiarticular osteochondromas observed by the author have had their origin during childhood. As growth occurs in the host bone the osteochondromas retain a constant relationship to the epiphysis. In contrast, the metaphyseal osteochondromas change their relative position by being left behind as length growth occurs in the host bone.

The mother tissue for the tumors lies in the deeper layers of the articular cartilage. So long as this tissue proliferates the process of enchondral ossification persists, thus giving rise to growth of the tumor. By the time the host bone has received its full growth most of the growth of the epiarticular osteochondromas ceases.

Free osseo-cartilaginous bodies in this entity undergo the same changes and have similar fates as do synovial osteochondromas.

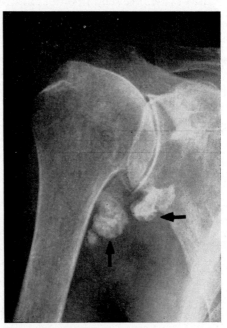

FIGURE 453. Epiarticular osteochondromas of the shoulder joint (arrows). (Los Angeles County Hospital.)

The synovialis in epiarticular osteochondromas shows no alteration beyond those incident to the trauma inflicted by the osteochondromas. A careful study of the synovial membrane from several cases failed to disclose evidence that any of the joint bodies were of synovial origin.

Histopathology

During growth of the osteochondromas, active enchondral ossification can be seen, the rate of growth being indicated by the distance the intratrabecular islands of calcified cartilage are detected from the enchondral line (Fig. 452F). Considerable variation is found in the orderliness of the enchondral ossification, the variation being from primitive to the high degree of orderliness seen at epiphyseal plates. When growth ceases a thin bony trabecular plate caps the zone of provisional calcification. Marrow spaces in the bone element of the tumor are usually filled with fibrous tissue. The cartilaginous cap, often thick and hyaline during growth of the tumor becomes thin and fibrocartilaginous after growth ceases.

Clinical Features

Most cases are seen in older children and young adults. Seldom is more than one joint involved, and seldom is there a history of significant trauma. The etiology is unknown. A family history has not been elicited.

As can be imagined, the function of the joint is seriously impaired in most instances. Episodes of locking of the involved joint are the rule.

The treatment is surgical and consists of the removal of the accessible free and attached osteochondromas. An arthrodesis may become necessary.

DIFFERENTIAL DIAGNOSIS: Osteoarthritis causes localized reactivation of enchondral ossification but involves an older age group, and causes exostoses to form only at the periphery. The cartilage space is narrowed in osteoarthritis and frequently widened in epiarticular osteochondromas.

A Charcot joint can cause large exostoses to form but is identified with older patients and generally with signs of tabes dorsalis.

Osteochondromatosis of synovial origin leaves articular cortices, and cartilage spaces intact. Epiarticular osteochondromas disrupt the articular cortex, and the cartilage space.

A chondrosarcoma of the joint often invades the epiphysis and joint capsule and does not tend to form multiple joint bodies.

MALIGNANT TUMORS OF JOINTS
SYNOVIOMA

Synovioma is decidedly the most common primary malignant tumor of joints. Except for the synoviomas, primarily malignant tumors of joints are extremely rare.

Smith's report in 1927 was the first comprehensive discussion of synovioma from this country.

In 1944 Haagensen and Stout screened medical literature, and found 95 definite cases; these were analyzed and nine new cases added. Bennett, in a recent report (1947) described 32 cases from military medical records. These and other excellent articles of the past two decades have served to make us conscious of the existence and the highly malignant character of this important entity.

The incidence of synoviomas is highest in young adults; in the Haagensen-Stout series the mean age was 32 years. There was a preponderance of males in the proportion of three to two. The lower extremity joints were involved in 79 percent of the cases, and the upper extremity joints in 21 percent. In nearly half of the series, the knee

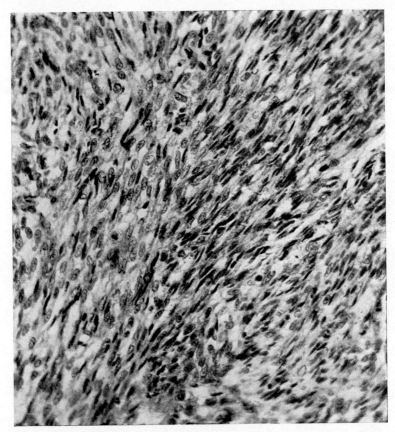

FIGURE 454. Synovioma. Photomicrographs of typical fields. (Courtesy, A. Purdy Stout, M.D.) A. Fibrosarcomatous area. The larger portion of the tumor is composed of this type of tissue.

region was the site of the tumor. Contrary to a widespread assumption, the tumor seldom develops within the synovial membrane proper. The usual location of the tumor mass is adjacent to a joint. A neighboring bursa or tendon sheath may be the site or origin or there may be no gross evidence of intimacy with any of the synovial structures.

Gross Pathology

The tumor mass is generally spherical, vascular, possesses a nodular,

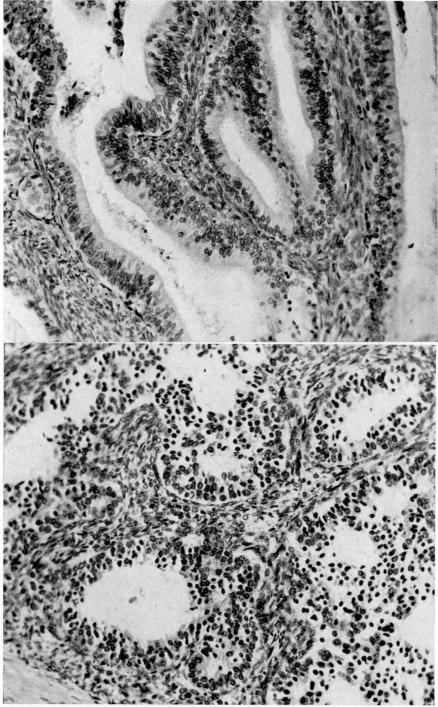

FIGURE 454. (Continued) B. (Above), C. (Below), D. (Opposite page). Synovial or adenomatous areas. Such fields as these must be present to make the diagnosis of synovioma.

well demarcated outline, a firm consistency, and a pseudocapsule, but no true tumor capsule. Firmness is contributed to the tumor mass by a preponderance of the fibrosarcomatous element in proportion to the synovial element and by islands of calcification or ossification.

Growth of the tumor is by expansion, and the rate of growth is slow. Metastatic spread, a late occurrence, generally takes place by way of the blood stream (pulmonary); however, a lymphatic extension has not been rare.

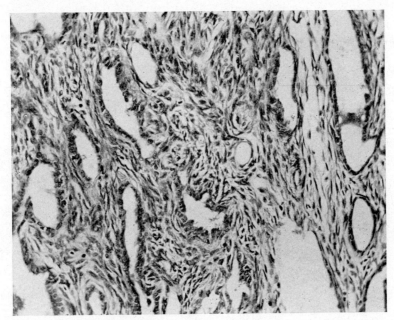

FIGURE 454. *(Continued)* D. See opposite page for description.

Histopathology

The preponderance of sheets of moderately anaplastic spindle cells has often led to the erroneous diagnosis of fibrosarcoma. Two types of tissue characterize the synovioma, fibrosarcomatous and synovial or adenomatous. While these two tissues vary widely in their relative proportions they must both be present to warrant the diagnosis of synovioma. The fibrosarcomatous element far exceeds the synovial; in fact, it is necessary in many instances to make sections from several parts of the tumor in order to avoid missing a sparce synovial element.

FIBROSARCOMA ELEMENT: This portion of the tumor is highly cellular, but is composed of fairly well differentiated spindle cells and not uncommonly, of collagen bundles (Fig. 454A). Reticulin fibers are always present in the fibrosarcoma portion of the tumor and a silver reticulin stain should be employed routinely to identify these fibers (Fig. 454E). Small deposits of calcium and a few trabeculae of fibrous bone are occasionally encountered in synoviomas.

SYNOVIAL ELEMENT: The synovial or adenomatous element of the tumor appears to represent the attempt by the tumor to reproduce a synovial membrane. This effort is manifest by the formation of clefts

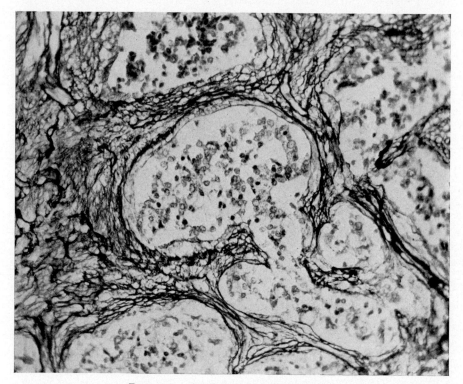

FIGURE 454. *(Continued)* E. Reticulin stain.

and oval spaces lined with cuboidal, spindle, or columnar synovial cells (Figs. 454B, C & D). Cells lining the splits and spaces often secrete an acidophilic mucinous material that takes a red stain with mucicarmine. Reticulin fibers do not appear in relation to the synovial cells. The number of mitotic figures seen varies widely. Bennett doubts that the frequency of mitotic figures is a reliable index to the degree of malignancy of this tumor.

Clinical features

Synoviomas must be carefully differentiated from xanthomatous giant cell tumors and from inflammatory hyperplasias. The treatment of these lesions has no common ground with that of synovioma.

Follow-up studies of synoviomas emphasize the catastrophic character of this tumor. In the Haagensen-Stout survey only one patient had survived eight years. (At the end of ten years post-amputation this patient was again examined and found to have pulmonary metastases.) Of the 101 patients of the series the total mean duration of the disease was 5.7 years. Only three of the patients survived as much as five years following therapy of the tumor.

Radiation therapy was "singularly futile." No evidence was found that it was even of palliative value.

Surgeons must not indulge in preliminary minor surgical procedures or even local excision of the tumor mass if the present mortality rate is to be lowered. The treatment of choice is an incisional biopsy followed by a high amputation or a disarticulation as soon as permanent histologic sections of the tumor have been carefully studied. Frozen sections are not recommended. It is the advice of Haagensen and Stout that a resection of the regional lymph nodes should be seriously considered in addition to the amputation.

CHONDROSARCOMA

Chondrosarcoma has been observed as a primary tumor of a joint but as such is extremely rare. Rupture of the tumor through the joint capsule and the articular surface has been the rule. Histologically joint chondrosarcomas have the same features as have chondrosarcomas of the bones.

REFERENCES

XANTHOMATOUS TUMORS OF JOINTS

BLANCO, P.: Giant cell tumor of the knee joint. *J. Orthop. Surg.*, *3*:156, 1921.
DESANTO, D. A. and WILSON, P. D.: Xanthomatous tumors of joints. *J. Bone & Joint Surg.*, *21*:531, 1939.
GALLOWAY, J. D. B., BRODERS, A. C., and GHORMLEY, R. K.: Xanthoma of the tendon sheaths and synovial membranes. *Arch. Surg.*, *40*:485, 1940.
HARBITZ, F.: Tumors of the tendon sheaths, joint capsules, and multiple xanthoma. *Arch. Path.*, *4*:507, 1927.
HERZMARK, M. H.: Giant cell synovial tumor of the knee. *J. Bone & Joint Surg.*, *23*:684, 1941.
MORTON, J. J.: Tumors of the tendon sheaths. Their close biological relationship to tumors of the joints and bursae. *Surg., Gynec. & Obst.*, *59*:441, 1934.
WIER, R. F.: On fatty and sarcomatous tumors of the knee joint. *Med. Record*, *29*:725, 1886.

HEMANGIOMA

BENNETT, G. E. and COBEY, M. C.: Hemangioma of joints. *Arch. Surg.*, *28*:487, 1939.
COBEY, M. C.: Hemangioma of joints. *Arch. Surg.*, *46*:465, 1943.
KLEINBERG, S.: Angioma of the foot. *J. Bone & Joint Surg.*, *24*:367, 1942.
OSGOOD, R. A.: Angioma of the knee. *S. Clin. North Am.*, *1*:681, 1921.

WEAVER, J. B.: Hemangiomata of the lower extremities, with special reference to those of the knee joint capsule and the phenomenon of spontaneous obliteration. *J. Bone & Joint Surg., 20*:731, 1938.

LIPOMA

GHORMLEY, R. K.: Lipoma of the capsule of the joint removed successfully: Presentation of three cases. *Minnesota Med., 17*:62, 1934.
SUTHERLAND, C. G.: A radiologic study of soft tissue tumors. *Radiology, 3*:420, 1924.
WEITZNER, I.: Unusually located lipoma complicated by foreign body. *Am. J. Roentgenol., 27*:267, 1932.

OSTEOCHONDROMAS

BRODIE, B.: *Pathological and Surgical Observations on the Diseases of the Joints.* Longman, London, 1836.
FALKNER, D. M.: Primary synovial membrane tumors of the joints. *Surg., Gynec. & Obst., 53*:189, 1933.
FALKNER, D. M.: Primary synovial membrane tumors of joints. *Surg., Gynec. & Obst., 53*:189, 1931.
FREUND, E.: Chondromatosis of joints. *Arch. Surg., 34*:670, 1937.
HALSTEAD, A. E.: Floating bodies in joints. *Ann. Surg., 22*:327, 1895.
HARTMAN, F. W.: Synovial membrane tumors of joints. *Surg., Gynec. & Obst., 34*:161, 1922.
JONES, H. T.: Loose body formation; synovial osteochondromatosis, with special reference to the etiology and pathology. *J. Bone & Joint Surg., 6*:407, 1924.
LEXER, E.: *Deutsche Ztschr. f. Chir., 88*:311, 1907.
OTTOLENGHI, C. E. and MUSCOLO, D. T.: Osteochondromatosis of the knee. *Revista de ortop. Y. traumatol., 5*:70, 1935.
RAZEMON, P. and BIZARD, G.: Les tumerus primitives des articulationn. *Rev. de chir., Paris, 50*:229, 1931.
REICHEL: *Arch. f. klin. Chir., 61*: 1900.
VINCENT, G. and VINCENT, J.: L'osteochondromatose synoviale du genou. *J. d. Sc. med. de Lille, 49*:405, 1931.
WILMONTH, C. L.: Osteochondromatosis. *J. Bone & Joint Surg., 23*:367, 1941.

EPIARTICULAR OSTEOCHONDROMAS

BOLOGNESI, G.: Sul mixoma articulare. *Chir. d. org. di movimento, 6*:17, 1922.
CONTINI, V.: Tumori primitivi delle articolazioni. *Chir. d. org. di movimento, 24*:529, 1939.
FREUND, E.: Unusual cartilaginous tumor formation of the skeleton. *Arch. Surg., 33*:1054, 1936.
GRABOWSKI, L.: Benign tumor diseases of the joints. *Roentgenpraxis, 9*:799, 1937.
LIEBERMAN, C. A.: Benign intraarticular growths as seen in roentgenograms. *Trood. po Roentgenol., 2*:9, 1936.

SYNOVIOMA

AITKIN, F. E.: Roentgenographic recognition of synovioma. *J. Bone & Joint Surg., 23*:950, 1941.
COLEY, B. L. and PIERSON, J. C.: Synovioma: Report of 15 cases with review of the literature. *Surgery, 1*:113, 1947.
DESANTO, D. A., TENNANT, R., and ROSAHN, P. D.: Synovial sarcomas in joints, bursae, and tendon sheaths: Clinical and pathologic study of 16 cases. *Surg., Gynec. & Obst., 72*:951, 1941.
FISHER, H. R.: Synovial sarcomesothelioma (sarcoendothelioma). *Am. J. Path., 18*:529, 1942.
GROSS, P. and CAMERON, D. W.: Synovioma. Case report. *Arch. Path., 33*: 1941.
HAAGENSEN, C. D. and STOUT, A. P.: Synovial sarcoma. *Ann. Surg., 120*:826, 1944.

HAGGART, G. E.: Synovioma of the knee joint. *J. Bone & Joint Surg.*, April, 1942.

HODGSON, F. G. and BISHOP, E. L.: Malignant synovioma of the knee joint. *J. Bone & Joint Surg.*, *17*:184, 1935.

HUTCHINSON, C. W. and KLING, D. H.: Malignant synovioma. *Am. J. Cancer, 40*:78, 1940.

KNOX, L. C.: Synovial sarcoma. *Am. J. Cancer, 28*:461, 1936.

LEWIS, R. W.: Roentgen recognition of synovioma. *Am. J. Roentgenol., 44*:170, 1941.

LEWIS, R. W.: Roentgen recognition of synovioma. *Am. J. Roentgenol., 44*:170, 1940.

MURRAY, M. R., STOUT, A. P., and POGOGEFF, I. A.: Synovial sarcoma and normal synovial tissue cultivated in Vitro. *Ann. Surg., 120*:843, 1944.

SMITH, L. W.: Synoviomata. *Am. J. Path., 3*:355, 1927.

STANFORD, S. and HORNE, E. A.: Malignant synovioma. *J. Bone & Joint Surg., 25*:883, 1943.

Index

This Book

BONE AND JOINT
DISEASES

By

J. VERNON LUCK

M.S. (Ortho.), M.D., F.A.C.S., F.I.C.S.

was set and printed by The Ovid Bell Press, Inc., of Fulton, Missouri. The binding was done by the Becktold Company of St. Louis, Missouri. The engravings were made by G. R. Grubb & Company of Champaign, Illinois. The type face is Baskerville, set 11 point on 13 point. The type page is 29 x 48 picas. The text paper is 70-pound Oxford Mainefold Enamel. The binding cloth is Du Pont Fabrikoid, Quality 700, Color 5027, Grain 0-7 (Roller), Medium Pliability, Finish SB.

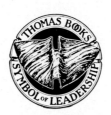

With THOMAS BOOKS *careful attention is given to all details of manufacturing and design. It is the Publisher's desire to present books that are satisfactory as to their physical qualities and artistic possibilities and appropriate for their particular use.* THOMAS BOOKS *will be true to those laws of quality that assure a good name and good will.*